Modern Critical Care Endocrinology

Editor

RINALDO BELLOMO

CRITICAL CARE CLINICS

www.criticalcare.theclinics.com

Consulting Editor
JOHN A. KELLUM

April 2019 • Volume 35 • Number 2

ELSEVIER

1600 John F. Kennedy Boulevard • Suite 1800 • Philadelphia, Pennsylvania, 19103-2899

http://www.theclinics.com

CRITICAL CARE CLINICS Volume 35, Number 2
April 2019 ISSN 0749-0704, ISBN-13: 978-0-323-67791-2

Editor: Colleen Dietzler
Developmental Editor: Casey Potter

Critical Care Clinics (ISSN: 0749-0704) is published quarterly by Elsevier Inc., 360 Park Avenue South, New York, NY 10010-1710. Months of issue are January, April, July, and October. Business and Editorial Offices: 1600 John F. Kennedy Blvd., Suite 1800, Philadelphia, PA 19103-2899. Customer Service Office: 6277 Sea Harbor Drive, Orlando, FL 32887-4800. Periodicals postage paid at New York, NY and additional mailing offices. Subscription prices are $243.00 per year for US individuals, $650.00 per year for US institution, $100.00 per year for US students and residents, $285.00 per year for Canadian individuals, $815.00 per year for Canadian institutions, $315.00 per year for international individuals, $815.00 per year for international institutions and $150.00 per year for Canadian and foreign students/residents. To receive student/resident rate, orders must be accompanied by name of affiliated institution, date of term, and the signature of program/residency coordinator on institution letterhead. Orders will be billed at individual rate until proof of status is received. Foreign air speed delivery is included in all *Clinics* subscription prices. All prices are subject to change without notice. POSTMASTER: Send address changes to *Critical Care Clinics*, Elsevier Periodicals Customer Service, 11830 Westline Industrial Drive, St. Louis, MO 63146. **Customer Service: 1-800-654-2452 (US). From outside of the US, call 1-314-447-8871. Fax: 1-314-447-8029. E-mail: journalscustomerservice-usa@ elsevier.com (for print support) or journalsonlinesupport-usa@elsevier.com (for online support).**

Reprints. For copies of 100 or more of articles in this publication, please contact the Commercial Reprints Department, Elsevier Inc., 360 Park Avenue South, New York, NY 10010-1710. Tel.: 212-633-3874; Fax: 212-633-3820; E-mail: reprints@elsevier.com.

Critical Care Clinics is also published in Spanish by Editorial Inter-Medica, Junin 917, 1er A, 1113, Buenos Aires, Argentina.

Critical Care Clinics is covered in *MEDLINE/PubMed (Index Medicus), EMBASE/Excerpta Medica, Current Concepts/ Clinical Medicine, ISI/BIOMED,* and *Chemical Abstracts.*

Contributors

CONSULTING EDITOR

JOHN A. KELLUM, MD, MCCM
Professor, Critical Care Medicine, Medicine, Bioengineering and Clinical and Translational Science, Director, Center for Critical Care Nephrology, Vice Chair for Research, Department of Critical Care Medicine, University of Pittsburgh School of Medicine, Pittsburgh, Pennsylvania, USA

EDITOR

RINALDO BELLOMO, AO, MBBS (Hons), MD, PhD, FRACP, FCICM, FAAHMS
Professor of Intensive Care, The University of Melbourne, Honorary Professor of Medicine, Monash University, Honorary Professor of Critical Care Medicine, University of New South Wales, Honorary Fellow, Howard Florey Institute of Physiology, NHMRC Practitioner Fellow and Co-director ANZ Intensive Care Research Centre, Editor-in-Chief, Critical Care and Resuscitation, Director of Intensive Care Research, Austin Hospital, Director of Data Analytics Research and Evaluation (DARE) Centre, Co-director of Centre for Integrated Critical Care, Melbourne University, Senior Research Advisor, The Royal Melbourne Hospital, Staff Specialist in Intensive Care, Austin Hospital, The Royal Melbourne Hospital, and Warringal Private Hospital, Department of Medicine, Radiology and Critical Care, Centre for Integrated Critical Care, The University of Melbourne, Melbourne, Victoria, Australia

AUTHORS

JAMES R. ANSTEY, MBBS, FRACP, FCICM
Intensive Care Unit, The Royal Melbourne Hospital, Parkville, Victoria, Australia

KARIM ASEHNOUNE, MD, PhD
EA3826 Thérapeutiques Anti-Infectieuses, Institut de Recherche en Santé 2 Nantes Biotech, Medical University of Nantes, Surgical Intensive Care Unit, Hotel Dieu, CHU Nantes, Nantes, France

ANCA BALINTESCU, MD
Department of Clinical Science and Education Södersjukhuset, Section of Anaesthesia and Intensive Care, Karolinska Institutet, Södersjukhuset, Stockholm, Sweden

BLAIRE BEERS-MULROY, MS
La Jolla Pharmaceutical Company, San Diego, California, USA

LAURENT BITKER, MD, MSc
Department of Intensive Care, ICU Research Office, Austin Hospital, Heidelberg, Victoria, Australia

LOUISE M. BURRELL, MBChB, MRCP, MD, FRACP
Department of Medicine, The University of Melbourne, Austin Health, Heidelberg, Victoria, Australia

LAURENCE W. BUSSE, MD
Assistant Professor, Division of Pulmonary, Critical Care, Allergy and Sleep Medicine, Emory University School of Medicine, Emory St. Joseph's Hospital, Atlanta, Georgia, USA

LAKHMIR S. CHAWLA, MD
Department of Medicine, Veterans Affairs Medical Center, La Jolla, California, USA; La Jolla Pharmaceutical Company, San Diego, California, USA

JEREMY COHEN, PhD
Deputy Director, Department of Intensive Care, The Wesley Hospital, Senior Specialist, Department of Intensive Care, The Royal Brisbane and Women's Hospital, Associate Professor, University of Queensland, Queensland, Australia; Honorary Professorial Fellow, Division of Critical Care, The George Institute for Global Health, Sydney, New South Wales, Australia

ADAM M. DEANE, MBBS, PhD
Staff Specialist, Associate Professor, Intensive Care Unit, The Royal Melbourne Hospital, Principal Research Fellow Intensive Care, University of Melbourne, Parkville, Victoria, Australia

ELIF I. EKINCI, MBBS, FRACP, PhD
Associate Professor, Sir Edward Dunlop Medical Research Foundation, Principal Research Fellow in Metabolic Medicine, Departments of Medicine and Endocrinology, The University of Melbourne, Director of Diabetes, Austin Health, Heidelberg West, Melbourne, Victoria, Australia

CRAIG FRENCH, MBBS, FANZCA, FCICM
Director of Intensive Care, Western Health, Footscray Hospital, Clinical Associate Professor, The University of Melbourne, Parkville, Victoria, Australia; Adjunct Associate Professor, Monash University, School of Public Health and Preventive Medicine, Melbourne, Victoria, Australia

ANATOLE HARROIS, MD, PhD
Intensive Care Unit, The Royal Melbourne Hospital, Parkville, Victoria, Australia; Department of Anesthesiology and Surgical Intensive Care, Hôpitaux Universitaires Paris Sud, Assistance Publique-Hôpitaux de Paris (AP-HP), Université paris Sud, Université Paris Saclay, Le Kremlin Bicêtre, France

CHRISTOPHER PATRICK HENSON, DO
Department of Anesthesiology, Division of Anesthesiology Critical Care Medicine, Vanderbilt University Medical Center, Nashville, Tennessee, USA

JEROEN HERMANIDES, MD, PhD
Staff Specialist, Department of Anaesthesiology, Amsterdam UMC, University of Amsterdam, Amsterdam, The Netherlands

ASHISH K. KHANNA, MD, FCCP, FCCM
Assistant Professor of Anesthesiology and Vice-Chief for Research, Department of General Anesthesiology, Anesthesiology Institute, Department of Outcomes Research, Center for Critical Care, Cleveland Clinic Foundation, Cleveland, Ohio, USA; Associate Professor of Anesthesiology, Wake Forest University School of Medicine, Winston-Salem, North Carolina, USA

MARK A. KOTOWICZ, MBBS, FRACP
Professor, University Hospital Geelong, Barwon Health, School of Medicine, Deakin University, Geelong, Australia; Department of Medicine, Melbourne Medical School-Western Campus, The University of Melbourne, St Albans, Australia

RENATA LIBIANTO, MBBS, BMedSci
Department of Medicine, The University of Melbourne, Austin Health, Heidelberg West, Melbourne, Victoria, Australia

JOHAN MÅRTENSSON, MD, PhD
Department of Physiology and Pharmacology, Section of Anaesthesia and Intensive Care, Karolinska Institutet, Function Perioperative Medicine and Intensive Care, Karolinska University Hospital, Stockholm, Sweden

MATTHEW J. MAIDEN, BSc, BMBS, PhD, FCICM, FACEM
Intensive Care Unit, Royal Adelaide Hospital, Adelaide, South Australia, Australia; Intensive Care Unit, Barwon Health, Geelong, Victoria, Australia; Discipline of Acute Care Medicine, University of Adelaide, Adelaide, South Australia, Australia

ANNACHIARA MARRA, MD, PhD
Department of Neurosciences, Reproductive and Odontostomatological Sciences, University of Naples, Federico II, Naples, Italy

TRACY J. McGRANE, MD, MPH
Department of Anesthesiology, Division of Anesthesiology Critical Care Medicine, Vanderbilt University Medical Center, Nashville, Tennessee, USA

HELEN INGRID OPDAM, MD, MBBS, FCICM, FRACP
Department of Intensive Care, Austin Hospital, Heidelberg, Victoria, Australia

NEIL R. ORFORD, MBBS, FCICM, PhD
Associate Professor, University Hospital Geelong, Barwon Health, School of Medicine, Deakin University, Geelong, Australia; Australian and New Zealand Intensive Care Research Centre (ANZIC-RC), Department of Epidemiology and Preventive Medicine (DEPM), Monash University, Melbourne, Australia

PRATIK P. PANDHARIPANDE, MD, MSCI, FCCM
Department of Anesthesiology, Division of Anesthesiology Critical Care Medicine, Vanderbilt University Medical Center, Nashville, Tennessee, USA

JULIE A. PASCO, BSc (Hons), DipEd, PhD, MEpi
Professor, University Hospital Geelong, Barwon Health, School of Medicine, Deakin University, Geelong, Australia; Department of Epidemiology and Preventive Medicine (DEPM), Monash University, Melbourne, Australia; Department of Medicine, Melbourne Medical School-Western Campus, The University of Melbourne, St Albans, Australia

MARK P. PLUMMER, MBBS, PhD
Senior Registrar, Intensive Care Unit, The Royal Melbourne Hospital, Parkville, Victoria, Australia

ANTOINE ROQUILLY, MD, PhD
EA3826 Thérapeutiques Anti-Infectieuses, Institut de Recherche en Santé 2 Nantes Biotech, Medical University of Nantes, Surgical Intensive Care Unit, Hotel Dieu, CHU Nantes, Nantes, France

GEORGE F. TIDMARSH, MD, PhD
La Jolla Pharmaceutical Company, San Diego, California, USA; Department of Pediatrics, Stanford University School of Medicine, Palo Alto, California, USA

DAVID J. TORPY, MBBS, PhD, FRACP
Endocrine and Metabolic Unit, Royal Adelaide Hospital, Adelaide, South Australia, Australia

IDA-FONG UKOR, MBBS, FANZCA, FCICM
Division of Critical Care Medicine and Centre for Heart Lung Innovation, University of British Columbia, Vancouver, British Columbia, Canada

BALASUBRAMANIAN VENKATESH, MD
Director, Department of Intensive Care, The Wesley Hospital, Pre-eminent Specialist, Princess Alexandra Hospital, Professor, Department of Intensive Care, University of Queensland, Queensland, Australia; Professorial Fellow, Division of Critical Care, The George Institute for Global Health, Honorary Professor, University of New South Wales, New South Wales, Australia

MICKAEL VOURC'H, MD, PhD
EA3826 Thérapeutiques Anti-Infectieuses, Institut de Recherche en Santé 2 Nantes Biotech, Medical University of Nantes, Surgical Intensive Care Unit, Hotel Dieu, CHU Nantes, Nantes, France

BRETT J. WAKEFIELD, MD
Anesthesiology Resident, Department of General Anesthesiology, Anesthesiology Institute, Cleveland Clinic, Cleveland, Ohio, USA; Critical Care Medicine Fellow, Department of Anesthesiology, Division of Critical Care Medicine, Washington University School of Medicine, St Louis, Missouri, USA

KEITH R. WALLEY, MD
Division of Critical Care Medicine and Centre for Heart Lung Innovation, University of British Columbia, Vancouver, British Columbia, Canada

Contents

Diabetes insipidus and the syndrome of inappropriate antidiuretic hormone secretion lie at opposite ends of the spectrum of disordered renal handling of water. Whereas renal retention of water insidiously causes hypotonic hyponatremia in syndrome of inappropriate antidiuretic hormone secretion, diabetes insipidus may lead to free water loss, hypernatremia, and volume depletion. Hypernatremia and hyponatremia are associated with worse outcomes and longer intensive care stays. Moreover, pathologies causing polyuria and hyponatremia in patients in intensive care may be multiple, making diagnosis challenging. We provide an approach to the diagnosis and management of these conditions in intensive care patients.

Low-dose hydrocortisone reduces the dose of vasopressors and hospital length of stay; it may also decrease the rate of hospital-acquired pneumonia and time on ventilator. No major side effect was reported, but glycemia and natremia should be monitored. Progesterone did not enhance outcome of trauma patients. A meta-analysis suggested that oxandrolone was associated with shorter length of stay and reduced weight loss. Erythropoietin did not enhance neurologic outcome of traumatic brain-injured patients; such treatment, however, could reduce the mortality in subgroups of patients. This review focuses mainly on glucocorticoids, which are the most extensively investigated treatments in hormone therapy.

Classic and nonclassic renin-angiotensin systems (RAS) are 2 sides of an ubiquitous endocrine/paracrine cascade regulating blood pressure and homeostasis. Angiotensin II and angiotensin-converting enzyme (ACE) levels are associated with severity of disease in the critically ill, and are central to the physiology and the pathogenesis of circulatory shock. Angiotensin (1–7) and ACE2 act as an endogenous counterregulatory arm to the angiotensin II/ACE axis. The tissue-based RAS has paracrine effects dissociated from those of the circulating RAS. Exogenous angiotensin II or ACE2 may improve the outcome of septic shock and acute respiratory distress syndrome, respectively.

Glycated hemoglobin A1c can be used to assess intensive care unit patients' level of chronic glycemic control. Compared with patients with normal glycated hemoglobin A1c, patients with elevated glycated hemoglobin A1c seem to better tolerate hyperglycemia and large glucose fluctuations during critical illness. The risks associated with hypoglycemia are markedly greater among patients with elevated glycated hemoglobin A1c. Observational studies suggest that more liberal targets further decrease the occurrence of hypoglycemia in patients with diabetes with elevated glycated hemoglobin A1c. Whether glycated hemoglobin A1c should be used to individualize glucose control during critical illness should be assessed in randomized trials.

Improved survival after critical illness has led to recognition of impaired recovery following critical illness as a major public health problem. A consistent association between critical illness and accelerated bone loss has been described, including changes in bone turnover markers, bone mineral density, and fragility fracture rate. An association between accelerated bone turnover and increased mortality after critical illness is probable. Assessment of the effect of antifracture agents on fracture rate and mortality in the high-risk population of postmenopausal women with prolonged ventilation is warranted.

The Renaissance of glucose-lowering therapies has arrived with multiple agents that lower blood glucose and demonstrate cardiovascular and renal benefits in people with type 2 diabetes. This article summarizes these new classes of therapies, including the sodium glucose co-transporter-2 inhibitors, glucagon-like peptide-1 agonists, and dipeptidyl peptidase-4 inhibitors. Their cardiovascular safety profile, effects on glycemic, weight, and renal outcomes are discussed. As more options become available to treat type 2 diabetes, clinicians need to be aware of the advantages of each class of medications, beyond their glycemic lowering effects. The safety profiles are summarized in this article.

Melatonin is involved in regulation of a variety of physiologic functions, including circadian rhythm, reproduction, mood, and immune function. Exogenous melatonin has demonstrated many clinical effects. Numerous clinical studies have documented improved sleep quality following administration of exogenous melatonin. Recent studies also demonstrate the analgesic, anxiolytic, antiinflammatory, and antioxidative effects of

CRITICAL CARE CLINICS

SERIES OF RELATED INTEREST

Emergency Medicine Clinics
Available at: https://www.emed.theclinics.com/

THE CLINICS ARE AVAILABLE ONLINE!
Access your subscription at:
www.theclinics.com

Preface

Modern Critical Care Endocrinology and Its Impact on Critical Care Medicine

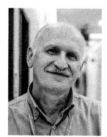

Rinaldo Bellomo, AO, MBBS (Hons), MD, PhD, FRACP, FCICM, FAAHMS
Editor

Endocrinology and issues related to the role of hormones in critical care medicine remain a dominant component of physiologic investigations, pathophysiologic manipulation, and treatment in patients admitted to intensive care units (ICUs) worldwide. As an example, only in the last 12 months, three major multicenter phase 3 randomized controlled trials (RCTs) have been published, which involved the assessment of hormonal therapy (hydrocortisone and angiotensin II) in patients with septic shock.[1–5]

However, until now, there has not been any dedicated attempt to introduce critical care physicians to modern ideas and recent evidence in this rapidly evolving field. This issue of *Critical Care Clinics* aims to do just that, by taking clinicians into a critical care endocrinology world many would not be familiar with. Yet, this is a world that brings important new pathophysiologic insights and promising new therapies into the field. Such insights and therapies should already shape the practice of intensive care medicine and may well shape much of the future treatment of our patients.

For the purpose of this issue, we have specifically chosen aspects of critical care endocrinology that have seen major changes in our understanding of how specific hormones work, how disorders of hormonal function should be diagnosed, and how hormones should be used for therapy in the ICU. We have started from issues related to the inadequate and/or excessive antidiuretic hormone secretion (ADH),[6] where modern endocrinology has delivered new diagnostic tools to our understanding of ADH (vasopressin) pathophysiology and where RCTs have provided new information about its use in septic shock[7] and the possible beneficial renal effects of ADH in this setting. We have then focused on emerging evidence for the possible role of hormone therapy in the management of trauma.[8] However, the most dramatic new entrant in critical care endocrinology has been the arrival of angiotensin II therapy and its Food and Drug

Crit Care Clin 35 (2019) xiii–xvi
https://doi.org/10.1016/j.ccc.2019.01.001
0749-0704/19/© 2019 Published by Elsevier Inc.

Administration approval as therapeutic agent after the completion and publication of the ATHOS-3 trial.[9] Accordingly, two articles in this issue are dedicated to angiotensin II. One is focused on new insights into the physiology and pathophysiology of angiotensin II, angiotensin-converting enzyme (ACE) and ACE2, and the growing family of angiotensin hormones.[10] The other is focused on its use for the treatment of vasodilatory shock.[11] Given the approval of this agent for the treatment of refractory vasodilatory shock, such articles are mandatory reading for critical care physicians. Similarly, a reassessment of another treatment of septic vasodilatory shock comes from the AD-RENAL and APROACCHSS trials,[1,3] which together randomized more than 5000 patients with septic shock. In this issue, the primary investigators of the ADRENAL trial review the powerful evidence derived from such studies and highlight their implications for clinical practice.[12]

The interaction between hormonal therapy and trauma is further developed in an article dedicated to the therapeutic potential and RCT data regarding erythropoietin (EPO) therapy for trauma and traumatic brain injury, where strong biological data, RCT-derived data, and meta-analytical data show a clear signal that EPO treatment might increase survival in trauma patients.[13]

The management of hyperglycemia in critically ill patients has been a major field of investigation for almost two decades, with multiple studies and several major RCTs. However, the field is now focusing on diabetic patients as a unique group of critically ill patients where the lessons learned from undifferentiated cohorts of critically ill patients may not apply, especially when preadmission glycemia (assessed by HbA1 levels) has been poorly controlled.[14,15] In this group of patients, permissive hyperglycemia may be both a rational approach and one capable of delivering significant benefits.[15] This is especially true as new technologies of semicontinuous glucose monitoring are becoming available for diabetic patients.[16] This controversial but rapidly evolving area is reviewed in a dedicated article.[17] However, these are not the only changes sweeping through the world of diabetes management. Several large RCTs have now established the potential for novel oral hypoglycemic agents to modify the risk of major adverse clinical outcomes in patients with diabetes. In particular, two classes of agents have now become widely used as a result of such trials: the sodium-glucose 2 cotransporter inhibitors (so called "flozins") and the dipeptidyl peptidase-4 inhibitors (so-called "gliptins"). These new drugs and the evidence behind their use are presented in this issue,[18] together with a review of a new class of hormones (the "incretins")[19] that appear to have a powerful role in regulating glucose absorption and blood glucose concentration.[20]

Other areas of ICU endocrinology are rapidly expanding. The regulation of disturbed sleep and the prevention of delirium have become major priorities in the care of ICU patients. Accordingly, the use of melatonin and melatonin receptor agonists has grown and has attracted attention as a novel pharmacologic development in intensive care treatment.[21]

Novel insights into the regulation of iron movement in and out of cells and the role of iron as a catalyst for oxygen radical species generation have led to renewed interest in hormones that regulate its extracellular availability. Of these, hepcidin, the master regulator of iron fluxes, is the most important. It role in physiology and pathophysiology and the potential for its therapeutic effects are a crucial new development of great interest to ICU clinicians.[22]

Finally, studies on the role of thyroid hormones[23] in the ICU, hormonal manipulation of organ donors,[24] and hormonal manipulation to prevent post-ICU accelerated osteoporosis[25] have markedly expanded our understanding of their pathophysiology and therapeutic potential. The implications of such new insights are reviewed in three key articles in this issue.

In summary, critical care endocrinology is a fundamental area of intensive care practice and is rapidly expanding in its knowledge base and therapeutic implications. Critical care physicians have a unique opportunity to update their knowledge and understanding through this dedicated issue of *Critical Care Clinics*. I am sure they will find it stimulating, provocative, and with multiple implications for their clinical practice.

Rinaldo Bellomo, AO, MBBS (Hons), MD, PhD, FRACP, FCICM, FAAHMS
Department of Medicine
Radiology and Critical Care
Centre for Integrated Critical Care
The University of Melbourne
Melbourne, VIC 3084, Australia

E-mail address:
Rinaldo.bellomo@austin.org.au

REFERENCES

1. Venkatesh B, Finfer S, Cohen J, et al. Adjunctive glucocorticoid therapy in patients with sepsis shock. N Engl J Med 2018;378:797–808.
2. Billot L, Venkatesh B, Myburgh J, et al. Statistical analysis plan for the adjunctive corticosteroid treatment in critically ill patients with septic shock (ADRENAL) trial. Crit Care Resusc 2017;19:183–91.
3. Annane D, Renault A, Brun-Buisson B, et al. Hydrocortisone plus fludrocortisone for adults with septic shock. N Engl J Med 2018;378:809–18.
4. Bellomo R, Hilton A. The ATHOS-3 trial, angiotensin II and the three musketeers. Crit Care Resusc 2017;19:1–4.
5. Chawla LS, Russell JA, Bagsahw SM, et al. Angiotensin II for the treatment of high-output shock 3 (ATHOS-3): protocol for a phase II, double-blind, randomised controlled trial. Crit Care Resusc 2017;19:43–9.
6. Harrois A, Anstey JR. Diabetes insipidus and syndrome of inappropriate antidiuretic hormone in critically ill patients. Crit Care Clin 2019;35(2):187–200.
7. Ukor IF, Walley KR. Vasopressin in vasodilatory shock. Crit Care Clin 2019;35(2):247–61.
8. Asehnoune K, Vourch'h M, Roquilly A. Hormone therapy in trauma patients. Crit Care Clin 2019;35(2):201–11.
9. Khanna A, English SW, Wang XS, et al. Angiotensin II for the treatment of vasodilatory shock. N Engl J Med 2017;377:419–30.
10. Bitker L, Burrell LM. Classic and nonclassic renin-angiotensin systems in the critically ill. Crit Care Clin 2019;35(2):213–27.
11. Wakefield BJ, Busse LW, Khanna AK. Angiotensin II in vasodilatory shock. Crit Care Clin 2019;35(2):229–45.
12. Venkatesh B, Cohen J. Hydrocortisone in vasodilatory shock. Crit Care Clin 2019;35(2):263–75.
13. French C. Erythropoietin in critical illness and trauma. Crit Care Clin 2019;35(2):277–87.
14. Plummer MP, Finnis ME, Horsfall M, et al. Prior exposure to hyperglycemia attenuates the relationship between glycaemic variability during critical illness and mortality. Crit Care Resusc 2016;18:189–97.
15. Martensson J, Bailey M, Venkatesh B, et al. Intensity of early correction of hyperglycemia and outcome of critically ill patients with diabetic ketoacidosis. Crit Care Resusc 2017;19:266–73.

16. Ancona P, Eastwood G, Lucchetta L, et al. The performance of flash glucose monitoring in critically ill patients with diabetes. Crit Care Resusc 2016;18: 167–74.
17. Balintescu A, Mårtensson J. Hemoglobin A1c and permissive hyperglycemia in patients in the intensive care unit with diabetes. Crit Care Clin 2019;35(2): 289–300.
18. Libianto R, Ekinci EI. New agents for the treatment of type 2 diabetes. Crit Care Clin 2019;35(2):315–28.
19. Plummer MP, Hermanides J, Deane AM. Incretin physiology and pharmacology in the intensive care unit. Crit Care Clin 2019;35(2):341–55.
20. Miller A, Deane AM, Plummer MP, et al. Exogenous glucagon-like peptide-1 attenuates glucose absorption and reduces blood glucose concentration after small intestinal glucose delivery in critical illness. Crit Care Resusc 2016;19: 37–42.
21. Marra A, McGrane TJ, Henson CP, et al. Melatonin in critical care. Crit Care Clin 2019;35(2):329–40.
22. Chawla LS, Beers-Mulroy B, Tidmarsh GF. Therapeutic opportunities for hepcidin in acute care medicine. Crit Care Clin 2019;35(2):357–74.
23. Maiden MJ, Torpy DJ. Thyroid hormones in critical illness. Crit Care Clin 2019; 35(2):375–88.
24. Opdam HI. Hormonal therapy in organ donors. Crit Care Clin 2019;35(2): 389–405.
25. Orford NR, Pasco JA, Kotowicz MA. Osteoporosis in the critically ill patient. Crit Care Clin 2019;35(2):301–13.

Diabetes Insipidus and Syndrome of Inappropriate Antidiuretic Hormone in Critically Ill Patients

Anatole Harrois, MD, PhD[a,b,]*, James R. Anstey, MBBS, FRACP, FCICM[a]

KEYWORDS

- Diabetes insipidus • Syndrome of inappropriate antidiuretic hormone (SIADH)
- Desmopressin • Hypernatremia • Hyponatremia • Fluid restriction • Oral urea
- Vaptans

KEY POINTS

- Diabetes insipidus can be diagnosed in the setting of hypotonic polyuria (urine output of >300 mL/h and urine osmolality of <300 mOsm/kg), leading to hypernatremia and volume depletion.
- Desmopressin is the standard replacement treatment to prevent free water loss in diabetes insipidus. The rate of correction of hypernatremia by hypotonic fluid warrants careful attention, principally to prevent neurologic complications.
- The syndrome of inappropriate antidiuretic hormone secretion can be diagnosed in the setting of inappropriately concentrated urine (>100 mOsm/kg) and urine sodium of greater than 30 mEq/L, leading to plasma hypoosmolality (<275 mOsm/kg) with clinical euvolemia.
- Management of the syndrome of inappropriate antidiuretic hormone secretion is guided by the severity of neurologic symptoms. Severe symptoms warrant emergent treatment with hypertonic saline. Although fluid restriction is effective in many cases, in patients in intensive care, this may not be feasible, and enteral urea or vaptans may be considered.

INTRODUCTION

Diabetes insipidus (DI) and the syndrome of inappropriate antidiuretic hormone secretion (SIADH) lie at opposite ends of the spectrum of disordered renal handling of water.

[a] Intensive Care Unit, Royal Melbourne Hospital, 300 Grattan Street, Parkville, Victoria 3050, Australia; [b] Department of Anesthesiology and Surgical Intensive Care, Hôpitaux Universitaires Paris Sud, Assistance Publique-Hôpitaux de Paris (AP-HP), Université Paris Sud, Université Paris Saclay, 78 rue du Général Leclerc, 94270 Le Kremlin Bicêtre, France
* Corresponding author. Intensive Care Unit, Royal Melbourne Hospital, 300 Grattan Street, Parkville, Victoria 3050, Australia.
E-mail address: harroisanatole@yahoo.fr

Crit Care Clin 35 (2019) 187–200
https://doi.org/10.1016/j.ccc.2018.11.001
0749-0704/19/© 2018 Elsevier Inc. All rights reserved.

At one end, DI occurs when there is a partial or complete absence of antidiuretic hormone (ADH) secretion, or limited renal response to this hormone, leading to renal loss of water. At the other end, SIADH is due to inappropriately high secretion of ADH, leading to renal retention of water. Although SIADH may present more insidiously and leads to hypotonic hyponatremia, DI may rapidly lead to severe free water loss, hypernatremia, and volume depletion if not treated.

Pathologies causing polyuria and hyponatremia in patients in the intensive care unit (ICU) may be multiple, making the diagnosis challenging in this setting. Herein, we provide an approach to the diagnosis and management of these conditions in ICU patients.

DIABETES INSIPIDUS

DI is defined by polyuria in the setting of hypotonic urine (osmolality <300 mOsm/kg H_2O), and polydipsia to compensate for the excessive urine output.[1] However, compensatory polydipsia is often absent in patients in the ICU because of an inability to sense or respond to thirst (eg, sedation, cerebral disease, inability to drink). Subsequently, in ICU patients who develop DI are particularly vulnerable to hypernatremia, and prompt diagnosis and intervention are important.

Some common causes of polyuria in patients in the ICU include diuretics, because of an osmotic load to the kidney (glycosuria, mannitol, urea), after excess administered salt or water, postobstructive diuresis, and in the recovery phase of critical illness. Unfortunately, given that polyuria is relatively common in patients in the ICU, DI may not be recognized until significant salt and water disturbance have occurred.

Etiologies

There are 4 etiologic categories of DI:

- Central (or neurogenic) DI is caused by a loss of the production of ADH (arginine vasopressin [AVP]), and is the most common etiology in patients in the ICU. A central cause occurs in the setting of injury to the posterior pituitary or hypothalamic median eminence. Early experiments suggested that 80% to 90% of magnocellular neurons in the hypothalamus need to be damaged before DI becomes manifest.[2] Central DI cases may occur in the setting of traumatic brain injury, after 20% to 30% cases of pituitary surgery,[3] and in about 50% of cases of brain death.[4] Less commonly, insidious cerebral diseases such as tumor, inflammatory disease (granulomatosis), or infectious diseases may also lead to a loss of ADH secretion. These conditions may not necessarily be obvious when a patient is admitted to the ICU and might need additional assessment (eg, MRI) to identify the pathology.
- Nephrogenic DI is caused by a loss of sensitivity of the kidney to ADH. However, these patients usually maintain some ability to form hypertonic urine, and as such polyuria seldom exceeds 3 to 4 L/d.[3] Medications and hypercalcemia are the most common causes.[5] Among medications known to induce nephrogenic DI, lithium therapy is the most common, and DI is seen in about 10% to 20% of patients treated long term.[6] Of note, it may occur at therapeutic lithium concentrations.[7] Genetic causes, usually presenting in childhood, are far less common.
- Primary polydipsia is seen in patients with increased thirst sensation and/or psychiatric disorders that lead to excessive water intake and subsequent diminished ADH secretion. Oral dryness from certain medications (eg, antidepressant medications) or advice to increase water consumption may similarly lead to polydipsia. Unlike other forms of DI, where the serum sodium is normal or high

once water is restricted, these patients may present to the ICU with severe hyponatremia. This condition develops owing to a combination of ingestion of large volumes of water, impairment of the diluting ability of the kidney (often from medications), and often low solute intake.[8]

- Gestational DI is due to excessive ADH degradation by a placentally-produced enzyme. However, ADH levels are often normal, suggesting a likely underlying deficiency.[9] This disorder is rarely encountered in the ICU.

Consequences of Diabetes Insipidus

Patients with DI produce an inappropriately large volume of hypotonic urine. Although a small proportion of ICU patients might be able to compensate for water loss by increasing fluid oral intake (ie, after pituitary surgery with preserved awareness), most patients in the ICU are unable to do so. As a result, hypernatremia can ensue rapidly. Intravascular depletion may rapidly lead to poor organ perfusion.

Hypernatremia (Na of $\geq$145 mmol/L) leads to a shift of free water from the intracellular space to the extracellular space. In patients in the ICU, serum sodium values of greater than 148 mmol/L are independently associated with mortality.[4,10–12] The link between hypernatremia and mortality is stronger in patients with acute cerebral disease than other patients in the ICU.[4] In traumatic brain injury, DI is associated with a mortality of 70%[13,14] and is in itself an independent risk factor for mortality.[15,16] More severe hypernatremia (>160 mmol/L) is an additional risk factor for death.[14]

In brain dead patients, several studies have suggested that severe hypernatremia (Na of 155–160 mmol/L) has detrimental effects on graft function after liver[17] and kidney transplantation.[18] Although this finding has been recently challenged[19] and hypernatremia of greater than 160 mmol/L is no longer an absolute contraindication to liver donation, significant hypernatremia remains undesirable in brain dead donors.

Diagnosis

Classical criteria to diagnose DI rely on the combination of a high urine output (>3 L/24 h), hypotonic urine (<300 mOsm/kg), and polydipsia.[1] However, the need for timely intervention in patients who cannot respond to thirst makes these diagnostic criteria unsafe in the ICU setting. Thus, central DI in patients in the ICU should be considered in any patient with a high urine output and a serum sodium concentration that is increasing beyond the normal range, especially in the setting of a likely cause such as acute cerebral injury. When there is a total absence of ADH release, extremely high urine outputs may be seen, often in the order of 400 mL/h to 1 L/h in the adult patient. These patients will typically have extremely hypotonic urine (<150 mOsm/kg). However, in partial ADH deficiency, urine outputs of as low as 3 L/d may be seen with urine osmolality between 200 and 300 mOsm/kg. In these cases, an unexplained increasing serum sodium may be the main clue.

DI diagnosis relies on 3 major elements in patients in the ICU:

1. *Polyuria*: Arbitrarily, an urine output of greater than 300 mL/h for at least 2 hours is consistent with this diagnosis,[15,16,20] although urine outputs ranging from 2 to 5 mL/kg/h have been proposed[14,21] in post neurosurgery or neurointensive care patients.
2. *Hypotonic urine*: A urine osmolality of less than 300 mOsm/kg (**Fig. 1**).[3]
   Urine osmolarity is essential to distinguish DI from polyuria owing to a solute (osmotic) diuresis. Glucose, urea, ethanol, mannitol, and sodium (from excess crystalloid) are common causes of a solute diuresis and in these cases the urine osmolality will be greater than 300 mOsm/kg. Some teams report the usefulness of measuring

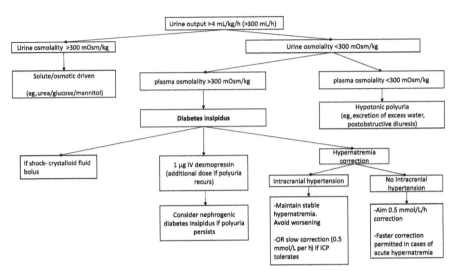

Fig. 1. An approach to the patient with possible central diabetes insipidus. ICP, intracranial pressure; IV, intravenous.

urine density and have suggested that a urine gravity of less than 1.005[14] or less than 1.003[20] fulfills the criteria of hypotonic urine. However, measuring urine gravity with a densitometer, refractometer, or reagent strips may lead to unreliable results. Indeed, these techniques are not identical[22] and measured urine density does not correlate well with urine osmolality. A recent study showed that about 28% of urine densities that are less than 1.010 had an osmolality of greater than 350 mOsm/kg, and a 1.005 threshold led to similar inaccuracy.[23] For this reason, a definitive diagnosis should rely on a laboratory measurement rather than urine dipsticks.

3. *Plasma hyperosmolality*: Because serum sodium is the major determinant of serum osmolality, a serum sodium concentration of greater than 145 mmol/L,[14,16] corresponding with a serum osmolality of greater than 300 mOsm/kg[14,16] may be used in the diagnosis of DI (see **Fig. 1**). However, an increase in serum sodium, rather than the absolute level, might be more relevant in patients in the ICU, where serum sodium may already be increased before the onset of DI. Therefore, we would suggest that an increase of 2 to 3 mmol/L in serum sodium (above the normal serum sodium range), associated with hypotonic urine, might be used to diagnose DI in patients in the ICU, when combined with the other 2 criteria.
Importantly, this picture should be distinguished from the entirely appropriate diuresis of hypotonic urine seen with water overload (eg, after consumption or administration of excess water), similarly associated with increasing serum sodium. Here, the response is physiologic and the serum sodium concentration would be expected to move back toward the normal range, not above it. As such, these patients would fulfill only the first 2 criteria.

Other tests

AVP measurement has been proposed for DI diagnosis, but remains technically difficult owing to the short half-life of the molecule.[24] More recently, measuring levels of copeptin, a glycoprotein of the AVP prohormone, and a stable surrogate for endogenous plasma AVP, has shown promising results.[25] In patients who have undergone pituitary surgery, copeptin concentrations of less than 2.5 pmol/L had a specificity of

97% for DI diagnosis. In a series of 92 patients with severe hypernatremia (Na of >155 mmol/L) of whom 54% were admitted to ICU, copeptin values of less than 4.4 pmol/L had a 100% sensitivity and 99% specificity to predict central DI. Of note, a urea lower than 5.05 mmol/L performed similarly well.[26] More recently, in an outpatient setting,[27] investigated the accuracy of hypertonic saline-stimulated plasma copeptin in the diagnosis of diabetes insipidus in 141 patients with hypotonic polyuria. A cutoff level of plasma copeptin of 4.9 pmol/L had a diagnostic accuracy of 96.5%, which performed better than the water-deprivation test that is considered as the current reference standard to distinguish diabetes insipidus from primary polydipsia.[27] Further investigations are needed to explore the utility of plasma copeptin in the diagnosis of diabetes insipidus in ICU.

Treatment

Treatment of DI has two components:

1. Replacing ADH to prevent ongoing renal water loss, and
2. Replacing any water loss that has already occurred to correct hypernatremia.

While patients in the ICU with DI are being stabilized, we would recommend hourly urine measurements and serum sodium measurements, at least until polyuria is controlled and serum sodium levels have plateaued.

Substitution treatment of antidiuretic hormone

ADH permits free water reabsorption by the kidneys via V2 receptors located in renal epithelial cells of collecting ducts. By interacting with V2 receptors, ADH causes epithelial cells to express aquaporin 2 ducts, which allows transfer of water from collecting ducts to the interstitial space. ADH acts also on V1b receptors, which are present in many tissues, and leads to peripheral vasoconstriction.

D-deargino-vasopressin (desmopressin, DDAVP), a vasopressin analogue, has now become the treatment of choice for central DI (see **Fig. 1**). Indeed, DDAVP has less vasoconstricting effect than the native hormone (ADH), with subsequent less risk of hypertension, and has a more sustained antidiuretic effect than ADH. Initial doses of 0.5 to 2.0 μg are usually given intravenously[20,28–30] with an antidiuretic action of around 12 hours, although individual variations in antidiuretic response are reported.[31] We use an initial dose of 1 μg, aiming at decreasing urine output to a physiologic range (1–2 mL/kg/h). A second injection of desmopressin should be given after 2 hours if the first dose does not achieve this goal. Regular administration every 12 hours may not be necessary because DI may be transient.[32] Further doses should be guided by a protocol based on hourly urine output. Excessive administration may lead to water retention and hypoosmolarity, however.

Oral desmopressin is also effective; however, its low bioavailability requires higher doses than intravenous administration. Its duration of action is also shorter (6–8 hours). This formulation would only be suitable in a small proportion of conscious patients in the ICU (ie, post pituitary surgery patients) upon step-down to the ward.

FLUID RESUSCITATION AND HYPERNATREMIA CORRECTION

Hypovolemia and shock call for fluid resuscitation that aims at expanding extracellular volume; crystalloid solutions should be used (see **Fig. 1**). We believe that it is desirable to administer a solution well-matched to the patient's hyperosmolar state, to avoid further rapid shifts in osmolarity and possible cerebral edema. For example, in a patient whose serum sodium has increased to 155 mmol/L (ie, a serum osmolarity of approximately 330 mOsm/L), we would prefer 0.9% NaCl over other crystalloids (such as

Hartmann's solution) in the resuscitation phase. After volume resuscitation has occurred, because these patients sometimes lose significant intravascular volume before the diagnosis is made, ongoing hypotonic fluid administration should be administered to compensate for water loss. In severe cases, we use intravenous free water administered via a central line, before transitioning to enteral administration (nasogastric water). This avoids giving large volumes of dextrose solution, which can lead to glycosuria, ongoing water loss, and hypernatremia. In conscious patients (eg, post pituitary surgery patients), free access to water should be promoted with intake according to thirst.

Close attention should be paid to the rate of serum sodium correction in hypernatremia. For patients with hypernatremia for more than 48 hours, correction should be limited to 8 to 10 mmol/L per 24-hour period.[33,34] When a patient already has an increased intracranial pressure, the correction process of hypernatremia should be meticulous (see **Fig. 1**). In general, in patients with shorter-lived hypernatremia, slightly faster correction of acutely elevated serum sodium may be permissible (1–2 mmol/L per hour with maximum daily correction of 12 mmol/L), although similar precautions should be taken in patients with raised intracranial pressure.[33,34]

NEPHROGENIC DIABETES INSIPIDUS

Because nephrogenic DI is due to renal inability to respond completely to ADH, ADH administration is only partially effective in decreasing urinary free water loss. Although lithium is the leading cause of this condition, other drugs including amphotericin B, ofloxacin, and chemotherapy agents (ifosfamide, cisplatin) can also cause nephrogenic DI.[35,36] Hypokalemia, hypercalcemia, and some systemic diseases are sometimes implicated. Obstructive renal diseases are also commonly reported to cause nephrogenic DI, with high urinary tract pressure being thought to decrease aquaporin expression, which could explain excessive diuresis after relief of obstruction.[37] Occasionally, adjunctive therapies may be necessary to limit fluid loss. Chlorothiazide, amiloride, and indomethacin have been used and are reported to halve urine output and double urine osmolality in cases of nephrogenic diabetes.[1,36] Amiloride is the most appropriate drug to counteract lithium toxicity by decreasing epithelial sodium channel activity, which transports lithium into renal epithelial cells. Fluid compensation is also mandatory to maintain serum osmolality because the available treatments are at best only partially effective.

THE SYNDROME OF INAPPROPRIATE ANTIDIURETIC HORMONE SECRETION

SIADH is a hormone disorder in which abnormal water retention and excessive electrolyte excretion occur. Consequently, it leads to hypotonic hyponatremia and increased total body water. By "inappropriate," the diagnosis implies that physiologic triggers for ADH secretion—hypovolemia or hyperosmolarity (plasma osmolality <280 mOsm/kg)—are absent. Although water retention caused by ADH secretion initially leads to plasma dilution with subsequent hyponatremia, it also leads to low-level volume overload. The latter triggers renal electrolyte excretion, including sodium, and further worsens hyponatremia. An endocrine cause (hypoadrenalism or hypothyroidism) may cause the same clinical picture and should be excluded.

Etiologies

Many diseases can result in SIADH, including cancer, lung diseases, cerebral disease, and a large list of drugs (**Table 1**). Some of these diseases, principally malignancy, cause ectopic production of ADH. A second group is due to excessive ADH release from the pituitary gland (central nervous system diseases). A third group is due to

Table 1
Causes of syndrome of inappropriate antidiuretic hormone

Cancer	Drugs	Lung Disease	Central Nervous System Diseases	Transient
Carcinoma (SCLC, NSCLC, oropharyngeal, gastrointestinal, genitourinary) Mesothelioma Lymphoma Sarcoma	Selective serotonin reuptake inhibitors Tricyclic antidepressants Neuroleptics Clofibrate Carbamazepine Sodium valproate Chlorpropamide Antineoplastic drugs (ifosfamide, vincristine, cyclophosphamide) Nonsteroidal antiinflammatory drugs Nicotine Amiodarone Proton pump inhibitors Vasopressin analogues (desmopressin, oxytocin, terlipressin, vasopressin)	Infections (bacterial, viral, abscess, tuberculosis, aspergillosis) Cystic fibrosis Positive pressure ventilation	Infections (abscess, meningitis, encephalitis) Bleeding (subdural hematoma, subarachnoid hemorrhage, traumatic brain injury) Brain tumor Multiple sclerosis Thrombosis	General anesthesia Stress Pain Exercise

Abbreviations: NSCLC, non–small cell lung carcinoma; SCLC, small cell lung carcinoma.
From New Engl J Med, Ellison DG, Berl T, The Syndrome of Inappropriate Antidiuresis, 356:2064-2072. Copyright ©2007 Massachusetts Medical Society. Reprinted with permission from Massachusetts Medical Society.

excessive sensitivity to ADH of vasopressin receptors in the renal collecting ducts, which may be caused by certain drugs (carbamazepine, for instance). In a series of 600 patients from the emergency department or hospital wards with hyponatremia (<130 mmol/L) and a subsequent diagnosis of SIADH, it was reported that central nervous system diseases accounted for 26% of cases, lung diseases 19%, cancers 18%, and drugs 8%.[38] Pain is among the triggers of hypersecretion of ADH and can also lead to SIADH,[39] which is important in the postoperative setting.

Consequences

The major consequence of SIADH is hyponatremia, resulting in hypotonic plasma. This may be categorized as mild (plasma Na^+ of 130–135 mmol/L), moderate (Na^+ of 125–129 mmol/L), or severe (Na^+ of $\leq$124 mmol/L). Hypotonic hyponatremia results in the movement of water from the extracellular space to the intracellular space. In the brain, this increase in cellular volume may be life-threatening, with a risk of intracranial hypertension and brain herniation. Counterregulatory mechanisms may protect against intracellular volume increase, achieved by early electrolyte extrusion (chloride, potassium) from neurons and astrocytes, followed by osmolyte extrusion (eg, myoinositol, phosphocreatine) after 48 hours.[40] However, in rapidly-occuring hyponatremia, this adaptive system is likely to be overwhelmed, leading to uncontrolled cerebral edema.

Clinical symptoms of hyponatremia may include headaches, poor concentration, nausea, or muscle cramps. In its most severe stage, hyponatremia causes seizures, hemiplegia, coma, and death. Interestingly, even asymptomatic chronic hyponatremia is associated with an increased risk of falls in the elderly, and the wisdom of tolerating mild hyponatremia in the absence of clear symptoms has been questioned.[41]

Diagnosis

SIADH is a diagnosis of exclusion. First, it is important to confirm that hyponatremia is associated with a hypoosmolality of less than 275 mOsm/kg.[42] In contrast, pseudohyponatremia may occur in the presence of significant hyperlipidemia or hyperproteinemia, when laboratory measurement of sodium concentration, which relies on dilutional techniques, is used to determine the sodium concentration.[43] Blood gas measurements, which use a direct Na ion-specific electrode, overcome this problem.[43] Hypertonic hyponatremia mostly caused by severe hyperglycemia or exogenous solute intake (mannitol or ethylene glycol, for instance) can be ruled out by confirming plasma hypoosmolarity.

Classic teaching is that the next step in the evaluation of hyponatremia is volume status assessment.[44] However, clinical appraisal of volume status has been reported to perform poorly.[45–47] For this reason, European guidelines now recommend measuring urine sodium concentration and urine osmolality, instead of undertaking clinical assessment of volume status.[42]

The diagnostic criteria for SIADH are:

1. Plasma hypoosmolality (<275 mOsm/kg),
2. Inappropriately concentrated urine (>100 mOsm/kg, but usually higher than serum osmolality),
3. Clinical euvolemia,
4. Urine sodium greater than 30 mEq/L,[a] and
5. Normal adrenal and thyroid function.

Additional diagnostic tests, such as fractional excretion of sodium, urea, and uric acid, have been proposed to guide SIADH diagnosis, but they lack specificity.[8,48,49] Moreover, their diagnostic value has not been assessed in patients in the ICU to date. Plasma copeptin levels have been reported to be higher in hypovolemic and hypervolemic hyponatremia than in patients with SIADH (euvolemic), but this test remains insufficiently accurate to discriminate between conditions.[50] Further research is needed to propose an accurate biomarker to help in the diagnosis of SIADH.

Specific challenges in diagnosis in the intensive care unit

Patients in the ICU present multiple challenges when determining the cause of hyponatremia. First, several causes of hyponatremia may coexist. Second, renal dysfunction may alter sodium and water excretion, resulting in misinterpretations of urine biochemistry,[51] which also cannot be interpreted meaningfully after diuretics. Finally, the clinical assessment of volume status is problematic.

Cerebral salt wasting syndrome: a challenging differential diagnosis

Because SIADH and cerebral salt wasting may both lead to hyponatremia in the setting of a brain injury, brief mention of this condition is worthwhile. Cerebral salt

---

[a] The urine sodium concentration may be low; however, in the salt-depleted patient,[41] rarely an issue except at ICU admission.

wasting syndrome is defined as abnormally high renal sodium excretion resulting in hyponatremia with extracellular volume depletion. Although initially described in the context of cerebral disease, it has been seen in other settings, and is now increasingly known as renal salt wasting syndrome (RSW).[52] The reported prevalence of RSW ranges from 1% to 34% among hyponatremic patients with cerebral insults.[53–55] Theoretically, differentiating SIADH from RSW is of importance because the treatment of SIADH relies on fluid restriction, whereas the treatment of RSW requires salt and water replacement. However, overlapping clinical and biological signs make them extremely difficult to differentiate. Indeed, hyponatremia, concentrated urine, a urine sodium of greater than 30 mEq/L, increased fractional excretion of urate, and intracranial disease are common to both syndromes. The only difference between the two is that RSW leads to volume depletion, unlike SIADH, which does not. For this reason, if SIADH treatment fails with worsening hyponatremia and volume depletion after fluid restriction, one should favor a diagnosis of RSW.[56]

Treatment of Hyponatremia Owing to the Syndrome of Inappropriate Antidiuretic Hormone Secretion

We propose a treatment algorithm for SIADH according to the severity of symptoms in **Fig. 2**.

Emergency treatment of syndrome of inappropriate antidiuretic hormone secretion-associated hyponatremia with severe symptoms

Severe symptoms of hyponatremia usually occur at a level lower than 120 to 125 mmol/L.[44] Patients can tolerate even lower levels if the onset occurs more gradually. Once severe symptoms (ie, vomiting, cardiorespiratory distress, deep somnolence, seizures, Glasgow Coma Scale of ≤8, intracranial hypertension) develop that are attributable to hyponatremia, prompt infusion of 150 mL of 3% hypertonic saline over 20 minutes is recommended. A second dose of 150 mL is proposed to achieve an improvement of symptoms, or sufficient to increase the serum sodium concentration by 5 mmol/L, whichever comes first.[42]

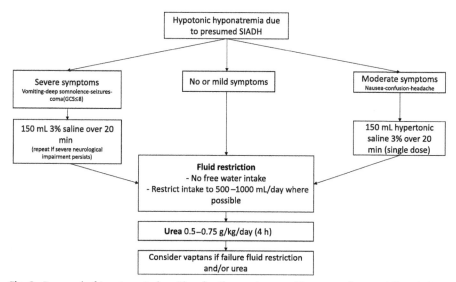

Fig. 2. Proposal of treatment algorithm for the syndrome of inappropriate antidiuretic hormone secretion (SIADH). GCS, Glasgow Coma Scale.

For moderate symptoms (nausea, confusion, or headache) that may also relate to brain edema, but are less likely to cause brain herniation, experts recommend 150 mL of a 3% hypertonic saline over 20 minutes once.[42]

Further correction of sodium concentration should occur at a rate not exceeding 8 to 10 mmol/L in the first 24 hours, or 18 mmol/L in the first 48 hours, to prevent osmotic demyelination.[57,58] This rate is all the more important in cases of chronic hyponatremia (>48 hours) owing to SIADH or in alcoholic patients who are more sensitive to large variations in plasma osmolality.[59] Frequent monitoring of serum sodium concentration is necessary.

In the event of excessively rapid correction of hyponatremia, we recommend relowering serum sodium concentration, an approach supported by experimental studies.[60] We achieve this by administering intravenous dextrose or enteral free water. In some cases, particularly when there is marked polyuria, we administer DDAVP (1–2 μg) to achieve control of the rapidly increasing serum sodium.

Ongoing treatment for the syndrome of inappropriate antidiuretic hormone secretion
Fluid restriction is generally the cornerstone of SIADH treatment. However, fluid restriction may not be possible in certain patients in the ICU owing to the administration of medications and enteral feeds. Moreover, fluid restriction may be undesirable in pathologies like subarachnoid hemorrhage if vasospasm has developed. Therefore, a second treatment is frequently required to correct hyponatremia.

In certain countries, enteral urea is available as a treatment, and enhances free water excretion and probably acts also by decreasing renal sodium excretion,[61] both resulting in an increase in serum sodium. Urea effectively corrected hyponatremia in 3 series of patients in the ICU who were diagnosed with euvolemic hyponatremia suggestive of SIADH. In mild to moderate hyponatremia (120–134 mmol/L), urea administration increased serum sodium by a mean of 7 mmol/L in 48 hours[61–63] and by about 10 mmol/L in patients with severe hyponatremia. Urea was also effective when fluid intake of 3000 mL of NaCl 0.9% and enteral feeding were maintained in patients with hyponatremia.[61] Enteral urea doses of 0.25 to 0.75 g/kg/d are recommended for this condition.[42,62]

Novel treatments
Vaptans, a recent class of vasopressin V2 receptor antagonists, have been proposed for the treatment of hyponatremia owing to SIADH in patients in the ICU. By promoting free water excretion, vaptans increase the serum sodium by approximately 5 to 8 mmol/L in first 24 hours when used in patients in the ICU.[64–67] Conivaptan can be administered intravenously (as a bolus of 20 mg sometimes followed by a 24-hour infusion of 20 mg); tolvaptan is an oral drug given at a dose of 15 mg/d. Although its use has been less reported in the ICU, tolvaptan leads to similar correction of hyponatremia[64,68]; however, one study reported a 20% rate of overcorrection.[64] In previous studies conducted in patients not in the ICU, vaptans led to a 60% increase in the risk of overcorrection when compared with placebo. This finding was confirmed in a recent study conducted by Tzoulis and colleagues[69] reporting a 20% rate of overcorrection with vaptans, although no cases of osmotic demyelination were described. Moreover, the US Food and Drug Administration has questioned tolvaptan's safety, because this agent has been reported to cause liver enzyme disturbances. For these reasons, European experts do not recommend their use in SIADH, although American experts consider their use second line and have suggested caution.[44] No study has ever compared urea with vaptans in the ICU. However, in an animal model of chronic hyponatremia, rapid correction of

hyponatremia with urea led to less brain histological changes and less neurologic impairment than with vaptans or hypertonic saline.[60]

A combination of low-dose loop diuretics and oral sodium intake has been proposed. Although a loop diuretic would be expected to lead to more free water excretion than salt administration, oral sodium intake compensates for the small amount of sodium loss induced by diuretics. However, the response to diuretics in SIADH is unpredictable, with the risk of intravascular volume depletion, and there are fewer data supporting this strategy than urea intake.

SUMMARY

Abnormal ADH secretion leads to acute natremia variations resulting in hypernatremia in DI, and hyponatremia in SIADH. Both hypernatremia and hyponatremia are associated with worse outcomes and longer ICU stays. Desmopressin is the key treatment in DI. Pitfalls relate to delays in diagnosis owing to multiple reasons for polyuria in patients in the ICU. The rate of correction of hypernatremia merits special attention, to prevent brain injury. A definitive diagnosis of SIADH may be difficult, because volume assessment can be unreliable, and this has been deemphasized in newer diagnostic approaches. Fluid restriction alone is often insufficient to manage SIADH, and a second treatment may be necessary, such as enteral urea. Although vaptans seem to be effective in achieving free water excretion, their benefit, as well as their safety, are yet to be confirmed.

REFERENCES

1. Robertson GL. Diabetes insipidus: differential diagnosis and management. Best Pract Res Clin Endocrinol Metab 2016;30:205–18.
2. Heinbecker P, White HL. The role of the pituitary gland in water balance. Ann Surg 1939;110:1037–49.
3. Fenske W, Allolio B. Clinical review: current state and future perspectives in the diagnosis of diabetes insipidus: a clinical review. J Clin Endocrinol Metab 2012;97:3426–37.
4. Imaizumi T, Nakatochi M, Fujita Y, et al. The association between intensive care unit-acquired hypernatraemia and mortality in critically ill patients with cerebrovascular diseases: a single-centre cohort study in Japan. BMJ Open 2017;7: e016248.
5. Moeller HB, Rittig S, Fenton RA. Nephrogenic diabetes insipidus: essential insights into the molecular background and potential therapies for treatment. Endocr Rev 2013;34:278–301.
6. Bendz H, Aurell M. Drug-induced diabetes insipidus: incidence, prevention and management. Drug Saf 1999;21:449–56.
7. Christensen S, Kusano E, Yusufi AN, et al. Pathogenesis of nephrogenic diabetes insipidus due to chronic administration of lithium in rats. J Clin Invest 1985;75: 1869–79.
8. Decaux G. The syndrome of inappropriate secretion of antidiuretic hormone (SIADH). Semin Nephrol 2009;29:239–56.
9. Ananthakrishnan S. Diabetes insipidus during pregnancy. Best Pract Res Clin Endocrinol Metab 2016;30:305–15.
10. Hu B, Han Q, Mengke N, et al. Prognostic value of ICU-acquired hypernatremia in patients with neurological dysfunction. Medicine (Baltimore) 2016;95:e3840.

11. Okazaki T, Hifumi T, Kawakita K, et al. Target serum sodium levels during intensive care unit management of aneurysmal subarachnoid hemorrhage. Shock 2017;48:558–63.

12. Darmon M, Timsit JF, Francais A, et al. Association between hypernatraemia acquired in the ICU and mortality: a cohort study. Nephrol Dial Transplant 2010;25: 2510–5.

13. Boughey JC, Yost MJ, Bynoe RP. Diabetes insipidus in the head-injured patient. Am Surg 2004;70:500–3.

14. Yang YH, Lin JJ, Hsia SH, et al. Central diabetes insipidus in children with acute brain insult. Pediatr Neurol 2011;45:377–80.

15. Hadjizacharia P, Beale EO, Inaba K, et al. Acute diabetes insipidus in severe head injury: a prospective study. J Am Coll Surg 2008;207:477–84.

16. Alharfi IM, Stewart TC, Foster J, et al. Central diabetes insipidus in pediatric severe traumatic brain injury. Pediatr Crit Care Med 2013;14:203–9.

17. Totsuka E, Fung U, Hakamada K, et al. Analysis of clinical variables of donors and recipients with respect to short-term graft outcome in human liver transplantation. Transplant Proc 2004;36:2215–8.

18. Kwiatkowska E, Bober J, Ciechanowski K, et al. Increased serum sodium values in brain-dead donor's influences its long-term kidney function. Transplant Proc 2013;45:51–6.

19. Khosravi MB, Firoozifar M, Ghaffaripour S, et al. Early outcomes of liver transplants in patients receiving organs from hypernatremic donors. Exp Clin Transplant 2013;11:537–40.

20. Guesde R, Barrou B, Leblanc I, et al. Administration of desmopressin in brain-dead donors and renal function in kidney recipients. Lancet 1998;352:1178–81.

21. Seckl J, Dunger D. Postoperative diabetes insipidus. BMJ 1989;298:2–3.

22. Dorizzi RM, Caputo M. Measurement of urine relative density using refractometer and reagent strips. Clin Chem Lab Med 1998;36:925–8.

23. Souza AC, Zatz R, de Oliveira RB, et al. Is urinary density an adequate predictor of urinary osmolality? BMC Nephrol 2015;16:46.

24. Balanescu S, Kopp P, Gaskill MB, et al. Correlation of plasma copeptin and vasopressin concentrations in hypo-, iso-, and hyperosmolar states. J Clin Endocrinol Metab 2011;96:1046–52.

25. Christ-Crain M, Fenske W. Copeptin in the diagnosis of vasopressin-dependent disorders of fluid homeostasis. Nat Rev Endocrinol 2016;12:168–76.

26. Nigro N, Winzeler B, Suter-Widmer I, et al. Copeptin levels and commonly used laboratory parameters in hospitalised patients with severe hypernatraemia - the "Co-MED study". Crit Care 2018;22:33.

27. Fenske W, Refardt J, Chifu I, et al. A copeptin-based approach in the diagnosis of diabetes insipidus. New Engl J Med 2018;379:428–39.

28. Chanson P, Salenave S. Treatment of neurogenic diabetes insipidus. Ann Endocrinol (Paris) 2011;72:496–9.

29. Juul KV, Bichet DG, Norgaard JP. Desmopressin duration of antidiuretic action in patients with central diabetes insipidus. Endocrine 2011;40:67–74.

30. Rembratt A, Graugaard-Jensen C, Senderovitz T, et al. Pharmacokinetics and pharmacodynamics of desmopressin administered orally versus intravenously at daytime versus night-time in healthy men aged 55-70 years. Eur J Clin Pharmacol 2004;60:397–402.

31. Juul KV, Erichsen L, Robertson GL. Temporal delays and individual variation in antidiuretic response to desmopressin. Am J Physiol Renal Physiol 2013;304: F268–78.

32. Sheehan JM, Sheehan JP, Douds GL, et al. DDAVP use in patients undergoing transsphenoidal surgery for pituitary adenomas. Acta Neurochir (Wien) 2006; 148:287–91.
33. Adrogue HJ, Madias NE. Hypernatremia. N Engl J Med 2000;342:1493–9.
34. Lindner G, Funk GC. Hypernatremia in critically ill patients. J Crit Care 2013;28: 216.e11-20.
35. Nigro N, Grossmann M, Chiang C, et al. Polyuria-polydipsia syndrome: a diagnostic challenge. Intern Med J 2018;48:244–53.
36. Bockenhauer D, Bichet DG. Pathophysiology, diagnosis and management of nephrogenic diabetes insipidus. Nat Rev Nephrol 2015;11:576–88.
37. Nielsen S, Frokiaer J, Marples D, et al. Aquaporins in the kidney: from molecules to medicine. Physiol Rev 2002;82:205–44.
38. Cuesta M, Garrahy A, Slattery D, et al. The contribution of undiagnosed adrenal insufficiency to euvolaemic hyponatraemia: results of a large prospective single-centre study. Clin Endocrinol (Oxf) 2016;85:836–44.
39. Shepshelovich D, Leibovitch C, Klein A, et al. The syndrome of inappropriate antidiuretic hormone secretion: distribution and characterization according to etiologies. Eur J Intern Med 2015;26:819–24.
40. Adrogue HJ, Madias NE. Hyponatremia. N Engl J Med 2000;342:1581–9.
41. Decaux G, Musch W. Clinical laboratory evaluation of the syndrome of inappropriate secretion of antidiuretic hormone. Clin J Am Soc Nephrol 2008;3:1175–84.
42. Spasovski G, Vanholder R, Allolio B, et al. Clinical practice guideline on diagnosis and treatment of hyponatraemia. Eur J Endocrinol 2014;170:G1–47.
43. Turchin A, Seifter JL, Seely EW. Clinical problem-solving. Mind the gap. N Engl J Med 2003;349:1465–9.
44. Verbalis JG, Goldsmith SR, Greenberg A, et al. Diagnosis, evaluation, and treatment of hyponatremia: expert panel recommendations. Am J Med 2013;126: S1–42.
45. McGee S, Abernethy WB 3rd, Simel DL. The rational clinical examination. Is this patient hypovolemic? JAMA 1999;281:1022–9.
46. Musch W, Thimpont J, Vandervelde D, et al. Combined fractional excretion of sodium and urea better predicts response to saline in hyponatremia than do usual clinical and biochemical parameters. Am J Med 1995;99:348–55.
47. Fenske W, Maier SK, Blechschmidt A, et al. Utility and limitations of the traditional diagnostic approach to hyponatremia: a diagnostic study. Am J Med 2010;123: 652–7.
48. Fenske W, Stork S, Koschker AC, et al. Value of fractional uric acid excretion in differential diagnosis of hyponatremic patients on diuretics. J Clin Endocrinol Metab 2008;93:2991–7.
49. Maesaka JK, Imbriano LJ, Miyawaki N. Application of established pathophysiologic processes brings greater clarity to diagnosis and treatment of hyponatremia. World J Nephrol 2017;6:59–71.
50. Nigro N, Winzeler B, Suter-Widmer I, et al. Evaluation of copeptin and commonly used laboratory parameters for the differential diagnosis of profound hyponatraemia in hospitalized patients: 'The Co-MED Study'. Clin Endocrinol (Oxf) 2017;86: 456–62.
51. Legrand M, Le Cam B, Perbet S, et al. Urine sodium concentration to predict fluid responsiveness in oliguric ICU patients: a prospective multicenter observational study. Crit Care 2016;20:165.
52. Maesaka JK, Imbriano LJ, Ali NM, et al. Is it cerebral or renal salt wasting? Kidney Int 2009;76:934–8.

53. Brimioulle S, Orellana-Jimenez C, Aminian A, et al. Hyponatremia in neurological patients: cerebral salt wasting versus inappropriate antidiuretic hormone secretion. Intensive Care Med 2008;34:125–31.

54. Kao L, Al-Lawati Z, Vavao J, et al. Prevalence and clinical demographics of cerebral salt wasting in patients with aneurysmal subarachnoid hemorrhage. Pituitary 2009;12:347–51.

55. Leonard J, Garrett RE, Salottolo K, et al. Cerebral salt wasting after traumatic brain injury: a review of the literature. Scand J Trauma Resusc Emerg Med 2015;23:98.

56. Taylor P, Dehbozorgi S, Tabasum A, et al. Cerebral salt wasting following traumatic brain injury. Endocrinol Diabetes Metab Case Rep 2017.

57. Sterns RH. Severe symptomatic hyponatremia: treatment and outcome. A study of 64 cases. Ann Intern Med 1987;107:656–64.

58. Sterns RH, Cappuccio JD, Silver SM, et al. Neurologic sequelae after treatment of severe hyponatremia: a multicenter perspective. J Am Soc Nephrol 1994;4:1522–30.

59. Gocht A, Colmant HJ. Central pontine and extrapontine myelinolysis: a report of 58 cases. Clin Neuropathol 1987;6:262–70.

60. Gankam Kengne F, Soupart A, Pochet R, et al. Re-induction of hyponatremia after rapid overcorrection of hyponatremia reduces mortality in rats. Kidney Int 2009;76:614–21.

61. Pierrakos C, Taccone FS, Decaux G, et al. Urea for treatment of acute SIADH in patients with subarachnoid hemorrhage: a single-center experience. Ann Intensive Care 2012;2:13.

62. Decaux G, Andres C, Gankam Kengne F, et al. Treatment of euvolemic hyponatremia in the intensive care unit by urea. Crit Care 2010;14:R184.

63. Coussement J, Danguy C, Zouaoui-Boudjeltia K, et al. Treatment of the syndrome of inappropriate secretion of antidiuretic hormone with urea in critically ill patients. Am J Nephrol 2012;35:265–70.

64. Der-Nigoghossian C, Lesch C, Berger K. Effectiveness and tolerability of conivaptan and tolvaptan for the treatment of hyponatremia in neurocritically ill patients. Pharmacotherapy 2017;37:528–34.

65. Murphy T, Dhar R, Diringer M. Conivaptan bolus dosing for the correction of hyponatremia in the neurointensive care unit. Neurocrit Care 2009;11:14–9.

66. Marik PE, Rivera R. Therapeutic effect of conivaptan bolus dosing in hyponatremic neurosurgical patients. Pharmacotherapy 2013;33:51–5.

67. Wright WL, Asbury WH, Gilmore JL, et al. Conivaptan for hyponatremia in the neurocritical care unit. Neurocrit Care 2009;11:6–13.

68. Umbrello M, Mantovani ES, Formenti P, et al. Tolvaptan for hyponatremia with preserved sodium pool in critically ill patients. Ann Intensive Care 2016;6:1.

69. Tzoulis P, Waung JA, Bagkeris E, et al. Real-life experience of tolvaptan use in the treatment of severe hyponatraemia due to syndrome of inappropriate antidiuretic hormone secretion. Clin Endocrinol (Oxf) 2016;84:620–6.

Hormone Therapy in Trauma Patients

Karim Asehnoune, MD, PhD[a,b,]*, Mickael Vourc'h, MD, PhD[a,b],
Antoine Roquilly, MD, PhD[a,b]

KEYWORDS

- Corticosteroids • Low-dose hydrocortisone • Trauma patients • Critical illness
- Traumatic brain injury • Erythropoietin • Progesterone

KEY POINTS

- After trauma, a poor response of the pituitary-adrenal system alters the outcome. Hormone therapies have shown promises, but biomarkers are lacking to guide treatment.
- After trauma, corticosteroids could decrease organ failure when an inflammatory response is present. No major safety concern was recorded when a low dose was used.
- After TBI, progesterone and erythropoietin may improve outcome. The dose and the subgroup of TBI that should be treated remains unknown.

The metabolic adaptation to acute diseases is finely tuned by the hypothalamo-hypophyseal system.[1] In particular, poor response of the pituitary-adrenal system is associated with hospital-acquired infections, protracted organ failures including hemodynamic instability, and death. This review focuses mainly on glucocorticoids, which are the most extensively investigated treatments in hormone therapy.

GLUCOCORTICOIDS THERAPY
Pituitary-Adrenocortical Axis

Resting state
The morning peak of the hypothalamic cortico-releasing hormone (CRH) stimulates the pituitary secretion of adrenocorticotropin hormone (ACTH), which induces the release of cortisol. A negative feedback control of cortisol on CRH and ACTH prevents hypercorticism. The night-day rhythm of cortisol secretion, characterized by a peak at

Disclosure Statement: K. Asehnoune declares personal fees from Fisher Paykel Healthcare, Baxter, LFB, Fresenius. A. Roquilly declares personal fees from MSD. M. Vourc'h declares personal fees from MSD, Pfizer, Baxter, grants from Fischer Paykel, outside the submitted work.
[a] EA3826 Thérapeutiques Anti-Infectieuses, Institut de Recherche en Santé 2 Nantes Biotech, Medical University of Nantes, 21 boulevard Benoni Goullin, Nantes 44000, France; [b] Surgical Intensive Care Unit, Hotel Dieu, CHU Nantes, 1 place alexis ricordeau, Nantes 44093, France
* Corresponding author. Department of Anesthesia Critical Care and Pain Medicine, University Hospital of Nantes, Place Alexis Ricordeau, Nantes 44000 France.
E-mail address: karim.asehnoune@chu-nantes.fr

Crit Care Clin 35 (2019) 201–211
https://doi.org/10.1016/j.ccc.2018.11.009
0749-0704/19/© 2018 Elsevier Inc. All rights reserved.

8:00 AM and a valley at night, is as important as the blood level of the hormone to regulate immunity and organ functions (**Fig. 1**).[2]

It is important to differentiate 2 periods of endocrine dysfunctions after trauma: early days are characterized by a peripheral resistance to steroids, whereas late adrenal insufficiency is induced by a central deficit of corticotropin hormones.

Response to stress: the early phase

The early phase lasts for 1 to 2 weeks. Inflammatory cytokines released by leukocytes in responses to cellular damages (such as interleukin-6 [IL-6]) activate the pituitary-adrenal axis and abolish daily oscillations of the secretion of cortisol. In critically ill patients, suppressed activity of cortisol-metabolizing enzymes and decreased level of cortisol blinding globulin participate to the elevation of free cortisol.[3,4] These high cortisol levels initiate a period of catabolism characterized by proteolysis, lipolysis, and gluconeogenesis to release amino acids, fatty acids, and glucose. Catabolism enables the provision of endogenous energetic substrates to injured tissues and organs with poor stock of energy (brain, heart).[5] Cortisol also ensures optimal arterial pressure and organ perfusion by sensitizing peripheral receptors to vasoactive amines[6] and inducing water and sodium retention.[7] High cortisol levels are, therefore, a physiologic phenomenon of adaptation to trauma.

In critically ill patients, disease severity is correlated with the level of the initial peak of cortisolemia. Critical illness–related corticosteroid insufficiency,[8] which is defined as an insufficient elevation of cortisolemia in response to stress, is observed in up to 65% of severe trauma patients.[9]

Critical illness–related corticosteroid insufficiency is associated with overwhelming inflammatory response, hemodynamic instability, hospital-acquired pneumonia, and risk of death.[7,10,11]

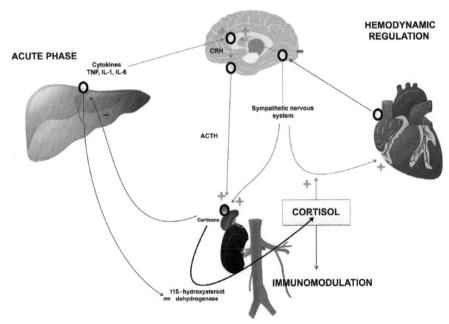

Fig. 1. Activation of the pituitary-adrenocortical axis after severe trauma. ACTH, adrenocorticotropic hormone; CRH, corticotropin-releasing hormone; TNF, tumor necrosis factor.

Response to stress: the late phase

This period is characterized by persistent high blood levels of cortisol independent from ACTH but mediated by endogenous endothelin.[12] During this late period, high cortisol levels contribute of delayed healing due to sustained catabolism.

Diagnosis of Critical Illness–Related Corticosteroid Insufficiency in Trauma Patients

The loss of the night-day rhythm allows clinicians to test adrenal function without the usual time constraints. The level of the free cortisol, the active form of the hormone, has been proposed as a marker,[4] but its measurement is not routinely available in clinical practice and there is no consensus definition of adrenal insufficiency in intensive care unit (ICU) based on its level. Adrenal function in trauma patients is usually tested by a standard stimulation test with Synacthen (measure of total cortisolemia at T0 and T30–60 minutes after an intravenous (IV) injection of 250 µg of ACTH). This supraphysiologic dose of ACTH evaluates the adrenal reserve in cortisol production even in the case of peripheral resistance to ACTH. A decreased response to ACTH means that the adrenal glands are exhausted and will not be able to handle a new stress. Most published studies define the critical illness–related corticosteroid insufficiency as a baseline total cortisol concentration of less than 15 µg/dL and/or an increase of less than 9 µg/dL after stimulation.[13] These thresholds are likely to vary depending on the intensity of the systemic inflammatory response,[14] and the results of the corticotrophin test have been proposed as a method to enhance the selection of patients requiring stress doses of glucocorticoids.

Limits of assessment methods in critically ill patients

It is important to note that many drugs can disrupt ACTH test results. Etomidate, which is frequently used for the rapid sequence induction of anesthesia in trauma patients, inhibits the synthesis of cortisol, limiting the interpretation of a Synacthen test for 8 to 72 hours.[15,16]

Indications of Glucocorticoids

Mortality and in-ICU complications are correlated with the response to a standard Synacthen test in septic shock and in trauma patients.[7,9,17] This observation has led to the concept of "critical illness–related corticosteroid insufficiency" in which ICU patients may benefit from corticotherapy even if the blood level of cortisol is increased.[18] The effects of prolonged (7–10 days) low doses of hydrocortisone (200 mg/d) have been tested in numerous randomized clinical trials.[19–21] The effects of hydrocortisone on mortality range from a small reduction (relative risk [RR] of death 0.88 [95% confidence interval [CI], 0.78–0.99][21] to no effect, 1.09; [0.77–1.52]).[22] Recent meta-analyses conclude that hydrocortisone decreases the early risk of death at day 28, but has no effect on mortality at 6 months.[23,24] However, the incidence of side effects with the treatment was low in all the published randomized studies, and hydrocortisone accelerated the weaning of vasoactive amines. Hydrocortisone induces hyperglycemia and sodium retention, but neither intensive insulin therapy nor the addition of mineralocorticoid alters mortality of septic patients.[25]

This abundant literature in sepsis has paved the way for the administration of steroids to a wide range of medical conditions. Critical illness–related corticosteroid insufficiency has notably been found in other ICU populations, such as trauma,[7] including traumatic brain injury (TBI),[9] and cardiac surgery patients.[8] After trauma, severe burn injury, and major surgery, hydrocortisone reduces the duration of vasopressor support and hospital length of stay.[7,26,27] Dexamethasone also prevents postoperative atrial fibrillation after cardiac surgery.[28] Steroid therapy may reduce the risk of long-term psychological disorder, such as posttraumatic stress disorder, which is frequently observed in critically ill patients.[29,30]

In severe traumatic brain–injured patients,[31] and in ventilated trauma patients,[32] prolonged low dose of hydrocortisone prevents hospital-acquired pneumonia and accelerates the weaning from mechanical ventilation. This counterintuitive effect is explained by the modulation of inflammation induced by hydrocortisone.[33,34] Moreover, hydrocortisone limits the development of critical illness–related immunosuppression, a prolonged state of immunosuppression associated with secondary infections.[35–37] In septic patients, hydrocortisone increased both in vitro phagocytosis and the blood level of the cytokine IL-12, at the same time IL-10 blood level decreased, suggesting that immunity was somehow enhanced.[38] In mice models of trauma hemorrhage or of viral pneumonia, hydrocortisone decreased the formation of immunosuppressive IL-10$^+$ natural killer cells[34] and prevented overwhelming lung inflammatory response during secondary bacterial pneumonia.[39]

Finally, corticosteroids have been recently recommended as adjunctive therapy in several nonseptic inflammatory conditions.[40] When analyzing the effects of steroids in critically ill patients, it is necessary to consider both the regimen dose and the duration of the treatment. Indeed, in the setting of septic shock, prolonged (7–10 days) low doses (200 mg/d) of hydrocortisone reduce the rate of mortality in septic patients, whereas a short course (2 days) of high doses is ineffective to prevent death.[41]

SAFETY CONCERNS

It remains unclear if low-dose corticosteroid therapy increases the risk of complications described with higher dose or long-term treatment. In a recent meta-analysis, the need for treatment of hyperglycemia increased by 6%, without long-term adverse consequences in patients with community-acquired pneumonia.[42] In the same context, a trial did not report any significantly increased risk for diabetes or use of glycemic agents 30 days after presentation.[43] Another systematic review evaluated corticosteroids for treating sepsis (33 trials, n = 4268 participants). No major adverse events (superinfection, gastrointestinal bleeding, neuromuscular weakness) were recorded, but increased metabolic disorders (hyperglycemia and hypernatremia) were reported.[24] Finally, in the 2 multicenter randomized controlled double-blind studies available to date evaluating low dose of hydrocortisone versus placebo in severe trauma patients and in TBI patients, no major side effect was reported, but the need for insulin and the rate of hypernatremia were enhanced in the treated group.[31,32] It should be kept in mind that moderate hypernatremia could be advantageous in the specific context of TBI.

In summary, in response to trauma, the pituitary-adrenocortical axis initiates an intense degree of catabolism and a state of acquired immunosuppression, both of which are associated with hospital-acquired infections, protracted organ failures, and death. However, it is important to understand the mechanisms of critical illness–related corticosteroid insufficiency to adequately treat patients. Initially, corticotropin is actively secreted, but peripheral tissues are resistant to cortisol. In a later period, the hypothalamic production of ACTH drops, and the blood levels of cortisol are low. Finally, the treatment of critically ill patients with prolonged low dose of hydrocortisone is probably beneficial, independently from any biological assessment of the adrenal function, particularly in cases of refractory shock, high risk of posttraumatic pneumonia, or high risk of death in septic patients.

OTHER HORMONES THERAPIES
Sex Steroid Hormones

The impact of gender on outcomes after trauma has been demonstrated both in animal models and in severe trauma patients. Gender dimorphism in outcomes following trauma was described with men having higher mortalities than women.[44] It is therefore suggested that sex steroid hormones play an important role in outcomes.[45] In a study of 681,000 trauma patients, men had higher mortality and more complications than women.[46] A meta-analysis confirmed that male gender was associated with increased mortality and higher incidence of complications.[47] In addition, male gender seems to be a risk factor for infections and multiple organ dysfunctions.[48]

Progesterone
Progesterone has been shown to have neuroprotective properties in several models of brain injury (**Table 1**). Its effects include inhibition of inflammatory cytokines, reduction of apoptosis, and better control of vasogenic edema.[49–51] Importantly, the progesterone receptor plays a key role in the described neuroprotective effects.[52] Two phase 2 randomized controlled clinical trials showed a clinical benefit when using progesterone.[53,54] Collectively, these positive results triggered the performance of 2 phase 3 multicenter, double-blind controlled randomized studies, the SYNAPSE and PROTECT III trial. In the latter trial,[55] patients with moderate to severe TBI (Glasgow

Table 1
Randomized controlled trial studies evaluating progesterone in patients with traumatic brain injury

Reference	Patients	Intervention	Main Results
Wright et al,[54] 2007	100 TBI	Progesterone vs placebo IV infusion 0.71 mg/kg for 1 h and 0.5 mg/kg/h for 11 h, then 0.5 mg/kg every 12 h for 60 h	No difference in adverse event Trends to lower mortality in interventional group, RR 0.43, CI 95% (0.18–0.99)
Xiao,[66] 2007	56 TBI	Progesterone vs no treatment Intramuscular injection of 80 mg every 12 h for 5 d	No difference in mortality
Xiao et al,[53] 2008	159 TBI	Progesterone vs placebo IV infusion 1 mg/kg every 12 h during 5 d	GOS score was improved in patients receiving PG compared with placebo
Aminmansour,[67] 2012	40 TBI	Progesterone vs progesterone + vitamin D vs placebo intramuscular 1 mg/kg every 12 h for 5 d	PG + Vitamin D Improved GCS score and GOS score at 3 mo
Shakeri,[68] 2013	76 TBI	Progesterone vs no treatment Oral administration 1 mg/kg per 12 h for 5 d	Favorable GOS was more frequent in PG group than in control group
Skolnick et al,[56] 2014	1179 TBI	Progesterone vs Placebo IV infusion of 0.71 mg/kg for 1 h and 0.5 mg/kg per hour for 119 h	No difference between PG and placebo
Wright et al,[55] 2014	882 TBI	Progesterone vs placebo IV infusion 0.71 mg/kg for 1 h and 0.5 mg/kg/h for 71 h, then 0.125 mg/kg every 8 h for 96 h	No difference between PG and placebo Trends toward an increased thrombophlebitis rate in PG group

Coma Score [GCS] of 4–12) were included. The treatment (progesterone or placebo) was allocated very early (within 4 hours after the injury) and administered for 96 hours. The primary outcome was neurologic recovery defined by an improvement of the Extended Glasgow Outcome Scale (GOS-E) at 6 months. The study was negative because there was no difference between the progesterone and the placebo group regarding the proportion of patients with a favorable outcome (relative benefit of progesterone, 0.95; 95% CI, 0.85–1.06; $P = .35$). Also, thrombophlebitis was more frequent in the progesterone group (RR, 3.03; CI, 1.96–4.66). No significant difference was apparent in the other safety outcomes. It should be mentioned that the study was stopped for futility after 882 out of 1140 planned patients were randomized. In the multinational SYNAPSE randomized placebo-controlled trial, 1195 adult patients with severe TBI (GCS ≤8) were randomized.[56] The primary outcome measure was the Glasgow Outcome Scale (GOS) at 6 months after TBI. There was no benefit in the treatment group as compared with placebo group (odds ratio, 0.96; CI, 0.77–1.18). The mortality was not different between groups, and no safety issue was reported. Despite the great enthusiasm toward progesterone after great results were published in animal models and single-center trials, the 2 large multicenter studies failed to show any improvement in patient outcome when using progesterone in TBI patients. Several points, however, should be emphasized. First, TBI is a complex, heterogenous pathologic condition, and the inclusion criteria were different in SYNAPSE and PROTECT III hampering any global conclusion. The clinical effect of higher doses than those used in the SYNAPSE and PROTECT III trial remains uncertain. Finally, current approaches characterizing TBI are unidimensional based only on GCS scores or Marshall Classification for the computed tomographic scan.

Oxandrolone

Oxandrolone is an anabolic androgenic steroid derived from testosterone. Oxandrolone is able to improve prognosis of catabolic conditions like severe burns and trauma.[57] Oxandrolone is the only anabolic androgenic steroid approved by the Food and Drug Administration for weight restitution following severe trauma and major surgery. One multicenter randomized controlled double-blind study demonstrated that oxandrolone decreased the length of hospital stay, and this decrease was even higher when hospital stay was indexed to burn size and when deaths were excluded.[58] A meta-analysis of 15 randomized controlled trials suggested that oxandrolone use was associated with shorter length of stay by 3 days, reduced weight loss by 5 kg, and nitrogen loss by 8.19 g/d. Also, when used in the rehabilitation phase, oxandrolone was associated with reduced weight loss and lean body mass by 6 and 12 months, respectively, after severe thermal injury.[59] In pediatric burn patients, the use of oxandrolone was associated with improvement in bone mineral content and density.[60]

Sex-hormone therapy in trauma represents a novel therapeutic strategy, but apart from oxandrolone that was studied in burn-injured patients, and progesterone in severe trauma patients (with TBI mainly), no strong clinical data are currently available in patients.

Erythropoietin

Erythropoietin (EPO), which is a very well-known glycoprotein hormone, displays neuroprotective effects.[61] These effects are independent of erythropoiesis and could alter the outcomes of patients with TBI.[61,62] Indeed, EPO has shown neuroprotective properties and increased functional outcome in animal studies.[63] In a large multicenter randomized control trial in ICU patients, EPO decreased the mortality in the subgroup of severe trauma patients, but the rate of venous thromboembolism was increased.[64] A double-blind, placebo-controlled (EPO-TBI) study randomized 606 TBI patients to receive either EPO or placebo.[65] The primary outcome was improvement in the neurologic status defined as a reduction in the proportion of patients with a GOS-E of 1 to 4 (death, vegetative state, and severe disability). EPO did not alter the primary outcome as compared with placebo. The results of the adjusted 6-month mortality suggest a potential reduction of mortality with EPO in patients with diffuse TBI: 9% (22/241) for EPO compared with 15% (36/237) for placebo (absolute risk reduction 6.1% [95% CI, 0.2–11.9], $P = .04$). However, in the overall population, EPO did not modify the mortality at 6 months versus placebo (32 [11%] of 305 patients died in the EPO group vs 46 [16%] of 297 [16%] in the placebo group; RR 0·68 [95% CI 0·44–1·03], $P = .07$). There was no safety issue because the rate of deep venous thrombosis of the lower limbs was not increased in the treatment group as compared with the placebo group. In conclusion, EPO did not reduce the proportion of patients with poor neurologic outcome, but the treatment could reduce the mortality in specific subgroups of patients, and future studies are needed to delineate more precisely the role that EPO might play in TBI patients.

SUMMARY

The failure of many hormone therapies despite a strong rationale for use should stimulate a rethinking of drug development and a reappraisal of the overall trauma (with or without TBI) treatment paradigm. In addition, the lack of reliable biomarkers to guide hormone therapy or any neuroprotective therapy can be considered a major issue. These considerations explain that appropriate targeted therapy is not available, and multidimensional approaches are warranted for a better characterization of trauma in a way that permits individualized therapy.

REFERENCES

1. Van den Berghe G. On the neuroendocrinopathy of critical illness. Perspectives for feeding and novel treatments. Am J Respir Crit Care Med 2016;194(11): 1337–48.
2. Shimba A, Cui G, Tani-Ichi S, et al. Glucocorticoids drive diurnal oscillations in T cell distribution and responses by inducing interleukin-7 receptor and CXCR4. Immunity 2018;48(2):286–98.e6.
3. Boonen E, Vervenne H, Meersseman P, et al. Reduced cortisol metabolism during critical illness. N Engl J Med 2013;368(16):1477–88.
4. Hamrahian AH, Oseni TS, Arafah BM. Measurements of serum free cortisol in critically ill patients. N Engl J Med 2004;350(16):1629–38.
5. Van den Berghe G, de Zegher F, Bouillon R. Clinical review 95: acute and prolonged critical illness as different neuroendocrine paradigms. J Clin Endocrinol Metab 1998;83(6):1827–34.
6. Hoen S, Mazoit J-X, Asehnoune K, et al. Hydrocortisone increases the sensitivity to alpha 1-adrenoceptor stimulation in humans following hemorrhagic shock. Crit Care Med 2005;33(12):2737–43.
7. Hoen S, Asehnoune K, Brailly-Tabard S, et al. Cortisol response to corticotropin stimulation in trauma patients: influence of hemorrhagic shock. Anesthesiology 2002;97(4):807–13.
8. Marik PE. Critical illness-related corticosteroid insufficiency. Chest 2009;135(1): 181–93.
9. Cohan P, Wang C, McArthur DL, et al. Acute secondary adrenal insufficiency after traumatic brain injury: a prospective study. Crit Care Med 2005;33(10):2358–66.

10. Woiciechowsky C, Schöning B, Lanksch WR, et al. Mechanisms of brain-mediated systemic anti-inflammatory syndrome causing immunodepression. J Mol Med 1999;77(11):769–80.
11. Woiciechowsky C, Schöning B, Cobanov J, et al. Early IL-6 plasma concentrations correlate with severity of brain injury and pneumonia in brain-injured patients. J Trauma 2002;52(2):339–45.
12. Roth-Isigkeit A, Dibbelt L, Eichler W, et al. Blood levels of atrial natriuretic peptide, endothelin, cortisol and ACTH in patients undergoing coronary artery bypass grafting surgery with cardiopulmonary bypass. J Endocrinol Invest 2001; 24(10):777–85.
13. Annane D, Maxime V, Ibrahim F, et al. Diagnosis of adrenal insufficiency in severe sepsis and septic shock. Am J Respir Crit Care Med 2006;174(12):1319–26.
14. Torres A, Sibila O, Ferrer M, et al. Effect of corticosteroids on treatment failure among hospitalized patients with severe community-acquired pneumonia and high inflammatory response: a randomized clinical trial. JAMA 2015;313(7): 677–86.
15. Asehnoune K, Mahe PJ, Seguin P, et al. Etomidate increases susceptibility to pneumonia in trauma patients. Intensive Care Med 2012;38(10):1673–82.
16. Vinclair M, Broux C, Faure P, et al. Duration of adrenal inhibition following a single dose of etomidate in critically ill patients. Intensive Care Med 2007;34(4):714–9.
17. Annane D, Sebille V, Troche G, et al. A 3-level prognostic classification in septic shock based on cortisol levels and cortisol response to corticotropin. JAMA 2000; 283(8):1038–45.
18. Annane D, Pastores SM, Arlt W, et al. Critical Illness-related corticosteroid insufficiency (CIRCI): a narrative review from a multispecialty task force of the society of critical care medicine (SCCM) and the European Society of Intensive Care Medicine (ESICM). Crit Care Med 2017;45(12):2089–98.
19. Annane D, Sebille V, Charpentier C, et al. Effect of treatment with low doses of hydrocortisone and fludrocortisone on mortality in patients with septic shock. JAMA 2002;288(7):862–71.
20. Sprung CL, Annane D, Keh D, et al. Hydrocortisone therapy for patients with septic shock. N Engl J Med 2008;358(2):111–24.
21. Annane D, Renault A, Brun-Buisson C, et al. Hydrocortisone plus fludrocortisone for adults with septic shock. N Engl J Med 2018;378(9):809–18.
22. Venkatesh B, Finfer S, Cohen J, et al. Adjunctive glucocorticoid therapy in patients with septic shock. N Engl J Med 2018;378(9):797–808.
23. Gibbison B, López-López JA, Higgins JPT, et al. Corticosteroids in septic shock: a systematic review and network meta-analysis. Crit Care 2017;21(1):78.
24. Annane D, Bellissant E, Bollaert P-E, et al. Corticosteroids for treating sepsis. Cochrane Database Syst Rev 2015;(12):CD002243.
25. COIITSS Study Investigators, Annane D, Cariou A, Maxime V, et al. Corticosteroid treatment and intensive insulin therapy for septic shock in adults: a randomized controlled trial. JAMA 2010;303(4):341–8.
26. Weis F, Beiras-Fernandez A, Schelling G, et al. Stress doses of hydrocortisone in high-risk patients undergoing cardiac surgery: effects on interleukin-6 to interleukin-10 ratio and early outcome*. Crit Care Med 2009;37(5):1685–90.
27. Venet F, Plassais J, Textoris J, et al. Low-dose hydrocortisone reduces norepinephrine duration in severe burn patients: a randomized clinical trial. Crit Care 2015;19(1):21.

28. Halonen J, Halonen P, Järvinen O, et al. Corticosteroids for the prevention of atrial fibrillation after cardiac surgery: a randomized controlled trial. JAMA 2007; 297(14):1562–7.
29. McFarlane AC, Atchison M, Yehuda R. The acute stress response following motor vehicle accidents and its relation to PTSD. Ann N Y Acad Sci 1997;821:437–41.
30. Delahanty DL, Raimonde AJ, Spoonster E. Initial posttraumatic urinary cortisol levels predict subsequent PTSD symptoms in motor vehicle accident victims. Biol Psychiatry 2000;48(9):940–7.
31. Asehnoune K, Seguin P, Allary J, et al. Hydrocortisone and fludrocortisone for prevention of hospital-acquired pneumonia in patients with severe traumatic brain injury (Corti-TC): a double-blind, multicentre phase 3, randomised placebo-controlled trial. Lancet Respir Med 2014;2(9):706–16.
32. Roquilly A, Mahe PJ, Seguin P, et al. Hydrocortisone therapy for patients with multiple trauma: the randomized controlled HYPOLYTE study. JAMA 2011;305(12): 1201–9.
33. Lepelletier Y, Zollinger R, Ghirelli C, et al. Toll-like receptor control of glucocorticoid-induced apoptosis in human plasmacytoid predendritic cells (pDCs). Blood 2010;116(18):3389–97.
34. Roquilly A, Broquet A, Jacqueline C, et al. Hydrocortisone prevents immunosuppression by interleukin-10+ natural killer cells after trauma-hemorrhage. Crit Care Med 2014;42(12):e752–61.
35. Roquilly A, Villadangos JA. The role of dendritic cell alterations in susceptibility to hospital-acquired infections during critical-illness related immunosuppression. Mol Immunol 2015;68(2 Pt A):120–3.
36. Hotchkiss RS, Monneret G, Payen D. Sepsis-induced immunosuppression: from cellular dysfunctions to immunotherapy. Nat Rev Immunol 2013;13(12):862–74.
37. Venet F, Monneret G. Advances in the understanding and treatment of sepsis-induced immunosuppression. Nat Rev Nephrol 2018;14(2):121–37.
38. Keh D. Immunologic and hemodynamic effects of "low-dose" hydrocortisone in septic shock: a double-blind, randomized, placebo-controlled, crossover study. Am J Respir Crit Care Med 2002;167(4):512–20.
39. Jamieson AM, Yu S, Annicelli CH, et al. Influenza virus-induced glucocorticoids compromise innate host defense against a secondary bacterial infection. Cell Host Microbe 2010;7(2):103–14.
40. Pastores SM, Annane D, Rochwerg B, Corticosteroid Guideline Task Force of SCCM and ESICM. Guidelines for the diagnosis and management of critical illness-related corticosteroid insufficiency (CIRCI) in critically ill patients (Part II): society of critical care medicine (SCCM) and European Society of Intensive Care Medicine (ESICM) 2017. Intensive Care Med 2018;44(4):474–7.
41. Annane D, Bellissant E, Bollaert P-E, et al. Corticosteroids in the treatment of severe sepsis and septic shock in adults: a systematic review. JAMA 2009;301(22): 2362–75.
42. Siemieniuk RAC, Meade MO, Alonso-Coello P, et al. Corticosteroid therapy for patients hospitalized with community-acquired pneumonia. Ann Intern Med 2015; 163(7):519–28.
43. Blum CA, Nigro N, Briel M, et al. Adjunct prednisone therapy for patients with community-acquired pneumonia: a multicentre, double-blind, randomised, placebo-controlled trial. Lancet 2015;385(9977):1511–8.
44. Chaudry IH, Bland KI. Cellular mechanisms of injury after major trauma. Br J Surg 2009;96(10):1097–8.

45. Angele MK, Frantz MC, Chaudry IH. Gender and sex hormones influence the response to trauma and sepsis: potential therapeutic approaches. Clinics (Sao Paulo) 2006;61(5):479–88.

46. Haider AH, Crompton JG, Oyetunji T, et al. Females have fewer complications and lower mortality following trauma than similarly injured males: a risk adjusted analysis of adults in the National Trauma Data Bank. Surgery 2009;146(2): 308–15.

47. Liu T, Xie J, Yang F, et al. The influence of sex on outcomes in trauma patients: a meta-analysis. Am J Surg 2015;210(5):911–21.

48. Gannon CJ, Pasquale M, Tracy JK, et al. Male gender is associated with increased risk for postinjury pneumonia. Shock 2004;21(5):410–4.

49. VanLandingham JW, Cekic M, Cutler S, et al. Neurosteroids reduce inflammation after TBI through CD55 induction. Neurosci Lett 2007;425(2):94–8.

50. He J, Hoffman SW, Stein DG. Allopregnanolone, a progesterone metabolite, enhances behavioral recovery and decreases neuronal loss after traumatic brain injury. Restor Neurol Neurosci 2004;22(1):19–31.

51. Cutler SM, Cekic M, Miller DM, et al. Progesterone improves acute recovery after traumatic brain injury in the aged rat. J Neurotrauma 2007;24(9):1475–86.

52. Liu A, Margaill I, Zhang S, et al. Progesterone receptors: a key for neuroprotection in experimental stroke. Endocrinology 2012;153(8):3747–57.

53. Xiao G, Wei J, Yan W, et al. Improved outcomes from the administration of progesterone for patients with acute severe traumatic brain injury: a randomized controlled trial. Crit Care 2008;12(2):R61.

54. Wright DW, Kellermann AL, Hertzberg VS, et al. ProTECT: a randomized clinical trial of progesterone for acute traumatic brain injury. Ann Emerg Med 2007; 49(4):391–402, 402.e1–2.

55. Wright DW, Yeatts SD, Silbergleit R, et al. Very early administration of progesterone for acute traumatic brain injury. N Engl J Med 2014;371(26):2457–66.

56. Skolnick BE, Maas AI, Narayan RK, et al. A clinical trial of progesterone for severe traumatic brain injury. N Engl J Med 2014;371(26):2467–76.

57. Orr R, Fiatarone Singh M. The anabolic androgenic steroid oxandrolone in the treatment of wasting and catabolic disorders: review of efficacy and safety. Drugs 2004;64(7):725–50.

58. Wolf SE, Edelman LS, Kemalyan N, et al. Effects of oxandrolone on outcome measures in the severely burned: a multicenter prospective randomized double-blind trial. J Burn Care Res 2006;27(2):131–9 [discussion: 140–1].

59. Li H, Guo Y, Yang Z, et al. The efficacy and safety of oxandrolone treatment for patients with severe burns: a systematic review and meta-analysis. Burns 2016;42(4):717–27.

60. Reeves PT, Herndon DN, Tanksley JD, et al. Five-year outcomes after long-term oxandrolone administration in severely burned children: a randomized clinical trial. Shock 2016;45(4):367–74.

61. Lykissas MG, Korompilias AV, Vekris MD, et al. The role of erythropoietin in central and peripheral nerve injury. Clin Neurol Neurosurg 2007;109(8):639–44.

62. Coleman T, Brines M. Science review: recombinant human erythropoietin in critical illness: a role beyond anemia? Crit Care 2004;8(5):337–41.

63. Bramlett HM, Dietrich WD. Pathophysiology of cerebral ischemia and brain trauma: similarities and differences. J Cereb Blood Flow Metab 2004;24(2): 133–50.

64. Corwin HL, Gettinger A, Fabian TC, et al. Efficacy and safety of epoetin alfa in critically ill patients. N Engl J Med 2007;357(10):965–76.

65. Nichol A, French C, Little L, et al. Erythropoietin in traumatic brain injury (EPO-TBI): a double-blind randomised controlled trial. Lancet 2015;386(10012): 2499–506.
66. Xiao GM, Wei J, Wu ZH, et al. [Clinical study on the therapeutic effects and mechanism of progesterone in the treatment for acute severe head injury]. Zhonghua Wai Ke Za Zhi 2007;45(2):106–8.
67. Aminmansour B, Nikbakht H, Ghorbani A, et al. Comparison of the administration of progesterone versus progesterone and vitamin D in improvement of outcomes in patients with traumatic brain injury: A randomized clinical trial with placebo group. Advanced Biomedical Research 2012;1(1):58.
68. Shakeri M, Boustani MR, Pak N, et al. Effect of progesterone administration on prognosis of patients with diffuse axonal injury due to severe head trauma. Clinical Neurology and Neurosurgery 2013;115(10):2019–22.

Classic and Nonclassic Renin-Angiotensin Systems in the Critically Ill

Laurent Bitker, MD, MSc[a],*,
Louise M. Burrell, MBChB, MRCP, MD, FRACP[b]

KEYWORDS

- Acute kidney injury • Acute respiratory distress syndrome • Angiotensin
- Angiotensin-converting enzyme • Sepsis • Inflammation • Septic shock • Renin

KEY POINTS

- Activation of the endocrine renin-angiotensin system (RAS) cascade induces immediate metabolic, hemodynamic, and renal responses, in response to changes in blood pressure and homeostasis.
- Renin and angiotensin II are upregulated in the setting of sepsis and septic shock. Higher renin and angiotensin II and lower circulating angiotensin-converting enzyme levels are associated with worse survival.
- Classic and nonclassic RASs modulate the inflammatory and immune responses. The angiotensin II axis stimulates a proinflammatory beneficial antibacterial response.
- In patients with vasoplegic shock, the infusion of exogenous angiotensin II lowers vasopressor requirements, and improves renal-related outcomes.
- Experimental evidence supports the direct role of classic RAS in the pathophysiology of acute respiratory distress syndrome, whereas clinical data suggest a lung protective effect of angiotensin-converting enzyme 2 administration.

INTRODUCTION

The renin-angiotensin systems (RASs) regulate blood pressure, kidney function, and salt and water homeostasis. Modulation of RAS is central in the intensive care unit spectrum of diseases (eg, hemodynamic failure) and is associated with patient outcomes.[1–7] The RASs are enzymatic cascades implicating sequential peptide

Disclosure Statement: The authors declare that they have no conflicts of interest.
[a] Department of Intensive Care, ICU Research Office, Austin Hospital, 145 Studley Road, Heidelberg, Victoria 3084, Australia; [b] Department of Medicine, University of Melbourne, Austin Health, Austin Hospital, 145 Studley Road, Heidelberg, Victoria 3084, Australia
* Corresponding author.
E-mail address: laurent.bitker@austin.org.au

cleavage, leading to angiotensin generation by angiotensin-converting enzymes (ACEs).[8] RAS also modulates inflammation and immune responses.[8,9]

The angiotensin (Ang) (1–7)/ACE2 cascade is known as the nonclassic RAS, which acts as an endogenous counterregulatory arm to the angiotensin II (Ang II)/ACE axis.[10] Both classic and nonclassic RAS have been identified at the tissue level, with paracrine effects dissociated from those of the circulating system.[11]

Better understanding of RAS physiology has led to the development of high-potential therapies, of interest to the intensivist. Administration of exogenous Ang II in vasoplegic shock alleviated vasopressor requirements, and was associated with improved survival in patients with severe acute kidney injury (AKI).[2,7] On the other hand, exogenous infusion of recombinant human ACE2 has demonstrated exciting lung protective properties in the context of the acute respiratory distress syndrome (ARDS).[3]

The scope of this review was to describe the classic and nonclassic RASs, and their physiologic effects, with an emphasis on their respective pathogenic and/or therapeutic roles in the context of critical illness.

THE CIRCULATING CLASSIC RENIN-ANGIOTENSIN SYSTEM

Two enzymatic cascades lead to the generation of the main endocrine agents of the classic and nonclassic RASs (see **Fig. 2**). Both arms exist as an endocrine (circulating) and a paracrine (tissue-based) system, with paracrine and autocrine effects independent of the systemic systems.[11,12] The organ localizations of the RASs are presented in **Fig. 1**.

Peptides

Angiotensinogen is a glycosylated protein, produced by the hepatic lobules.[13] Plasma levels are stable, and in excess when compared with circulating renin concentrations. Local generation of angiotensinogen also exists in the renal epithelium, brain, heart, adrenal, endothelial, and intestinal tissue.[11,12] Ang I is a biologically inactive decapeptide generated by the proteolysis of angiotensinogen by renin.[9]

Ang II is the pivotal peptide of the classic RAS. This octapeptide is the product of the cleavage of Ang I by ACE, but may also be generated under the action of other enzymes.[9] Plasma Ang II is rapidly degraded into Ang III, IV, or Ang (1–7), under the action of various enzymes (**Fig. 2**).

Ang III is the product of the cleavage of Ang II by aminopeptidase A, or by the cleavage of Ang (1–9) under the action of ACE.[9] Like Ang II, Ang III is a potent vasopressor, a thirst and salt appetite stimulant, and an activator of aldosterone secretion.[14] Ang IV mainly modulates cerebral blood flow and cognition, increases renal blood flow (RBF), and decreases water and sodium reabsorption in the renal epithelium.[15,16]

Enzymes

Renin is an aspartyl-protease released by the juxta-glomerular apparatus, and is the key rate-limiting factor of Ang II generation.[8] Its secretion is regulated by renal perfusion, sodium-chloride balance, sympathetic nervous tone, and Ang II (**Box 1**).[17–19] Renin has also been identified in the proximal tubule and distal nephron, the brain, and in some immune system circulating elements.[20,21]

ACE is a dicarboxypeptidase metalloenzyme that generates Ang II, via a zinc-dependent shedding of a C-terminal dipeptide from Ang I. ACE also generates Ang (1–7) from Ang (1–9), and inactivates bradykinin, a natriuretic and vasodilator

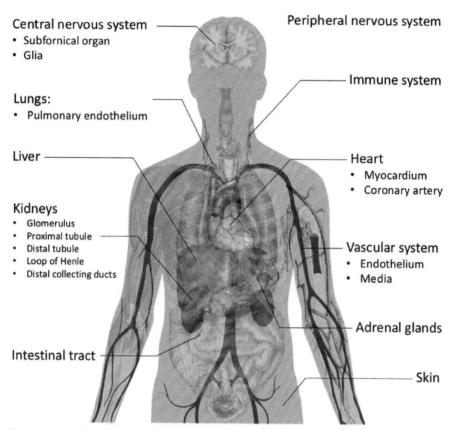

Fig. 1. Localization of RASs. Presented here are the organs or tissues in which at least 1 component of classic and/or nonclassic systems have been identified and are considered as being locally generated and/or secreted.

peptide.[22] The protein is a transmembrane ecto-enzyme found mainly in the pulmonary endothelium, where most of the Ang II is generated, but also in the brain, heart, and renal endothelium, and immune system cellular components.[23–25]

Receptors

Ang II receptors are G protein–coupled transmembrane proteins with 7 membrane-spanning domains.[26]

Angiotensin type 1 receptor (AT$_1$R) represents the principal transductor of Ang II into its main physiologic responses.[26] AT$_1$R is found in the endothelium (smooth muscular cells), kidneys (glomeruli and proximal tubule), adrenal glands, heart, lymphocytes, and granocytes.[27–29] Ang II-AT$_1$R binding induces the activation of multiple intracellular secondary messenger cascade, including intracellular Ca^{2+}, nuclear factor (NF) κB, phospholipase C and Janus kinase families.[27]

Angiotensin type 2 receptor (AT$_2$R) presents a 34% homology with AT$_1$R and is similarly structured.[26] It is found in the endothelium, heart, brain, kidneys and adrenal glands. AT$_2$R main actions antagonize those of AT1R. *Angiotensin type 4 receptor* (AT$_4$R) is principally located in the brain, and to a lesser extent in the renal artery, and binds Ang IV.[15]

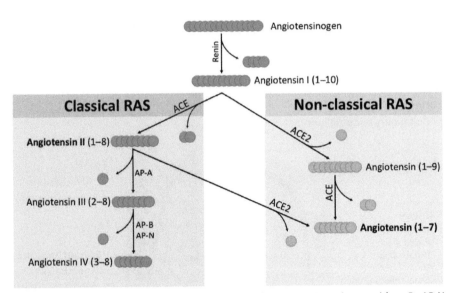

Fig. 2. RASs enzymatic cascades. AP-A, aminopeptidase A; AP-B, aminopeptidase B; AP-N, aminopeptidase N.

PHYSIOLOGY OF THE CIRCULATING CLASSIC RENIN-ANGIOTENSIN SYSTEM

The physiologic effects of classic RAS upregulation are summarized in **Fig. 3.**

Renal Physiology

Regulation of renal blood flow and glomerular filtration rate
Ang II augments glomerular filtration rate (GFR) and RBF, by increasing the vasomotor tone of efferent renal arterioles, acting alongside with myogenic reflex activation and

Box 1 Mechanisms leading to renin release by the juxta-glomerular apparel	
Physiologic Trigger	**Description**
Renal perfusion pressure	Baroreceptors in the juxta-glomerular apparel are sensitive to changes in renal perfusion pressure below 90 mm Hg.
Na+ and Cl− delivery to the macula densa	This effect is immediately transduced to the juxta-glomerular cells, due to their intimate contact with the *macula densa,* forming the juxta-glomerular apparatus. Evidence suggest that this effect is mainly due to chloride depletion.
Adrenergic activation	The sympathetic autonomous neural system, through a dense population of ß1- noradrenergic nerves, directly stimulates renin release by the juxta-glomerular apparel. These effects are dissociated from those induced by changes in renal perfusion pressure.
Angiotensin II: acute stimulus	Negative short-loop biofeedback by Ang II binding of AT_1R present in the juxta-glomerular cell membrane.
Angiotensin II: chronic stimulus	This compensatory mechanism, named juxta-glomerular recruitment, increases the number of renin-secreting cells in upregulated Ang II environments.
Abbreviations: Ang II, angiotensin II; AT_1R, angiotensin II type 1 receptor.	

Angiotensin II   Angiotensin (1–7)

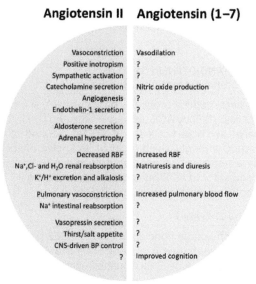

Angiotensin II	Angiotensin (1–7)
Vasoconstriction	Vasodilation
Positive inotropism	?
Sympathetic activation	?
Catecholamine secretion	Nitric oxide production
Angiogenesis	?
Endothelin-1 secretion	?
Aldosterone secretion	?
Adrenal hypertrophy	?
Decreased RBF	Increased RBF
Na$^+$,Cl- and H$_2$O renal reabsorption	Natriuresis and diuresis
K$^+$/H$^+$ excretion and alkalosis	?
Pulmonary vasoconstriction	Increased pulmonary blood flow
Na$^+$ intestinal reabsorption	?
Vasopressin secretion	?
Thirst/salt appetite	?
CNS-driven BP control	?
?	Improved cognition

Fig. 3. Mirrorlike physiologic effects of the pivotal peptides of the classic and nonclassic RASs. BP, blood pressure; CNS, central nervous system. The question mark indicates the unknown/unexplored effect of Angiotensin (1-7), in regard to that observed with Angiotensin II upregulation.

tubulo-glomerular feedback.[8,9,30] Its effects seem maximum when blood pressure is sufficiently low to stimulate renin release.[31] However, overstimulation by Ang II may decrease GFR due to excessive vasoconstriction.

Sodium homeostasis and acid-base balance regulation
Local and circulating Ang II stimulate the AT$_1$R-dependent reabsorption of sodium, chloride, and bicarbonate and excretion of potassium and protons by the renal epithelia.[9] It activates the apical Na$^+$/H$^+$ exchanger coupled with a basal Na$^+$/HCO$_3^-$ cotransporter in the proximal tubule and the ascending limb of the loop of Henle.[32] Ang II also activates Na$^+$/K$^+$ ATPase anti-transporters (leading to increased kaliuresis) and pendrin, a Cl$^-$/HCO$_3^-$ anti-transporter involved in chloride reabsorption.[33] Finally, aldosterone augments the recruitment of Na$^+$/K$^+$ ATPase and epithelial sodium channel transporters in the distal tubules and collecting ducts.[30]

Cardiovascular Physiology

Although the effects of Ang II on blood pressure are partly related to extracellular volume regulation, Ang II is a potent vasopressor agent, via an AT$_1$R-dependent influx of calcium into smooth muscular cells cytoplasm, but is downregulated by Ang II/AT$_2$R-dependent NO endothelial production and bradykinin generation[34,35]; however, vasomotor modulation may vary between and within organs.[36] Suvannapura and Levens[37] observed splanchnic vasoconstriction at normal Ang II circulating levels, whereas none was observed on RBF. Finally, Ang II increases blood pressure by upregulating adrenergic stimulation and endothelin 1 (ET-1) transcription.[38,39] Finally, Ang II increases cardiac output by inhibiting the vagal tone and upregulating ET-1.[40]

Other Effects

Ang II (and Ang III) stimulates adrenal synthesis and release of aldosterone and of catecholamines, and induces adrenal hypertrophy.[39] In the brain, circulating and locally produced Ang II stimulates thirst and salt-seeking behavior, vasopressin release by the posterior hypophysis, and acts as a central stimulant of sympathetic nervous tone.[9,14,27,41,42]

THE NONCLASSIC RENIN-ANGIOTENSIN SYSTEM
Nonclassic Renin-Angiotenin System Angiotensins

Angiotensin (1–7) is a heptapeptide produced by the proteolysis of Ang II by ACE2 (see **Fig. 2**).[10] Cleavage of Ang (1–9) by ACE also generates Ang (1–7). Ang (1–7) is found in the plasma, heart, renal, and brain tissues, and may be excreted in the urine. Ang (1–7) binds the Mas receptor, through which most of its known effects are mediated.[43] Angiotensin (1–9) is a nonapeptide generated by the ACE2-related breakdown of Ang I, acting as a competitor to ACE-related generation of Ang II.[44] It is a potent cardioprotective antifibrotic agent that binds the AT_2R.[44,45]

Angiotensin-Converting Enzyme 2

ACE2 is the pivotal enzyme of the nonclassic RAS.[10] ACE2 is transmembrane monocarboxypeptidase that converts Ang II into Ang (1–7) and Ang I into Ang (1–9). ACE2 was simultaneously discovered by 2 independent groups, using 2 complementary DNA libraries (heart and lymphoma).[46,47] ACE2 is the receptor to the severe acute respiratory syndrome coronavirus, and has been identified in the kidneys, lungs, brain, heart, and testes.[10,48,49] Through the generation of Ang (1–7), and the degradation of Ang II, the effect of ACE2 is tissue-protective. Due to structural differences in the binding sites of ACE and ACE2, ACE inhibitors do not inhibit the activity of ACE2.[50]

The Mas Receptor

The *Mas receptor* is a G-protein–coupled transmembrane receptor with high affinity for Ang (1–7), and little affinity for Ang II.[43] The receptor is distributed along the intrarenal epithelium and vascular endothelium, in accordance with the renal and hemodynamic effects of Ang (1–7).[51]

Nonclassic Renin-Angiotensin System and the Cardiovascular System

Ang (1–7) induces systemic and local vasodilation, by upregulating NO production.[51] Ang (1–7) and ACE2 have demonstrated cardioprotective anti-inflammatory features in an experimental model of myocardial infarction and heart failure (decreased reactive oxygen species [ROS] production and fibroblasts recruitment).[52–57] However, these observations were contradicted by the observation of cardiac fibrosis after Ang (1–7) upregulation in experimental renal dysfunction, in relation to a compensatory increase in ACE.[58]

Nonclassic Renin-Angiotensin System and Renal Function

In the kidneys, the activation of the Mas receptor by Ang (1–7) increases RBF and GFR, natriuresis, and diuresis.[59,60] Ang (1–7) and ACE2 may also present renoprotective properties, although limited by the potential compensatory upregulation of Ang II.[60–63] The role of ACE2 circulating levels in the context of chronic kidney disease remains controversial.[64,65]

RENIN-ANGIOTENSIN SYSTEMS AND THE IMMUNE SYSTEM

Classic and nonclassic RAS modulate the innate and adaptive immune system responses, regulating inflammation, cell proliferation, fibrogenesis, and apoptosis (**Box 2**).[56,57,60,66,67] The Ang II/ACE axis potentiates bacterial clearance, by

Box 2 Immunomodulatory mechanisms and consequences of classic and nonclassic renin-angiotensin systems	
Angiotensin II/ACE/AT₁R axis	**Angiotensin (1–7)/ACE2/Mas axis**
NFκB upregulation	NFκB downregulation
Increase in production of ROS	Downregulation of ROS production
Increase in secretion of proinflammatory cytokines	Lower proinflammatory cytokine levels
Collagen production	Antiproliferative effect
Macrophages/neutrophils recruitment	Decrease macrophage tissue recruitment
Activation of fibroblasts	Decrease fibroblast activation
Fibrosis, apoptosis	Tissue protection

Abbreviations: ACE2, angiotensin-converting enzyme2; AT₁R, angiotensin II type 1 receptor; NFκB, nuclear factor κB; ROS, reactive oxygen species.

upregulating neutrophils and macrophages chemotaxis and activation, generation of ROS, and secretion of proinflammatory cytokines.[28,68,69] Yet, lymphocytic AT₁R activation inhibits CD8⁺ T-cell activation.[25,29] These phenomena modulate the NFκB cascade, a transcription factor involved in both the physiology and pathogenesis of septic shock and organ failure.[70–72] These effects also may be directly mediated by ACE, as suggested by the effects of ACE inhibitors but not by AT₁R antagonists on immunomodulation.[73] In sheer contrast, activation of the Ang (1–7)/ACE2 axis inhibits ROS production, downregulates proinflammatory cytokine secretion, and has immunomodulatory tissue-protective features (see **Box 2**).[60,62,66,74]

ANGIOTENSIN II IN VASODILATORY SHOCK AND SEPSIS

In the critical setting, the upregulation of the classic RAS is a physiologic and potentially life-saving response. Ang II and renin levels are increased in the context of sepsis and significantly associated with severity of disease.[1,6,75] Serum ACE concentration in patients with pulmonary sepsis were lower than in healthy volunteers, with reduced levels associated with increased mortality.[6,76] In line with our understanding of Ang II effects, recent data strongly suggest that exogenous Ang II infusion decreases vasopressor dose requirements in patients with vasodilatory shock, mirroring the physiologic effects of endogenous Ang II: increase in sympathetic tone, endogenous catecholamine and vasopressin release, and direct stimulation of vascular smooth muscle cells.[2]

During sepsis, Ang II upregulation may induce ROS generation and endothelial structural changes, both being pivotal physiologic responses to infection, yet also central in the pathogenesis of its most severe presentation, namely septic shock, where they become oxidative stress and endothelial dysfunction.[1] Historically, although meeting promising successes in animal models, ACE inhibition did not prove to attenuate the inflammatory response in healthy volunteers exposed to endotoxemia.[77,78] Furthermore, large observational evidence was not supportive of classic RAS downregulation having protective effects against sepsis.[79] Conversely, Ang II improved phagocytosis and inhibited abscess formation during experimental murine peritonitis.[80] In the ATHOS-3 trial, the vast majority of patients had confirmed or suspected sepsis. Ang II infusion at the acute phase of vasodilatory shock of septic origin also may contribute to an unknown degree of inflammation enhancement and bacterial clearance.

ANGIOTENSIN-CONVERTING ENZYMES IN ACUTE RESPIRATORY DISTRESS SYNDROME

ACE levels were respectively increased in the broncho-alveolar lavage and decreased in the serum of patients with ARDS, whereas higher circulating levels of Ang I were associated with mortality.[5,76,81] The epithelial and endothelial damage observed in the course of ARDS may create an imbalance favoring classic over nonclassic RAS pathways in the lungs.[82] Although little is known about Ang II in human ARDS, upregulation of the Ang II/ACE cascade in experimental ARDS worsens perfusion/ventilation mismatch, increases secretion of proinflammatory intracellular cascades and agents, and local production of ROS, all directly implicated in the disease's pathogenesis.[4] Classic RAS inhibition may limit the pulmonary inflammatory response and the extent of lung injury, but has been poorly evaluated in humans.[77,83,84]

In contrast, growing evidence suggests the pivotal role of nonclassic RAS in lung protection in the face of acute injury. First, ACE2 was identified as being the receptor to the severe acute respiratory syndrome coronavirus, via the Spike protein. Inhibition of ACE2-coronavirus binding effectively inhibited virus replication and limited RAS-dependent acute lung injury.[85] Then, experimental models of ARDS modulating Ang (1–7) and ACE2 activities have demonstrated significant lung protection (**Fig. 4**).[74,86,87] Ang (1–7) infusion in murine experimental ARDS decreased the proinflammatory response, improved lung injury scores and lung function, and decreased cellular infiltrate in piglets with acid aspiration.[74,82] These beneficial effects are mediated by downregulation of the intracellular proinflammatory NFκB cascade and increased NO synthesis.[51] A randomized controlled trial of recombinant human ACE2 in humans with ARDS showed it decreased Ang II levels and proinflammatory mediators, and augmented plasmatic surfactant protein D, with no hemodynamic side effects.[3,88] The effects of recombinant human ACE2 (rhACE2) may be principally mediated by its competing effects with ACE in limiting the generation of Ang II, while potentiating Ang (1–7) activity. Those findings demonstrate that ACE2-related immunomodulation in the context of ARDS may improve pulmonary outcomes, in

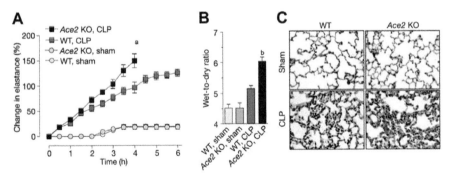

Fig. 4. ACE2 controls acute lung failure. Lung elastance (*A*) after acute lung injury in wild-type (WT) and Ace2 knockout (KO) mice induced by cecal ligation perforation (CLP). CLP-treated Ace2 KO mice had significantly higher elastance than CLP-treated WT mice ([a] P<.01). Wet-to-dry weight ratios of lungs (*B*) in CLP-treated Ace2 KO mice after 4 hours of ventilation was significantly increased, compared with CLP-treated WT and sham. Histopathology (*C*) showed increased lung edema and inflammatory infiltrate in CLP-treated Ace2 knockout mice, compared to CLP-treated WT and sham. [b] P<.05 between CLP-treated WT and Ace2 KO mice. (*From* Imai Y, Kuba K, Rao S, et al. Angiotensin-converting enzyme 2 protects from severe acute lung failure. Nature 2005;436:114; with permission.)

congruence with what we know of the downregulating effect of nonclassic RAS on the inflammatory response. Larger randomized controlled trails are necessary to confirm the promising lung protective properties of rhACE2.

PLACE OF RENIN-ANGIOTENSIN SYSTEMS IN ACUTE KIDNEY INJURY

Evidence in AKI suggests a complex picture. In patients with suspected acute tubular necrosis, angiotensinogen and Ang II expression and urinary secretion are increased, and associated with the severity of pathology and AKI risk.[89,90] However, whether the upregulation of the classic RAS is the cause or the consequence of AKI remains unknown and findings may be model-dependent. Ang II upregulation improves renal function, while not aggravating medullary hypoxia, in an experimental model of septic AKI, and attenuates intrarenal inflammation and apoptosis in murine ischemia/reperfusion-induced AKI.[91,92] Interaction of local and systemic systems may also be of importance. Renal injury may depend on renal cell AT_1R activation, whereas a reno-protective phenotype is observed if lymphocytes AT_1R are activated.[93] The Ang II/Ang (1–7) balance may also play a role, as ACE2 knockout mice with ischemia/reperfusion-induced AKI showed worsening renal function.[94] From a clinical perspective, exogenous Ang II administration in patients with vasoplegic shock and severe AKI was associated with higher survival and renal replacement therapy weaning rates.[7] The role of Ang II on renal recovery after AKI, well supported by experimental data, will require further evaluation in the critical setting.

INTEGRATION OF RENIN-ANGIOTENSIN SYSTEM PHYSIOLOGY IN CRITICAL ILLNESS

Description of the physiology of the classic and nonclassic RAS has direct implications in the setting of critical illness. On the one hand, increased Ang II activity is a life-saving response to hypotension and infection, with proven effects on cardiovascular physiology and renal outcomes in the context of vasoplegic shock.[2] It also implies that Ang II enhancement of hemodynamic management at the acute phase of septic shock may improve organ failure, including renal failure. Also, Ang II in the acute context may boost the proinflammatory response, with subsequent enhanced bacterial clearance, opposite to the deleterious effects of inflammation in the chronic setting. On the other hand, ACE2 enhancement decreases lung inflammation and improves lung hemodynamics and function in the setting of ARDS.[3] The control of pulmonary damage by the nonclassic RAS demonstrates the central role of

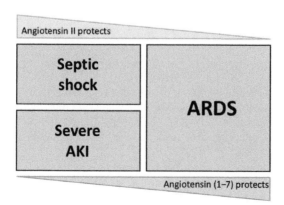

Fig. 5. The paradigm of classic and nonclassic RAS roles in critical illness.

immunomodulation in this potentially lethal inflammation-mediated disease. Those 2 pivotal trials convey highly encouraging changes in the treatment strategies of septic shock and ARDS. Yet, their individualization at the bedside is far from being achieved, as both targeted conditions may be simultaneously present in a given individual (**Fig. 5**). Better understanding of how local and systemic systems interact may help target which should be favored.

SUMMARY

Our knowledge of the RASs is growing exponentially and exposing their complexity. The RAS is more than an endocrine system, and exists in most organs, with local physiologic and biological effects dissociated from the classic circulating RAS. In the context of critical illness, the regulation of the classic/nonclassic RAS balance plays a unique role in the response to vasodilatory shock and ARDS. Rapidly evolving clinical data suggest that Ang II may save lives in vasodilatory shock and accelerate renal recovery in patients with severe AKI in this setting. Conversely, ACE2 may prove an important new protective therapy in ARDS. A new chapter of the RAS, now dealing with critical illness, is being written and opens the door to a new concept in the manipulation of this ubiquitous system: inhibition in the chronic setting but activation in the acute setting.

REFERENCES

1. Doerschug KC, Delsing AS, Schmidt GA, et al. Renin-angiotensin system activation correlates with microvascular dysfunction in a prospective cohort study of clinical sepsis. Crit Care 2010;14(1):R24.
2. Khanna A, English SW, Wang XS, et al. Angiotensin II for the treatment of vasodilatory shock. N Engl J Med 2017;377(5):419–30.
3. Khan A, Benthin C, Zeno B, et al. A pilot clinical trial of recombinant human angiotensin-converting enzyme 2 in acute respiratory distress syndrome. Crit Care 2017;21(1):234.
4. Cruces P, Diaz F, Puga A, et al. Angiotensin-converting enzyme insertion/deletion polymorphism is associated with severe hypoxemia in pediatric ARDS. Intensive Care Med 2012;38(1):113–9.
5. Annoni F, Orbegozo Cortés D, Irazabal M, et al. Angiotensin converting enzymes in patients with acute respiratory distress syndrome. Intensive Care Med Exp 2015;3(1):A91.
6. Zhang W, Chen X, Huang L, et al. Severe sepsis: low expression of the renin-angiotensin system is associated with poor prognosis. Exp Ther Med 2014;7(5):1342–8.
7. Tumlin JA, Murugan R, Deane AM, et al. Outcomes in patients with vasodilatory shock and renal replacement therapy treated with intravenous angiotensin II. Crit Care Med 2018;46(6):949–57.
8. Sparks MA, Crowley SD, Gurley SB, et al. Classical renin-angiotensin system in kidney physiology. Compr Physiol 2014;4(3):1201–28.
9. Ballermann BJ, Onuigbo MA. Angiotensins. Compr Physiol 2011;(Supplement 22):104–55.
10. Chappell MC. Nonclassical renin-angiotensin system and renal function. Compr Physiol 2012;2(4):2733–52.
11. Paul M, Poyan Mehr A, Kreutz R. Physiology of local renin-angiotensin systems. Physiol Rev 2006;86(3):747–803.

12. Yang T, Xu C. Physiology and pathophysiology of the intrarenal renin-angiotensin system: an update. J Am Soc Nephrol 2017;28(4):1040–9.
13. Matsusaka T, Niimura F, Shimizu A, et al. Liver angiotensinogen is the primary source of renal angiotensin II. J Am Soc Nephrol 2012;23(7):1181–9.
14. Wright JW, Bechtholt AJ, Chambers SL, et al. Angiotensin III and IV activation of the brain AT1 receptor subtype in cardiovascular function. Peptides 1996;17(8): 1365–71.
15. Kramar EA, Harding JW, Wright JW. Angiotensin II- and IV-induced changes in cerebral blood flow. Roles of AT1, AT2, and AT4 receptor subtypes. Regul Pept 1997;68(2):131–8.
16. Handa RK, Krebs LT, Harding JW, et al. Angiotensin IV AT4-receptor system in the rat kidney. Am J Physiol 1998;274(2 Pt 2):F290–9.
17. Bock HA, Hermle M, Brunner FP, et al. Pressure dependent modulation of renin release in isolated perfused glomeruli. Kidney Int 1992;41(2):275–80.
18. Thurau K, Schnermann J, Nagel W, et al. Composition of tubular fluid in the macula densa segment as a factor regulating the function of the juxtaglomerular apparatus. Circ Res 1967;21(1 Suppl 2):79–90.
19. Kirchheim HR, Ehmke H, Hackenthal E, et al. Autoregulation of renal blood flow, glomerular filtration rate and renin release in conscious dogs. Pflugers Arch 1987; 410(4–5):441–9.
20. Rohrwasser A, Morgan T, Dillon HF, et al. Elements of a paracrine tubular renin-angiotensin system along the entire nephron. Hypertension 1999;34(6):1265–74.
21. Mackins CJ, Kano S, Seyedi N, et al. Cardiac mast cell-derived renin promotes local angiotensin formation, norepinephrine release, and arrhythmias in ischemia/reperfusion. J Clin Invest 2006;116(4):1063–70.
22. Hornig B, Kohler C, Drexler H. Role of bradykinin in mediating vascular effects of angiotensin-converting enzyme inhibitors in humans. Circulation 1997;95(5): 1115–8.
23. Alhenc-Gelas F, Corvol P. Molecular and physiological aspects of angiotensin I converting enzyme. Compr Physiol 2011;(Supplement 22):81–103.
24. Bruneval P, Hinglais N, Alhenc-Gelas F, et al. Angiotensin I converting enzyme in human intestine and kidney. Ultrastructural immunohistochemical localization. Histochemistry 1986;85(1):73–80.
25. Coppo M, Bandinelli M, Chiostri M, et al. Persistent and selective upregulation of renin-angiotensin system in circulating T lymphocytes in unstable angina. J Renin Angiotensin Aldosterone Syst 2017;18(1). 1470320317698849.
26. Guthrie GP Jr. Angiotensin receptors: physiology and pharmacology. Clin Cardiol 1995;18(6 Suppl 3):III 29–34.
27. Allen AM, Zhuo J, Mendelsohn FA. Localization and function of angiotensin AT1 receptors. Am J Hypertens 2000;13(1 Pt 2):31S–8S.
28. Hernandez-Presa M, Bustos C, Ortego M, et al. Angiotensin-converting enzyme inhibition prevents arterial nuclear factor-kappa B activation, monocyte chemoattractant protein-1 expression, and macrophage infiltration in a rabbit model of early accelerated atherosclerosis. Circulation 1997;95(6):1532–41.
29. Zhang JD, Patel MB, Song YS, et al. A novel role for type 1 angiotensin receptors on T lymphocytes to limit target organ damage in hypertension. Circ Res 2012; 110(12):1604–17.
30. Taal MWB, Barry M. 1937-; Rector. In: Floyd C, editor. Brenner & Rector's the kidney. 9th edition. Philadelphia: Elsevier/Saunders; 2012.
31. Hall JE, Guyton AC, Cowley AW Jr. Dissociation of renal blood flow and filtration rate autoregulation by renin depletion. Am J Physiol 1977;232(3):F215–21.

32. Geibel J, Giebisch G, Boron WF. Angiotensin II stimulates both Na(+)-H+ exchange and Na+/HCO3− cotransport in the rabbit proximal tubule. Proc Natl Acad Sci U S A 1990;87(20):7917–20.

33. Wall SM, Lazo-Fernandez Y. The role of pendrin in renal physiology. Annu Rev Physiol 2015;77:363–78.

34. Hall JE, Guyton AC, Smith MJ Jr, et al. Blood pressure and renal function during chronic changes in sodium intake: role of angiotensin. Am J Physiol 1980;239(3): F271–80.

35. Heinemann A, Wachter CH, Holzer P, et al. Nitric oxide-dependent and -independent vascular hyporeactivity in mesenteric arteries of portal hypertensive rats. Br J Pharmacol 1997;121(5):1031–7.

36. Myers BD, Deen WM, Brenner BM. Effects of norepinephrine and angiotensin II on the determinants of glomerular ultrafiltration and proximal tubule fluid reabsorption in the rat. Circ Res 1975;37(1):101–10.

37. Suvannapura A, Levens NR. Local control of mesenteric blood flow by the renin-angiotensin system. Am J Physiol 1988;255(3 Pt 1):G267–74.

38. Rossi GP, Sacchetto A, Cesari M, et al. Interactions between endothelin-1 and the renin-angiotensin-aldosterone system. Cardiovasc Res 1999;43(2):300–7.

39. Peach MJ. Adrenal medullary stimulation induced by angiotensin I, angiotensin II, and analogues. Circ Res 1971;28(5 Suppl 2):107–17.

40. Cingolani HE, Villa-Abrille MC, Cornelli M, et al. The positive inotropic effect of angiotensin II: role of endothelin-1 and reactive oxygen species. Hypertension 2006;47(4):727–34.

41. Coble JP, Grobe JL, Johnson AK, et al. Mechanisms of brain renin angiotensin system-induced drinking and blood pressure: importance of the subfornical organ. Am J Physiol Regul Integr Comp Physiol 2015;308(4):R238–49.

42. Dendorfer A, Thornagel A, Raasch W, et al. Angiotensin II induces catecholamine release by direct ganglionic excitation. Hypertension 2002;40(3):348–54.

43. Santos RA, Simoes e Silva AC, Maric C, et al. Angiotensin-(1-7) is an endogenous ligand for the G protein-coupled receptor Mas. Proc Natl Acad Sci U S A 2003; 100(14):8258–63.

44. Flores-Munoz M, Smith NJ, Haggerty C, et al. Angiotensin1-9 antagonises pro-hypertrophic signalling in cardiomyocytes via the angiotensin type 2 receptor. J Physiol 2011;589(Pt 4):939–51.

45. Fattah C, Nather K, McCarroll CS, et al. Gene therapy with angiotensin-(1-9) preserves left ventricular systolic function after myocardial infarction. J Am Coll Cardiol 2016;68(24):2652–66.

46. Donoghue M, Hsieh F, Baronas E, et al. A novel angiotensin-converting enzyme-related carboxypeptidase (ACE2) converts angiotensin I to angiotensin 1-9. Circ Res 2000;87(5):E1–9.

47. Tipnis SR, Hooper NM, Hyde R, et al. A human homolog of angiotensin-converting enzyme. Cloning and functional expression as a captopril-insensitive carboxypeptidase. J Biol Chem 2000;275(43):33238–43.

48. Chappell MC. Emerging evidence for a functional angiotensin-converting enzyme 2-angiotensin-(1-7)-MAS receptor axis: more than regulation of blood pressure? Hypertension 2007;50(4):596–9.

49. Wiener RS, Cao YX, Hinds A, et al. Angiotensin converting enzyme 2 is primarily epithelial and is developmentally regulated in the mouse lung. J Cell Biochem 2007;101(5):1278–91.

50. Towler P, Staker B, Prasad SG, et al. ACE2 X-ray structures reveal a large hinge-bending motion important for inhibitor binding and catalysis. J Biol Chem 2004; 279(17):17996–8007.
51. Gwathmey TM, Westwood BM, Pirro NT, et al. Nuclear angiotensin-(1-7) receptor is functionally coupled to the formation of nitric oxide. Am J Physiol Renal Physiol 2010;299(5):F983–90.
52. Qi Y, Shenoy V, Wong F, et al. Lentivirus-mediated overexpression of angiotensin-(1-7) attenuated ischaemia-induced cardiac pathophysiology. Exp Physiol 2011; 96(9):863–74.
53. Grobe JL, Der Sarkissian S, Stewart JM, et al. ACE2 overexpression inhibits hypoxia-induced collagen production by cardiac fibroblasts. Clin Sci (Lond) 2007;113(8):357–64.
54. Burrell LM, Risvanis J, Kubota E, et al. Myocardial infarction increases ACE2 expression in rat and humans. Eur Heart J 2005;26(4):369–75 [discussion: 322–64].
55. Trask AJ, Groban L, Westwood BM, et al. Inhibition of angiotensin-converting enzyme 2 exacerbates cardiac hypertrophy and fibrosis in Ren-2 hypertensive rats. Am J Hypertens 2010;23(6):687–93.
56. Tallant EA, Ferrario CM, Gallagher PE. Angiotensin-(1-7) inhibits growth of cardiac myocytes through activation of the mas receptor. Am J Physiol Heart Circ Physiol 2005;289(4):H1560–6.
57. Patel VB, Bodiga S, Fan D, et al. Cardioprotective effects mediated by angiotensin II type 1 receptor blockade and enhancing angiotensin 1-7 in experimental heart failure in angiotensin-converting enzyme 2-null mice. Hypertension 2012; 59(6):1195–203.
58. Velkoska E, Dean RG, Griggs K, et al. Angiotensin-(1-7) infusion is associated with increased blood pressure and adverse cardiac remodelling in rats with subtotal nephrectomy. Clin Sci (Lond) 2011;120(8):335–45.
59. Heller J, Kramer HJ, Maly J, et al. Effect of intrarenal infusion of angiotensin-(1-7) in the dog. Kidney Blood Press Res 2000;23(2):89–94.
60. Pinheiro SV, Ferreira AJ, Kitten GT, et al. Genetic deletion of the angiotensin-(1-7) receptor Mas leads to glomerular hyperfiltration and microalbuminuria. Kidney Int 2009;75(11):1184–93.
61. Zhang J, Noble NA, Border WA, et al. Infusion of angiotensin-(1-7) reduces glomerulosclerosis through counteracting angiotensin II in experimental glomerulonephritis. Am J Physiol Renal Physiol 2010;298(3):F579–88.
62. Jin HY, Chen LJ, Zhang ZZ, et al. Deletion of angiotensin-converting enzyme 2 exacerbates renal inflammation and injury in apolipoprotein E-deficient mice through modulation of the nephrin and TNF-alpha-TNFRSF1A signaling. J Transl Med 2015;13:255.
63. Oudit GY, Liu GC, Zhong J, et al. Human recombinant ACE2 reduces the progression of diabetic nephropathy. Diabetes 2010;59(2):529–38.
64. Lely AT, Hamming I, van Goor H, et al. Renal ACE2 expression in human kidney disease. J Pathol 2004;204(5):587–93.
65. Reich HN, Oudit GY, Penninger JM, et al. Decreased glomerular and tubular expression of ACE2 in patients with type 2 diabetes and kidney disease. Kidney Int 2008;74(12):1610–6.
66. Bernstein KE, Khan Z, Giani JF, et al. Angiotensin-converting enzyme in innate and adaptive immunity. Nat Rev Nephrol 2018;14(5):325–36.
67. Sachse A, Wolf G. Angiotensin II-induced reactive oxygen species and the kidney. J Am Soc Nephrol 2007;18(9):2439–46.

68. Khan Z, Shen XZ, Bernstein EA, et al. Angiotensin-converting enzyme enhances the oxidative response and bactericidal activity of neutrophils. Blood 2017; 130(3):328–39.
69. Okwan-Duodu D, Datta V, Shen XZ, et al. Angiotensin-converting enzyme overexpression in mouse myelomonocytic cells augments resistance to *Listeria* and methicillin-resistant *Staphylococcus aureus*. J Biol Chem 2010;285(50): 39051–60.
70. Meng Y, Chen C, Liu Y, et al. Angiotensin II regulates dendritic cells through activation of NF-kappaB/p65, ERK1/2 and STAT1 pathways. Cell Physiol Biochem 2017;42(4):1550–8.
71. Abraham E. Nuclear factor-kappaB and its role in sepsis-associated organ failure. J Infect Dis 2003;187(Suppl 2):S364–9.
72. Ozawa Y, Kobori H. Crucial role of Rho-nuclear factor-kappaB axis in angiotensin II-induced renal injury. Am J Physiol Renal Physiol 2007;293(1):F100–9.
73. Shen XZ, Li P, Weiss D, et al. Mice with enhanced macrophage angiotensin-converting enzyme are resistant to melanoma. Am J Pathol 2007;170(6):2122–34.
74. Zambelli V, Bellani G, Borsa R, et al. Angiotensin-(1-7) improves oxygenation, while reducing cellular infiltrate and fibrosis in experimental acute respiratory distress syndrome. Intensive Care Med Exp 2015;3(1):44.
75. Hilgenfeldt U, Kienapfel G, Kellermann W, et al. Renin-angiotensin system in sepsis. Clin Exp Hypertens A 1987;9(8–9):1493–504.
76. Casey L, Krieger B, Kohler J, et al. Decreased serum angiotensin converting enzyme in adult respiratory distress syndrome associated with sepsis: a preliminary report. Crit Care Med 1981;9(9):651–4.
77. Shen L, Mo H, Cai L, et al. Losartan prevents sepsis-induced acute lung injury and decreases activation of nuclear factor kappaB and mitogen-activated protein kinases. Shock 2009;31(5):500–6.
78. Graninger M, Marsik C, Dukic T, et al. Enalapril does not alter adhesion molecule levels in human endotoxemia. Shock 2003;19(5):448–51.
79. Dial S, Nessim SJ, Kezouh A, et al. Antihypertensive agents acting on the renin-angiotensin system and the risk of sepsis. Br J Clin Pharmacol 2014;78(5): 1151–8.
80. Rodgers K, Xiong S, Espinoza T, et al. Angiotensin II increases host resistance to peritonitis. Clin Diagn Lab Immunol 2000;7(4):635–40.
81. Reddy LM, Baydur L, Liebler JM, et al. The role of renin-angiotensin peptides in the pathogenesis of acute respiratory distress syndrome. Am J Respir Crit Care Med 2017;195:A4773.
82. Wosten-van Asperen RM, Lutter R, Specht PA, et al. Acute respiratory distress syndrome leads to reduced ratio of ACE/ACE2 activities and is prevented by angiotensin-(1-7) or an angiotensin II receptor antagonist. J Pathol 2011;225(4): 618–27.
83. Raiden S, Nahmod K, Nahmod V, et al. Nonpeptide antagonists of AT1 receptor for angiotensin II delay the onset of acute respiratory distress syndrome. J Pharmacol Exp Ther 2002;303(1):45–51.
84. Wosten-van Asperen RM, Lutter R, Specht PA, et al. Ventilator-induced inflammatory response in lipopolysaccharide-exposed rat lung is mediated by angiotensin-converting enzyme. Am J Pathol 2010;176(5):2219–27.
85. Kuba K, Imai Y, Rao S, et al. A crucial role of angiotensin converting enzyme 2 (ACE2) in SARS coronavirus-induced lung injury. Nat Med 2005;11(8):875–9.
86. Imai Y, Kuba K, Rao S, et al. Angiotensin-converting enzyme 2 protects from severe acute lung failure. Nature 2005;436(7047):112–6.

87. Treml B, Neu N, Kleinsasser A, et al. Recombinant angiotensin-converting enzyme 2 improves pulmonary blood flow and oxygenation in lipopolysaccharide-induced lung injury in piglets. Crit Care Med 2010;38(2):596–601.

88. Haschke M, Schuster M, Poglitsch M, et al. Pharmacokinetics and pharmacodynamics of recombinant human angiotensin-converting enzyme 2 in healthy human subjects. Clin Pharmacokinet 2013;52(9):783–92.

89. Cao W, Jin L, Zhou Z, et al. Overexpression of intrarenal renin-angiotensin system in human acute tubular necrosis. Kidney Blood Press Res 2016;41(6):746–56.

90. Alge JL, Karakala N, Neely BA, et al. Urinary angiotensinogen and risk of severe AKI. Clin J Am Soc Nephrol 2013;8(2):184–93.

91. Lankadeva YR, Kosaka J, Evans RG, et al. Urinary oxygenation as a surrogate measure of medullary oxygenation during angiotensin II therapy in septic acute kidney injury. Crit Care Med 2018;46(1):e41–8.

92. Efrati S, Berman S, Hamad RA, et al. Effect of captopril treatment on recuperation from ischemia/reperfusion-induced acute renal injury. Nephrol Dial Transplant 2012;27(1):136–45.

93. Zhang J, Rudemiller NP, Patel MB, et al. Competing actions of type 1 angiotensin II receptors expressed on T lymphocytes and kidney epithelium during cisplatin-induced AKI. J Am Soc Nephrol 2016;27(8):2257–64.

94. Fang F, Liu GC, Zhou X, et al. Loss of ACE2 exacerbates murine renal ischemia-reperfusion injury. PLoS One 2013;8(8):e71433.

Angiotensin II in Vasodilatory Shock

Brett J. Wakefield, MD[a,b], Laurence W. Busse, MD[c], Ashish K. Khanna, MD[a,d,e],*

KEYWORDS

- Vasodilatory shock • Septic shock • Angiotensin II • Vasopressor • Blood pressure

KEY POINTS

- Vasodilatory shock, also known as distributive shock, is characterized by decreased systemic vascular resistance with impaired oxygen extraction leading to profound vasodilation.
- The Angiotensin II for the Treatment of Vasodilatory Shock (ATHOS-3) trial demonstrated the vasopressor and catecholamine-sparing effect of angiotensin II in patients with vasodilatory shock.
- Further studies suggest Angiotensin II may offer a benefit in patients with increased severity of illness, acute kidney injury requiring renal replacement therapy, severe acute respiratory distress syndrome and in brisk responders to minimal doses of therapy.

INTRODUCTION

Shock is common in the intensive care unit (ICU), and up to one-third of critically ill patients are admitted to the ICU with some form of shock.[1] Shock is defined as a pathologic condition of acute and life-threatening circulatory failure resulting in inadequate tissue oxygen utilization.[2] The tenets of management include treatment of the underlying cause and blood pressure support with fluid resuscitation and vasopressor

Conflict of Interest: Drs A.K. Khanna and L.W. Busse have received support from the La Jolla Pharmaceutical Company as consultants and speakers.
Funding: No funding was procured for this work.
[a] Department of General Anesthesiology, Anesthesiology Institute, Cleveland Clinic, 9500 Euclid Avenue, Cleveland, OH 44195, USA; [b] Department of Anesthesiology, Division of Critical Care Medicine, Washington University School of Medicine, 660 South Euclid Avenue, Campus Box 8054, St Louis, MO 63110, USA; [c] Division of Pulmonary, Critical Care, Allergy and Sleep Medicine, Emory University School of Medicine, Emory St. Joseph's Hospital, 5665 Peachtree Dunwoody Road, Atlanta, GA 30342, USA; [d] Center for Critical Care, Department of Outcomes Research, Cleveland Clinic, 9500 Euclid Avenue - G58, Cleveland, OH 44195, USA; [e] Department of Anesthesiology, Wake Forest University School of Medicine, Winston-Salem, NC, USA
* Corresponding author. Cleveland Clinic Foundation, 9500 Euclid Avenue - G58, Cleveland, OH 44195.
E-mail address: ashish@or.org

Crit Care Clin 35 (2019) 229–245
https://doi.org/10.1016/j.ccc.2018.11.003
0749-0704/19/© 2018 Elsevier Inc. All rights reserved.

criticalcare.theclinics.com

administration when required.[3] Previously, vasopressor options were limited to 2 broad classes of vasopressors: catecholamines (norepinephrine, epinephrine, and dopamine) and vasopressin. Recently, however, angiotensin II, a component of the renin–angiotensin–aldosterone system (RAAS), has been approved by the Food and Drug Administration (FDA) as the third class of vasopressor. Angiotensin II may play an important role in the treatment of difficult-to-manage vasodilatory shock.

VASODILATORY SHOCK

Vasodilatory shock, also known as distributive shock, is characterized by decreased systemic vascular resistance with impaired oxygen extraction leading to profound vasodilation.[4] The most common type of vasodilatory shock is septic shock, which represents 50% to 80% of all cases.[5,6] Other nonseptic causes of vasodilatory shock include postoperative vasoplegia, anaphylaxis, severe metabolic acidosis, pancreatitis, and chronic angiotensin-converting enzyme (ACE) inhibitor overdose.[5,7–10] The term "refractory" has been used in cases of vasodilatory shock in which there is a failure to maintain mean arterial pressure (MAP) despite volume resuscitation and the use of vasopressors.[11] A consensus definition for refractory vasodilatory shock has not been established; however, high-dose vasopressors defined at various thresholds are associated with substantial mortality.[12,13] The recently published Angiotensin II for the Treatment of High-Output Shock 3 (ATHOS-3) trial defined refractory vasodilatory shock as shock that required the use of greater than 0.2 mcg/kg/min of norepinephrine equivalent vasopressor doses in order to maintain an MAP of 65 mm Hg, a threshold that was used as enrollment criteria into this study.[14] This threshold is twice the threshold used in estimating a mortality of nearly 50% as part of the calculation of the Sequential Organ Failure Assessment (SOFA) score.[15] A threshold of 0.5 mcg/kg/min of norepinephrine or epinephrine has also been frequently used in clinical trials to define the threshold for refractory shock.[16–18] Benbenishty and colleagues[16] reported a sensitivity of 96% and specificity of 76% for prediction of mortality in patients receiving greater than 0.5 mcg/kg/min of norepinephrine, which has been confirmed in other analyses.[19] Furthermore, norepinephrine-equivalent vasopressor doses of greater than 1 mcg/kg/min are associated with a mortality of 80% or higher at 90 days.[12] Considering these observations, refractory vasodilatory shock may be present when (1) vasopressors fail to result in an adequate MAP response, (2) patients require additional or adjunctive therapies to support blood pressure, or (3) current levels of therapy are associated with a dose-dependent increase in mortality.[16–20]

HEMODYNAMIC TARGETS FOR MANAGEMENT OF VASODILATORY SHOCK

Ample evidence suggests that low blood pressure is associated with increased morbidity and mortality. An MAP less than 55 mm Hg for as little as 1 minute during the intraoperative period was found to be associated with acute kidney injury (AKI) and myocardial injury.[21] Similar analyses have found that as the time-weighted average of intraoperative MAP decreased from 80 to 50 mm Hg, the 30-day mortality more than tripled.[22] Khanna and colleagues[23] reported an almost 50% increase in mortality and myocardial injury with every 10 mm Hg difference (compared between patients) in the lowest MAP on any given day in critically ill postoperative patients. This relationship was seen at any MAP less than a threshold of 90 mm Hg.[24]

Blood pressure goals in septic shock are delineated in the Surviving Sepsis Campaign guidelines and describe a target MAP of at least 65 mm Hg as an initial resuscitative strategy.[25] This recommendation is supported in part by a large multicenter randomized controlled trial, which found no difference in mortality when comparing MAP targets of 80 to 85 mm Hg and 65 to 70 mm Hg in patients with septic shock.[26] This study and many other smaller studies have associated higher MAP targets with more cardiac arrhythmias and vasopressor use, but a similar serum lactate, regional blood flow, and mortality compared with lower blood pressure targets.[27–30]

Despite guideline recommendations, an MAP target of 65 mm Hg is often challenging to achieve consistently, and recent data has now questioned the sufficiency of this target in the ICU.[23,24,28,31] Nielsen and colleagues[32] found that among patients with septic shock who are on vasopressors, 62%, 37%, and 18% had MAP values below 65, 60, and 55 mm Hg, respectively, for greater than 2 hours and up to 4 hours. In addition, increased duration at these low MAP values was associated with increased mortality. A multivariable logistic regression analysis of nearly 9000 septic patients across 110 ICUs in the United States found the risks for mortality, AKI, and myocardial injury first developed at an MAP of 85 mm Hg, and the risk of mortality and AKI progressively worsened as MAP decreased from 85 to 55 mm Hg.[31]

The maintenance of a minimally acceptable MAP goal during resuscitation of septic shock needs to be understood in the context of the currently available vasopressor options. The surviving sepsis campaign guidelines recommend the use of norepinephrine as the first-line vasopressor, with the addition of epinephrine or vasopressin as adjunctive therapies.[25] However, the use of catecholamines and vasopressin at high doses are associated with poor outcomes and even risk of injury. By one estimate, only 17% of patients with septic shock requiring vasopressor therapy of greater than or equal to 1 mcg/kg/min of norepinephrine-equivalent dosing survive to 90 days.[12] In addition, high-dose catecholamine therapy has been shown to be independently predictive of mortality after controlling for many factors, including severity of illness.[33] Catecholamine monotherapy is also associated with significant cardiac side effects, morbidity, and mortality, an effect that is correlated with the cumulative dose of catecholamines, the number of different catecholamines used, and the duration of therapy.[34] Vasopressin has been shown to reduce the need for catecholamine therapy (a phenomenon commonly referred to as catecholamine-sparing) and is frequently deployed as a second-line agent in septic shock.[25,35] Although superiority of vasopressin has yet to be demonstrated, patients with less severe shock (lactate <1.4 mmol/L or norepinephrine dose <15 mcg/min) treated with vasopressin had better survival when compared with norepinephrine.[36] In addition, vasopressin has been associated with a reduced requirement for renal replacement therapy (RRT) in patients with septic shock.[37] However, vasopressin at high doses has also been associated with adverse outcomes including hyperbilirubinemia, increased liver enzymes, reduced platelet count, ischemic skin lesions, and mesenteric ischemia.[19,38,39] Moreover, less than half of patients with septic shock respond to vasopressin, highlighting the need for additional options.[40]

Angiotensin II, recently approved by the FDA, is a novel vasopressor agent that has been shown to increase blood pressure with a catecholamine-sparing effect in patients with vasodilatory shock.[14]

ANGIOTENSIN II PHYSIOLOGY

Angiotensin II is an essential component of the RAAS and is synthesized in the liver as angiotensinogen before being cleaved by renin into angiotensin I (**Fig. 1**). Renin is a carboxypeptidase released from the juxtaglomerular cells in response to reduced renal afferent arteriole pressure, increased sympathetic stimulation, and decreased sodium or chloride concentrations in the distal tubule.[41,42] Angiotensin I undergoes

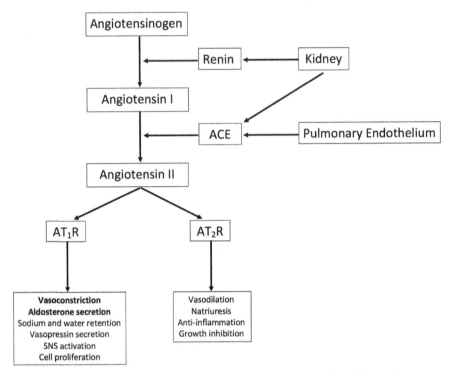

Fig. 1. The physiology of the renin-angiotensin system. AT1R, angiotensin type 1 receptor; AT2R, angiotensin type 2 receptor; SNS, sympathetic nervous system. (*Courtesy of* Brett J. Wakefield, MD, St Louis, MO.)

ACE-mediated hydrolysis into the octapeptide angiotensin II. ACE, a membrane-bound metalloproteinase, is located primarily on the surface of pulmonary capillary endothelial cells. Furthermore, it participates in the conversion of bradykinin to an inactive metabolite.[43,44] Angiotensin II acts primarily on the angiotensin type I receptor (AT1R) which is widely distributed throughout the body, including the vasculature, heart, kidney, brain, adrenal glands, and lung.[45] The AT1R is a transmembrane G protein–coupled receptor with multiple signaling pathways, including inositol 1,4,5-trisphosphate; MAP kinases; phospholipase C, A2, and D activation; calcium mobilization; and the JAK/STAT pathway, among others.[46] The downstream effects of the AT1R include vasoconstriction, sympathetic nervous system activation, secretion of aldosterone and vasopressin, increased cardiac contractility, and sodium and water retention in the kidneys.[47,48] Other renal effects of angiotensin II include preferential vasoconstriction of the efferent glomerular arterioles leading to an increased transglomerular pressure gradient and thus an increased glomerular filtration rate (GFR).[49] Animal studies have suggested that during sepsis, there is vasodilation of the renal efferent arterioles to a greater extent than the afferent arterioles.[50] Vasoconstriction of the efferent arterioles with angiotensin II may help restore hemostatic mechanisms. Wan and colleagues[51] found that although angiotensin II reduced renal blood flow in animals, it increased creatinine clearance and urine output. In addition, a study in septic ewes reported similar results.[51] This effect, however, has not manifested in human studies, and most of the investigations report a reduced GFR, decreased plasma flow, and antinatriuresis.[52] Another receptor in the angiotensin family is the angiotensin type II receptor (AT_2R). The AT_2R works in contradiction to the AT_1R causing physiologic responses including vasodilation and natriuresis.[53–55] Angiotensin II has a plasma half-life of 1 minute and is rapidly metabolized by aminopeptidase A and ACE 2 into the active metabolites angiotensin III, a weak vasoconstrictor, and angiotensin-(1–7), which has vasodilatory properties.[56] Angiotensin II metabolism occurs independently of renal and hepatic mechanisms.[57]

Abnormalities in the RAAS can occur during sepsis, and activation is known to occur with the onset of sepsis. However, reduced activity has also been reported.[58–61] Zhang and colleagues[59] evaluated RAAS activity in patients with sepsis and found that low angiotensin II (<86.1 ng/mL) and ACE (<39.2 ng/mL) levels were better predictors of mortality than the APACHE II or SOFA scores. Furthermore, downregulation of the AT_1R occurs during sepsis potentially due to proinflammatory cytokines and increased expression of nitric oxide.[60]

ANGIOTENSIN II USE IN VASODILATORY SHOCK

Angiotensin II (historically referred to as both hypertensin and angiotonin) was identified and isolated in the 1940s and found to produce a strong vasoconstrictive effect.[62] The octapeptide was synthesized in the 1950s and subsequently identified under a single nomenclature, angiotensin.[63–65] In the 1960s, various studies validated the vasopressor effect of angiotensin II in patients with vasodilatory shock and after cardiac surgery.[66,67] Norepinephrine and angiotensin II were compared directly by Cohn and Luria[68] who found that both agents increased blood pressure, but norepinephrine had a more significant impact on cardiac output (34% vs 15%). Multiple case reports were published throughout the 1990s describing the use of angiotensin II in vasodilatory shock.[69–71] In each case, angiotensin II was added to norepinephrine following the failure of norepinephrine to adequately increase blood pressure. In a series of 32 patients with refractory septic shock, 84% responded to angiotensin II; however, only 32% achieved rapid improvement with a sustained increase in systemic vascular resistance.[72] In addition, angiotensin II has been used for reversal of ACE inhibitor overdose.[73,74]

The Angiotensin II for the Treatment of High-Output Shock (ATHOS) pilot study (ClinicalTrials.gov #NCT01393782) evaluated the safety and efficacy of angiotensin II in humans with vasodilatory shock.[75] Twenty patients with high-output shock, defined as a cardiovascular SOFA score of 4 in addition to a cardiac index greater than 2.4 L/min/m^2, were randomized to receive either angiotensin II or placebo. The primary end point of the study was the catecholamine-sparing effect of angiotensin II on the background dose of norepinephrine-equivalent vasopressors required to maintain an MAP greater than 65 mm Hg. Angiotensin II resulted in norepinephrine-equivalent dose reduction in all patients. After 1 hour of drug infusion, the mean norepinephrine doses were 27.6 ± 29.3 mcg/min in the placebo arm and 7.4 ± 12.4 mcg/min in the angiotensin II group.

More recently, Khanna and colleagues[14] completed the Angiotensin II for the Treatment of Vasodilatory Shock (ATHOS-3) trial (ClinicalTrials.gov #NCT02338843) in 75 ICUs across 9 countries, which randomized 344 patients with refractory vasodilatory shock (defined as an MAP between 55 and 70 mm Hg with the support of >0.2 mcg/kg/min of norepinephrine-equivalent vasopressor dosing and either a cardiac index >2.3 L/min/m^2 or a central venous saturation >70% plus a central venous pressure >8 mm Hg) to receive angiotensin II or placebo. The primary end point was an MAP response at 3 hours or greater than or equal to 75 mm Hg or an increase of at least 10 mm Hg higher than the baseline MAP. Secondary endpoints evaluated differences in cardiovascular and total SOFA scores between the angiotensin II and placebo groups. Primary and secondary outcomes are presented in **Table 1**. More patients randomized to angiotensin II reached the primary end point than those in the placebo group (69.9% angiotensin II vs 23.4% placebo; odds ratio [OR] = 7.95; 95% confidence interval [CI] 4.76–13.3; $P<.001$) (**Fig. 2**A, **Table 2**). Patients receiving angiotensin II achieved a significantly greater reduction in cardiovascular SOFA scores (-1.75 ± 1.77 angiotensin II vs -1.28 ± 1.65 placebo; $P = .01$), whereas no difference was seen in overall scores (1.05 ± 5.50 angiotensin II vs 1.04 ± 5.34 placebo; $P = .49$). Importantly, there was a significant catecholamine-sparing effect on background vasopressors during the first 3 hours of study drug infusion in patients receiving angiotensin II, which was maintained consistently throughout the study period (**Fig. 2**B, see **Table 2**). There was no statistically significant difference in 7-day (29% angiotensin II vs 35% placebo; hazard ratio [HR] = 0.78; 95% CI 0.53–1.16; $P = .22$) and 28-day mortality (46% angiotensin II vs 54% placebo; HR = 0.78; 95% CI 0.57–1.07, $P = .12$). These results formed the basis for FDA approval of angiotensin II for use in septic and other forms of distributive shock.

Table 1
ATHOS-3 primary and secondary endpoints

End Point	Angiotensin II[a] (N = 163)	Placebo[a] (N = 158)	Odds or Hazard Ratio (95%)	P Value
Primary efficacy end point: MAP response at hour 3—no. (%)[b]	114 (69.9)	37 (23.4)	Odds ratio, 7.95 (4.76–13.3)	<.001
Secondary efficacy endpoints				
Mean change in cardiovascular SOFA score at hour 48[c]	-1.75 ± 1.77	-1.28 ± 1.65		.01
Mean change in total SOFA score at hour 48[d]	1.05 ± 5.50	1.04 ± 5.34		.49
Additional endpoints				
Mean change in norepinephrine-equivalent dose from baseline to hour 3[e]	-0.03 ± 0.10	0.03 ± 0.23		<.001
All-cause mortality at day 7—no. (%)	47 (29)	55 (35)	Hazard ratio, 0.78 (0.53–1.16)	.22
All-cause mortality at day 28—no. (%)	75 (46)	85 (54)	Hazard ratio, 0.78 (0.57–1.07)	.12

[a] Plus–minus values are means $\pm$ SD.
[b] Response with respect to mean arterial pressure at hour 3 after the start of infusion was defined as an increase from baseline of at least 10 mm Hg or an increase to at least 75 mm Hg, without an increase in the dose of background vasopressors.
[c] Scores on the cardiovascular Sequential Organ Failure Assessment range from 0 to 4, with higher scores indicating more severe dysfunction.
[d] The total SOFA score ranges from 0 to 20, with higher scores indicating more severe dysfunction.
[e] Data were missing for 3 patients in the angiotensin II group and for one patient in the placebo group.

Reprinted from Khanna A, English SW, Wang XS, et al. Angiotensin II for the treatment of vasodilatory shock. N Engl J Med 2017;377:426. Copyright © 2017 Massachusetts Medical Society; with permission.

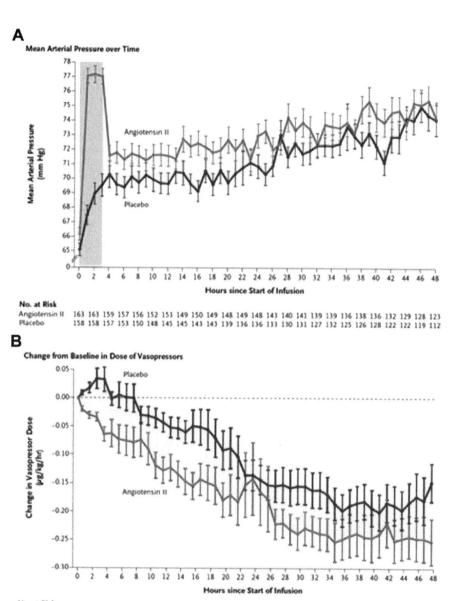

Fig. 2. ATHOS-3 angiotensin II treatment responses. (*A*) The higher mean arterial pressure achieved with angiotensin II. The difference in pressures was consistent over a 48-hour period and significant over the first 3 hours of angiotensin II infusion. (*B*) The catecholamine-sparing effect of angiotensin II with a significant drop in background vasopressor use over the first 3 hours and a consistent difference over a 48 hour period. (*Reprinted from* Khanna A, English SW, Wang XS, et al, Angiotensin II for the treatment of vasodilatory shock. N Engl J Med 2017;377:427. Copyright © 2017 Massachusetts Medical Society; with permission.)

Table 2
Inclusion and exclusion criteria for angiotensin II administration

Inclusion Criteria[c]	Exclusion Criteria
• 18 years or older • Vasodilatory shock[a] despite IV fluid resuscitation • High-dose vasopressors[b]	• Burns covering >20% BSA • Acute coronary syndrome • Bronchospasm • Liver failure • Mesenteric ischemia • Active bleeding • Abdominal aortic aneurysm • ANC <1000/mm³ • ECMO • High-dose glucocorticoids

Abbreviations: ANC, absolute neutrophil count; BSA, body surface area; ECMO, extracorporeal membrane oxygenation; IV, intravenous.
[a] Vasodilatory shock defined as cardiac index greater than 2.3 L/min/m² or central venous oxygen saturation greater than 70% with a central venous pressure greater than 8 mm Hg with an MAP of 55 to 70 mm Hg.
[b] High-dose vasopressors defined as greater than 0.2 mcg/kg/min norepinephrine or norepinephrine equivalent.
[c] Both criteria a and b had to be present for a minimum of 6 hours and a maximum of 48 hours before randomization.
Data from Khanna A, English SW, Wang XS, et al. Angiotensin II for the treatment of vasodilatory shock. N Engl J Med 2017;377(5):419–30.

ANGIOTENSIN II SAFETY PROFILE

Busse and colleagues[52] evaluated the safety profile of angiotensin II, at doses ranging from 0.5 ng/kg/min to 3780 ng/kg/min, in an analysis of 1124 studies describing 31,281 patients who received angiotensin II. Two deaths were reported due to angiotensin II, including one patient who suffered a hemorrhagic stroke while performing a Valsalva maneuver after 6 days of angiotensin II treatment and another patient with decompensated heart failure who failed to respond to angiotensin II for profound cardiogenic shock.[68,76] Further investigations of angiotensin II administration in cardiogenic shock are lacking. A review of 276 patients with various forms of shock receiving angiotensin II demonstrated a significant vasopressor response in most of the 38 patients with cardiogenic shock.[77] The 2 largest cohorts of cardiogenic shock patients (1963: 11 patients; 1964: 17 patients) found no adverse reactions due to the medication.[78,79] Angiotensin II has been found to increase pulmonary vascular resistance and pressure, but the effect on heart rate, cardiac output, and contractility have yielded conflicting results, possibly due to the varying effects of the different angiotensin II receptors.[80] Asthma exacerbations have been associated with angiotensin II administration; however, the cause has not been fully elucidated.[52,75] Angiotensin II administration has been shown to alter hormone levels in the RAAS, including an increase in aldosterone and a decrease in renin.[81,82] Studies have demonstrated increased plasma arginine vasopressin, endothelin, atrial natriuretic peptide, and erythropoietin. Increased glucose utilization and insulin secretion have been described, which is attributable to angiotensin II–mediated shunting of blood toward insulin-dependent tissues (skeletal muscle).[83] Angiotensin II has been shown to reduce GFR, decrease renal plasma flow, and decrease sodium excretion. Eleven studies reported reduced GFR, whereas an increased GFR was only found in 2. The reduced plasma flow and GFR has been attributed to increased vascular resistance and alterations in glomerular pore size. Adverse events seen in the ATHOS study included alkalosis and hypertension (with 2 patients experiencing a super response of MAP >90 mm Hg despite discontinuation of all vasopressors).[75] Patients treated with angiotensin II in the ATHOS-3 trial experienced an increased incidence of thromboembolic events (13% vs 5%) when compared with placebo.[57] Additional imbalances were seen with regard to delirium and fungal infection, the mechanisms for which have not been fully explored.[57]

ANGIOTENSIN II AND SPECIAL POPULATIONS

Analyses of the efficacy of angiotensin II have been described for several prespecified patient groups. Szerlip and colleagues[84] evaluated the subgroup of patients within ATHOS-3 with an increased severity of illness (demonstrated by either an APACHE II score >30 or a baseline MAP <65 mm Hg despite high-dose vasopressor requirements) and found that patients with high APACHE II scores who received angiotensin II experienced improved survival compared with placebo (28-day mortality: 51.8% vs 70.8%; HR = 0.62; 95% CI 0.39–0.98; P = .037). In addition, patients with baseline MAPs greater than 65 mm Hg despite high-dose vasopressors who received angiotensin II exhibited a trend toward improved survival compared with placebo (28-day mortality: 54.2% vs 70.4%; HR = 0.66; 95% CI 0.40–1.09; P = .10). The investigators suggest that exogenous angiotensin II may address a significant physiologic deficiency among patients with increased illness severity.

Angiotensin II may be useful in patients with vasodilatory shock and renal injury. Tumlin and colleagues[85] found that patients enrolled in ATHOS-3 with AKI requiring RRT had improved survival when treated with angiotensin II compared with placebo (53% [95% CI 38%–67%] vs 30% [95% CI19%–41%]; P = .012). In addition, those patients in the angiotensin II group discontinued RRT at a higher rate of 38% (95% CI 25%–54%) versus 15% (95% CI 8%–27%) on day 7 (P = .007). In contrast to the human studies described previously, these results support the earlier findings from animal models, which demonstrated the beneficial effects of angiotensin II on renal function.[86]

Damage or dysfunction of the pulmonary capillary endothelium may be associated with reduced ACE functionality and decreased conversion of angiotensin I to angiotensin II, resulting in a relative angiotensin II deficiency.[87] Acute respiratory distress syndrome (ARDS) is characterized by damage to the capillary endothelium and alveolar epithelium resulting in diffuse alveolar damage.[88] Previous studies have found decreased ACE levels in patients with sepsis and ARDS.[89] Busse and colleagues[90] evaluated the safety and efficacy of angiotensin II in a subgroup of the ATHOS-3 population with ARDS. Patients with severe ARDS (Pao_2/Fio_2 <100) experienced a greater MAP response than those with milder forms of ARDS (OR = 8.4 [95% CI 1.8–39.7] vs 6.6 [95% CI 2.8–15.9]). In addition, there was a trend toward improved 28-day mortality in patients with severe ARDS treated with angiotensin II compared with placebo (mortality of 50% [95% CI 30%–74%] vs 74% [95% CI 53%–90%]; P = .145).

The effects encountered in both the renal and pulmonary populations described earlier suggest that in patients in whom the RAAS is impaired, angiotensin II may confer clinical outcome benefits. It is hypothesized that RAAS dysfunction and subsequent angiotensin II deficiency may be a common finding in patients with septic shock and AKI or ARDS.[91] Angiotensin II deficiency, or the relative ratio of angiotensin I to angiotensin II, in patients with distributive shock has been evaluated.[92] A low angiotensin II state, calculated as an angiotensin I to angiotensin II ratio greater than 1.63 (the median ratio for the ATHOS-3 cohort), was associated with higher mortality (HR = 1.78; 95% CI: 1.25–2.53, P = .002). Furthermore, in patients with a ratio of greater than 1.63, a survival benefit was seen in patients receiving angiotensin II compared with placebo (HR = 0.64; 95% CI: 0.41–1.00, P = .047).

Another post hoc analysis evaluated the angiotensin II dose-response effect ($\leq$5 ng/kg/min vs >5 ng/kg/min) 30 minutes after initiation on mortality, safety, and tolerability.[93] Patients requiring lower doses of angiotensin II to achieve the target MAP experienced improved 28-day survival when compared with the higher dose treatment group (low dose: 67.1%; 95% CI 55.6%–76.3%; high dose: 41.4%; 95% CI 30.8%–51.7%; P = .0007). This effect was significant after multivariate adjustment for several disease covariates (HR = 2.19; 95% CI 1.32–3.64, P = .0026). The patients requiring lower doses of angiotensin II had a decreased incidence of adverse events and were more likely to achieve the target MAP at 3 hours. In addition, patients requiring lower doses of angiotensin II had significantly lower baseline levels of both angiotensin I and angiotensin II, suggesting to the investigators that angiotensin II deficiency may have contributed to these findings.

ILLUSTRATIVE CASE AND CONCEPTS ON THE PRACTICAL APPLICATION OF ANGIOTENSIN II
A Case of Septic Shock from Pneumococcal Pneumonia

A 65-year-old woman with a past medical history of hereditary hemorrhagic telangiectasia, chronic anemia, and chronic obstructive pulmonary disease on home oxygen therapy presented to the emergency department with 4 days of shortness of breath and a productive cough. A chest radiograph demonstrated a dense left-sided consolidation. Her laboratory results were notable for leukocytosis, a serum creatinine of 4.56 mg/dL, and a lactate of 3.4 mmol/L. She was admitted to the general medical ward for community-acquired pneumonia.

Her condition rapidly declined and she was transferred to the ICU for septic shock (ICU Day 0 at 21:45) within 2 hours of admission. Blood cultures were immediately obtained and the patient was started on broad spectrum antibiotics. Despite fluid administration and vasopressor (norepinephrine 0.5 mcg/kg/min, vasopressin 0.04 U/min) initiation, MAPs continued to fall short of the 65 mm Hg target. Epinephrine was started at 04:21 on ICU day 1 and rapidly titrated to 0.35 mcg/kg/min; however, MAPs continued to fluctuate between 55 and 73 mm Hg. A transthoracic echocardiogram demonstrated normal ventricular function. In addition, the patient was started on ascorbic acid, thiamine, and corticosteroids and was intubated for acute respiratory failure.

On ICU Day 1, the patient's family was counseled regarding her poor prognosis. The possibility of administering angiotensin II (Giapreza; La Jolla Pharmaceutical Company, La Jolla, California), which at the time was available through the manufacturer's compassionate use program, was approached with the family. Administration of angiotensin II through this mechanism required consent from the patient's legally authorized representative as well as adherence to prespecified inclusion and exclusion criteria (see **Table 2**).

The patient was enrolled in the manufacturer's compassionate use program and received her first dose of angiotensin II at 17:27PM on ICU Day 1. The doses of her other vasopressors at the time of initiation of angiotensin II were as follows: epinephrine at 0.18 mcg/kg/min, norepinephrine at 0.4 mcg/kg/min, and vasopressin at 0.04 U/min. With this level of support, the patient's MAP was recorded as 67 mm Hg but had been as low as 49 mm Hg in the previous 90 minutes. Notably, at the time of initiation of angiotensin II, the patient's serum creatinine remained elevated to 4.56 and the lactate had resolved to 1.6. Her blood cultures became positive for *Streptococcus pneumoniae*.

A detailed pictogram of the 48 hours following the initiation of angiotensin II is presented as **Fig. 3**. Angiotensin II had a profound effect on the concurrent doses of the patient's standard-of-care vasopressors. Angiotensin II was started at 5 ng/kg/min. Epinephrine was weaned off approximately 30 minutes after the initiation of angiotensin II. Over the next 9 hours (18:00 on ICU Day 1 to 03:00 on ICU Day 2), norepinephrine was titrated down from 0.4 mcg/kg/min to 0.1 mcg/kg/min, as angiotensin II was titrated up from 5 ng/kg/min to 20 ng/kg/min. Over the following 2 hours, vasopressin was discontinued and angiotensin II was decreased to 15 ng/kg/min. Starting at 07:00AM on ICU Day 2, both norepinephrine and angiotensin II levels were deescalated over the next 51 hours, until both infusions were discontinued at 10:26 on ICU Day 3. Importantly, during the angiotensin II infusion, the patient's MAP was rarely reduced to less than 65 mm Hg, only occurring on 3 occasions during vasopressor weaning.

At the time of vasoactive medication cessation, serum creatinine and lactate levels were noted to be 1.15 mg/dL and 0.9 mmol/L, respectively. On ICU Day 6 the patient was extubated. On ICU Day 10 she was transferred out of the ICU and she was discharged home 5 days later. Her ICU course was complicated by hypernatremia (>145 mmol/L at 07:14AM on ICU Day 4, after cessation of vasopressors) and thrombocytopenia (<140,000/mcL on ICU Day 2), both of which resolved spontaneously; however, the thrombocytopenia did not resolve until ICU Day 10.

Case discussion

This case illustrates the rapid resolution of septic shock through the use of multimodal therapy with angiotensin II as well as catecholamines and vasopressin. Similar findings were reported recently by Chow and colleagues, and the successful outcomes described earlier and in the case by Chow and colleagues[94] highlight some important aspects regarding the clinical use and utility of angiotensin II in septic shock. The hemodynamic homeostasis achieved by this patient may be related to synergistic mechanisms of the RAAS, the sympathetic nervous system, and the arginine-vasopressin system. There is evidence of a synergistic effect amongst these 3 systems in the

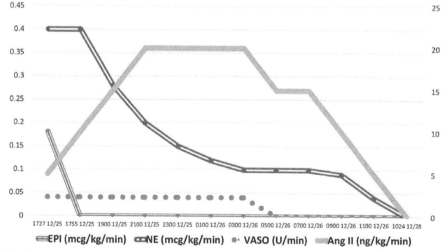

Fig. 3. Vasopressor doses over a 24-hour period in the patient with pneumococcal pneumonia and septic shock. Ang II, angiotensin II; EPI, epinephrine; NE, norepinephrine; VASO, vasopressin.

literature. Prejunctional angiotensin II receptors have been described, which facilitate norepinephrine release.[95] Furthermore, vasopressin hypersensitivity in patients with septic shock can occur and may be due to potentiation of catecholamine vasopressors.[96,97] In addition, once angiotensin II was started, MAPs in this patient rarely fell below 65 mm Hg. As previously mentioned, there is emerging evidence that even slight episodes of blood pressure less than this threshold are related to worse outcomes.[23,31,32] Finally, as previously mentioned, patients with AKI and severe lung pathology may preferentially benefit from angiotensin II, and both of these organ dysfunctions were present in the patient described herein. In summary, beneficial patient-centered outcomes may be a result of the deployment of angiotensin II as part of a multimodal balanced approach of vasopressor treatment, strict avoidance of hypotension, and selection of the right patient population.

SUMMARY

With recent FDA approval, the use of angiotensin II in vasodilatory shock is increasing, but questions remain as to when and how to best initiate therapy and which groups will uniquely benefit most from its specific use. Ongoing research is focused on specific subpopulations including patients with AKI, those with reduced pulmonary endothelial ACE activity in the setting of lung pathology (ARDS, severe pneumonia, cardiopulmonary bypass, or extracorporeal membrane oxygenation), patients with chronic ACE inhibitor use, angiotensin II low-dose responders, and patients with liver failure and a high-output vasodilated state. Further exploration into angiotensin II levels, angiotensin II dysfunction, and the angiotensin I/II ratio may also help to identify patients deficient in functional angiotensin II who would preferentially benefit from exogenous angiotensin II administration. Future analyses will also shed light on meaningful patient-centered outcomes and the role of angiotensin II within the accepted sepsis management guidelines. An earlier multi-modal and synergistic utilization of vasopressor therapy is the need of the hour to effectively and safely manage patients with severe vasodilatory shock.

REFERENCES

1. Sakr Y, Reinhart K, Vincent JL, et al. Does dopamine administration in shock influence outcome? Results of the Sepsis Occurrence in Acutely Ill Patients (SOAP) study. Crit Care Med 2006;34(3):589–97.
2. Cecconi M, De Backer D, Antonelli M, et al. Consensus on circulatory shock and hemodynamic monitoring. Task force of the European Society of intensive care medicine. Intensive Care Med 2014;40(12):1795–815.
3. Dellinger RP, Levy MM, Rhodes A, et al. Surviving sepsis campaign: international guidelines for management of severe sepsis and septic shock: 2012. Crit Care Med 2013;41(2):580–637.
4. Vincent JL, De Backer D. Circulatory shock. N Engl J Med 2013;369(18): 1726–34.
5. Vallabhajosyula A, Jentzer JC, Khanna AK. Vasodilatory shock in the ICU: perils, pitfalls and therapeutic options. Annual update in intensive care and emergency medicine 2018. 2018.
6. De Backer D, Biston P, Devriendt J, et al. Comparison of dopamine and norepinephrine in the treatment of shock. N Engl J Med 2010;362(9):779–89.
7. Valentine E, Gregorits M, Gutsche JT, et al. Clinical update in liver transplantation. J Cardiothorac Vasc Anesth 2013;27(4):809–15.

8. Fischer GW, Levin MA. Vasoplegia during cardiac surgery: current concepts and management. Semin Thorac Cardiovasc Surg 2010;22(2):140–4.

9. Landry DW, Oliver JA. The pathogenesis of vasodilatory shock. N Engl J Med 2001;345(8):588–95.

10. Brown SG. The pathophysiology of shock in anaphylaxis. Immunol Allergy Clin North Am 2007;27(2):165–75, v.

11. Jentzer JC, Vallabhajosyula S, Khanna AK, et al. Management of refractory vasodilatory shock. Chest 2018;154(2):416–26.

12. Brown SM, Lanspa MJ, Jones JP, et al. Survival after shock requiring high-dose vasopressor therapy. Chest 2013;143(3):664–71.

13. Auchet T, Regnier MA, Girerd N, et al. Outcome of patients with septic shock and high-dose vasopressor therapy. Ann Intensive Care 2017;7(1):43.

14. Khanna A, English SW, Wang XS, et al. Angiotensin II for the treatment of vasodilatory shock. N Engl J Med 2017;377(5):419–30.

15. Peres Bota D, Melot C, Lopes Ferreira F, et al. The Multiple Organ Dysfunction Score (MODS) versus the Sequential Organ Failure Assessment (SOFA) score in outcome prediction. Intensive Care Med 2002;28(11):1619–24.

16. Benbenishty J, Weissman C, Sprung CL, et al. Characteristics of patients receiving vasopressors. Heart Lung 2011;40(3):247–52.

17. Dunser MW, Mayr AJ, Ulmer H, et al. Arginine vasopressin in advanced vasodilatory shock: a prospective, randomized, controlled study. Circulation 2003; 107(18):2313–9.

18. Torgersen C, Luckner G, Schroder DC, et al. Concomitant arginine-vasopressin and hydrocortisone therapy in severe septic shock: association with mortality. Intensive Care Med 2011;37(9):1432–7.

19. Luckner G, Dunser MW, Jochberger S, et al. Arginine vasopressin in 316 patients with advanced vasodilatory shock. Crit Care Med 2005;33(11):2659–66.

20. Torgersen C, Dunser MW, Wenzel V, et al. Comparing two different arginine vasopressin doses in advanced vasodilatory shock: a randomized, controlled, open-label trial. Intensive Care Med 2010;36(1):57–65.

21. Walsh M, Devereaux PJ, Garg AX, et al. Relationship between intraoperative mean arterial pressure and clinical outcomes after noncardiac surgery: toward an empirical definition of hypotension. Anesthesiology 2013;119(3):507–15.

22. Mascha EJ, Yang D, Weiss S, et al. Intraoperative mean arterial pressure variability and 30-day mortality in patients having noncardiac surgery. Anesthesiology 2015;123(1):79–91.

23. Khanna AK, Guangmei M, Liu L, et al. 177: hypotension increases acute kidney injury, myocardial injury, and mortality in surgical critical care. Crit Care Med 2018;46(1 Suppl 1):71.

24. Sessler DI, Khanna AK. Perioperative myocardial injury and the contribution of hypotension. Intensive Care Med 2018;44(6):811–22.

25. Rhodes A, Evans LE, Alhazzani W, et al. Surviving sepsis campaign: international guidelines for management of sepsis and septic shock: 2016. Crit Care Med 2017;45(3):486–552.

26. Asfar P, Meziani F, Hamel JF, et al. High versus low blood-pressure target in patients with septic shock. N Engl J Med 2014;370(17):1583–93.

27. Bourgoin A, Leone M, Delmas A, et al. Increasing mean arterial pressure in patients with septic shock: effects on oxygen variables and renal function. Crit Care Med 2005;33(4):780–6.

28. Thooft A, Favory R, Salgado DR, et al. Effects of changes in arterial pressure on organ perfusion during septic shock. Crit Care 2011;15(5):R222.

29. Lamontagne F, Meade MO, Hebert PC, et al. Higher versus lower blood pressure targets for vasopressor therapy in shock: a multicentre pilot randomized controlled trial. Intensive Care Med 2016;42(4):542–50.

30. LeDoux D, Astiz ME, Carpati CM, et al. Effects of perfusion pressure on tissue perfusion in septic shock. Crit Care Med 2000;28(8):2729–32.

31. Maheshwari K, Nathanson BH, Munson SH, et al. The relationship between ICU hypotension and in-hospital mortality and morbidity in septic patients. Intensive Care Med 2018;44(6):857–67.

32. Nielsen ND, Zeng F, Gerbasi ME, et al. P104 treatment and outcomes of vasodilatory shock in an academic medical center. Presented at the 38th International Symposium on Intensive Care and Emergency Medicine. Brussels, Belgium, March 22, 2018.

33. Sviri S, Hashoul J, Stav I, et al. Does high-dose vasopressor therapy in medical intensive care patients indicate what we already suspect? J Crit Care 2014;29(1): 157–60.

34. Schmittinger CA, Torgersen C, Luckner G, et al. Adverse cardiac events during catecholamine vasopressor therapy: a prospective observational study. Intensive Care Med 2012;38(6):950–8.

35. Patel BM, Chittock DR, Russell JA, et al. Beneficial effects of short-term vasopressin infusion during severe septic shock. Anesthesiology 2002;96(3):576–82.

36. Russell JA, Walley KR, Singer J, et al. Vasopressin versus norepinephrine infusion in patients with septic shock. N Engl J Med 2008;358(9):877–87.

37. Gordon AC, Mason AJ, Thirunavukkarasu N, et al. Effect of early vasopressin vs norepinephrine on kidney failure in patients with septic shock: the VANISH randomized clinical trial. JAMA 2016;316(5):509–18.

38. Dunser MW, Mayr AJ, Tur A, et al. Ischemic skin lesions as a complication of continuous vasopressin infusion in catecholamine-resistant vasodilatory shock: incidence and risk factors. Crit Care Med 2003;31(5):1394–8.

39. van Haren FM, Rozendaal FW, van der Hoeven JG. The effect of vasopressin on gastric perfusion in catecholamine-dependent patients in septic shock. Chest 2003;124(6):2256–60.

40. Sacha GL, Lam SW, Duggal A, et al. Predictors of response to fixed-dose vasopressin in adult patients with septic shock. Ann Intensive Care 2018;8(1):35.

41. Aoi W, Henry DP, Weinberger MH. Evidence for a physiological role of renal sympathetic nerves in adrenergic stimulation of renin release in the rat. Circ Res 1976;38(2). UNKNOWN.

42. Skott O, Briggs JP. Direct demonstration of macula densa-mediated renin secretion. Science 1987;237(4822):1618–20.

43. Soubrier F, Wei L, Hubert C, et al. Molecular biology of the angiotensin I converting enzyme: II. Structure-function. Gene polymorphism and clinical implications. J Hypertens 1993;11(6):599–604.

44. Bernstein KE, Ong FS, Blackwell WL, et al. A modern understanding of the traditional and nontraditional biological functions of angiotensin-converting enzyme. Pharmacol Rev 2013;65(1):1–46.

45. Mehta PK, Griendling KK. Angiotensin II cell signaling: physiological and pathological effects in the cardiovascular system. Am J Physiol Cell Physiol 2007; 292(1):C82–97.

46. Kawai T, Forrester SJ, O'Brien S, et al. AT1 receptor signaling pathways in the cardiovascular system. Pharmacol Res 2017;125(Pt A):4–13.

47. Fyhrquist F, Saijonmaa O. Renin-angiotensin system revisited. J Intern Med 2008; 264(3):224–36.

48. Brewster UC, Perazella MA. The renin-angiotensin-aldosterone system and the kidney: effects on kidney disease. Am J Med 2004;116(4):263–72.
49. Heller J, Horacek V. Angiotensin II: preferential efferent constriction? Ren Physiol 1986;9(6):357–65.
50. Langenberg C, Wan L, Egi M, et al. Renal blood flow in experimental septic acute renal failure. Kidney Int 2006;69(11):1996–2002.
51. Wan L, Langenberg C, Bellomo R, et al. Angiotensin II in experimental hyperdynamic sepsis. Crit Care 2009;13(6):R190.
52. Busse LW, Wang XS, Chalikonda DM, et al. Clinical experience with IV angiotensin II administration: a systematic review of safety. Crit Care Med 2017; 45(8):1285–94.
53. Katada J, Majima M. AT(2) receptor-dependent vasodilation is mediated by activation of vascular kinin generation under flow conditions. Br J Pharmacol 2002; 136(4):484–91.
54. Padia SH, Howell NL, Siragy HM, et al. Renal angiotensin type 2 receptors mediate natriuresis via angiotensin III in the angiotensin II type 1 receptor-blocked rat. Hypertension 2006;47(3):537–44.
55. Carey RM, Padia SH. Angiotensin AT2 receptors: control of renal sodium excretion and blood pressure. Trends Endocrinol Metab 2008;19(3):84–7.
56. Bissell BD, Browder K, McKenzie M, et al. A blast from the past: revival of angiotensin II for vasodilatory shock. Ann Pharmacother 2018;52(9):920–7.
57. Giapreza (angiotensin II) [package insert]. San Diego, CA: La Jolla Pharmaceutical Company; 2018.
58. Salgado DR, Rocco JR, Silva E, et al. Modulation of the renin-angiotensin-aldosterone system in sepsis: a new therapeutic approach? Expert Opin Ther Targets 2010;14(1):11–20.
59. Zhang W, Chen X, Huang L, et al. Severe sepsis: low expression of the renin-angiotensin system is associated with poor prognosis. Exp Ther Med 2014; 7(5):1342–8.
60. Bucher M, Ittner KP, Hobbhahn J, et al. Downregulation of angiotensin II type 1 receptors during sepsis. Hypertension 2001;38(2):177–82.
61. Tamion F, Le Cam-Duchez V, Menard JF, et al. Erythropoietin and renin as biological markers in critically ill patients. Crit Care 2004;8(5):R328–35.
62. Bradley SE, Parker B. The hemodynamic effects of angiotonin in normal man. J Clin Invest 1941;20(6):715–9.
63. Braun-Menendez E, Page IH. Suggested revision of nomenclature–angiotensin. Science 1958;127(3292):242.
64. Bumpus FM, Schwarz H, Page IH. Synthesis and pharmacology of the octapeptide angiotonin. Science 1957;125(3253):886–7.
65. Basso N, Terragno NA. History about the discovery of the renin-angiotensin system. Hypertension 2001;38(6):1246–9.
66. Derrick JR, Anderson JR, Roland BJ. Adjunctive use of a biologic pressor agent, angiotensin, in management of shock. Circulation 1962;25:263–7.
67. Del Greco F, Johnson DC. Clinical experience with angiotensin II in the treatment of shock. JAMA 1961;178:994–9.
68. Cohn JN, Luria MH. Studies in clinical shock and hypotension. Ii. Hemodynamic effects of norepinephrine and angiotensin. J Clin Invest 1965;44:1494–504.
69. Wray GM, Coakley JH. Severe septic shock unresponsive to noradrenaline. Lancet 1995;346(8990):1604.
70. Yunge M, Petros A. Angiotensin for septic shock unresponsive to noradrenaline. Arch Dis Child 2000;82(5):388–9.

71. Thomas VL, Nielsen MS. Administration of angiotensin II in refractory septic shock. Crit Care Med 1991;19(8):1084–6.
72. Whiteley SM, Dade JP. Treatment of hypotension in septic shock. Lancet 1996; 347(9001):622.
73. Trilli LE, Johnson KA. Lisinopril overdose and management with intravenous angiotensin II. Ann Pharmacother 1994;28(10):1165–8.
74. Newby DE, Lee MR, Gray AJ, et al. Enalapril overdose and the corrective effect of intravenous angiotensin II. Br J Clin Pharmacol 1995;40(1):103–4.
75. Chawla LS, Busse L, Brasha-Mitchell E, et al. Intravenous angiotensin II for the treatment of high-output shock (ATHOS trial): a pilot study. Crit Care 2014; 18(5):534.
76. Ames RP, Borkowski AJ, Sicinski AM, et al. Prolonged infusions of angiotensin Ii and norepinephrine and blood pressure, electrolyte balance, and aldosterone and cortisol secretion in normal man and in cirrhosis with ascites. J Clin Invest 1965;44:1171–86.
77. Busse LW, McCurdy MT, Ali O, et al. The effect of angiotensin II on blood pressure in patients with circulatory shock: a structured review of the literature. Crit Care 2017;21(1):324.
78. Wedeen R, Zucker G. Angiotensin II in the treatment of shock. Am J Cardiol 1963; 11:82–6.
79. Beanlands DS, Gunton RW. Angiotensin Ii in the treatment of shock following myocardial infarction. Am J Cardiol 1964;14:370–3.
80. Capote LA, Mendez Perez R, Lymperopoulos A. GPCR signaling and cardiac function. Eur J Pharmacol 2015;763(Pt B):143–8.
81. Boyd GW, Adamson AR, Arnold M, et al. The role of angiotensin II in the control of aldosterone in man. Clin Sci 1972;42(1):91–104.
82. Weekley LB. Renal renin secretion rate and norepinephrine secretion rate in response to centrally administered angiotensin-II: role of the medial basal forebrain. Clin Exp Hypertens A 1992;14(5):923–45.
83. Buchanan TA, Thawani H, Kades W, et al. Angiotensin II increases glucose utilization during acute hyperinsulinemia via a hemodynamic mechanism. J Clin Invest 1993;92(2):720–6.
84. Szerlip H, Bihorac A, Chang S, et al. Effect of disease severity on survival in patients receiving angiotensin II for vasodilatory shock. Crit Care Med 2018;46(1):3.
85. Tumlin JA, Murugan R, Deane AM, et al. Outcomes in patients with vasodilatory shock and renal replacement therapy treated with intravenous angiotensin II. Crit Care Med 2018;46(6):949–57.
86. Lankadeva YR, Kosaka J, Evans RG, et al. Urinary oxygenation as a surrogate measure of medullary oxygenation during angiotensin II therapy in septic acute kidney injury. Crit Care Med 2018;46(1):e41–8.
87. Chawla LS, Busse LW, Brasha-Mitchell E, et al. The use of angiotensin II in distributive shock. Crit Care 2016;20(1):137.
88. Umbrello M, Formenti P, Bolgiaghi L, et al. Current concepts of ARDS: a narrative review. Int J Mol Sci 2016;18(1) [pii:E64].
89. Casey L, Krieger B, Kohler J, et al. Decreased serum angiotensin converting enzyme in adult respiratory distress syndrome associated with sepsis: a preliminary report. Crit Care Med 1981;9(9):651–4.
90. Busse L, Albertson T, Gong M, et al. P125 outcomes in patients with acute respiratory distress syndrome receiving angiotensin II for vasodilatory shock. Presented at the 38th International Symposium on Intensive Care and Emergency Medicine. Brussels, Belgium, March 22, 2018.

91. Bussard R, Busse LW. Angiotensin II: a new therapeutic option for vasodilatory shock. Ther Clin Risk Manag 2018;14:1287–98.
92. Wunderink RG, Albertson TE, Busse LW, et al. Baseline angiotensin levels and ACE effects in patients with vasodilatory shock treated with angiotensin II. Intensive Care Med Exp 2017;5(Suppl 2):358–9.
93. Khanna AK, McCurdy MT, Boldt DW, et al. Association of angiotensin II dose with all-cause mortality in patients with vasodilatory shock. Presented at the SOCCA 2018 Annual Meeting and Critical Care Update. Chicago, IL, April 27, 2018.
94. Chow JH, Galvagno SM Jr, Tanaka KA, et al. When all else fails: novel use of angiotensin II for vasodilatory shock: a case report. A A Pract 2018;11(7):175–80.
95. Clemson B, Gaul L, Gubin SS, et al. Prejunctional angiotensin II receptors. Facilitation of norepinephrine release in the human forearm. J Clin Invest 1994;93(2):684–91.
96. Landry DW, Levin HR, Gallant EM, et al. Vasopressin pressor hypersensitivity in vasodilatory septic shock. Crit Care Med 1997;25(8):1279–82.
97. Bartelstone HJ, Nasmyth PA. Vasopressin potentiation of catecholamine actions in dog, rat, cat, and rat aortic strip. Am J Physiol 1965;208:754–62.

Vasopressin in Vasodilatory Shock

Ida-Fong Ukor, MBBS, FANZCA, FCICM, Keith R. Walley, MD*

KEYWORDS

- Vasopressin • Antidiuretic hormone • Vasodilatory shock • Vasoplegia • Sepsis

KEY POINTS

- Vasodilatory shock is the final common pathway for all forms of severe shock.
- Vasopressin deficiency seems to play a significant role in vasodilatory shock.
- In contrast to catecholamines, vasopressin acts through alternate signaling pathways and uniquely modulates the pathophysiology of vasodilatory shock.

INTRODUCTION

Vasodilatory shock is characterized by a failure of peripheral vascular vasoconstriction in the face of low systemic arterial pressure, resulting in inadequate tissue perfusion.[1] Several causes have been identified that result in vasodilatory shock, the most common of these being sepsis, which is also the leading cause of mortality in hospitalized critically ill patients.[2] Vasoplegia, a subset of vasodilatory shock, is a phenomenon that encompasses not only a failure of vasoconstriction but also a diminished responsiveness to vasopressor therapy. Furthermore, it is well accepted that vasodilatory shock and vasoplegia are the common consequence of all prolonged states of severe shock of any etiology.[1]

Treatment of vasodilatory shock includes infusion of vasopressors. The most commonly used vasopressors are catecholamines, including norepinephrine (NE), epinephrine, and phenylephrine. It is increasingly clear, however, that the addition of noncatecholamine vasopressors, such as vasopressin (VP) and angiotensin II, may be helpful. These agents engage alternate signaling pathways resulting in a different spectrum of actions that may be usefully used in certain clinical situations. This article reviews the role of VP in the management of vasodilatory shock.

Disclosure Statement: The authors have no conflicts of interest with respect to this article. Support: Canadian Institutes of Health Research FDN 154311.

Division of Critical Care Medicine, Centre for Heart Lung Innovation, University of British Columbia, 1081 Burrard Street, Vancouver, British Columbia V6Z 1Y6, Canada
* Corresponding author.
E-mail address: Keith.Walley@hli.ubc.ca

Crit Care Clin 35 (2019) 247–261
https://doi.org/10.1016/j.ccc.2018.11.004
0749-0704/19/© 2018 Elsevier Inc. All rights reserved.

MECHANISMS OF VASODILATORY SHOCK AND VASOPLEGIA

The pathophysiology underlying vasodilatory shock and vasoplegia is incompletely elucidated. Several mechanisms have been shown to be contributory, involving an interplay between nitric oxide (NO)-mediated pathways; endothelium-derived hyperpolarizing factor (EDHF) activity; ATP-sensitive potassium (K_{ATP}) channel activation; down-regulation of vasopressor receptors, leading to vasopressor hyposensitivity; and deficiency of the neuropeptide hormone VP.[1,3]

Nitric Oxide–mediated Vasodilatation

Over-production of NO is a key component of the vasodilation and vasopressor refractoriness of vasodilatory shock.[4] The increase in NO synthesis results from up-regulation of the inducible form of NO synthase (iNOS), a calcium (Ca^{2+})-independent and calmodulin-independent isoform of NO synthase (NOS). Inflammatory cytokines, including interleukin-1β (IL-1β), tumor necrosis factor-α (TNF-α), interferon-γ, and bacterial lipopolysaccharide, are inducers of iNOS in vascular smooth muscle,[5,6] importantly via the inflammatory transcription factor nuclear factor (NF)-κB.[5,7] Endothelial NOS (eNOS) seems to play a facilitatory role in iNOS induction.[5]

NO produced as a result of increased iNOS activity leads to activation of soluble guanylyl cyclase (sGC), increased intracellular cyclic guanosine monophosphate (cGMP), and vascular smooth muscle relaxation.[8,9] Increased cGMP and the subsequent fall in intracellular calcium (Ca^{2+}_i) cause vasodilation through a combination of K_{ATP} channel and large-conductance Ca^{2+}-dependent potassium (K^+) channel activation. There is concurrent increased activity of small-conductance Ca^{2+}-dependent K^+ channels, also causing hyperpolarization of smooth muscle cells and vasodilation.[10] Typically, these channels open in response to raised Ca^{2+}_i and mitigate the effects of vasoconstrictors that raise Ca^{2+}_i, such as α-adrenergic stimulation of vascular smooth muscle.[1,11] Persistent activation of iNOS and sGC in this way contributes to profound vasodilation and the resultant state of shock.[12]

Endothelium-derived Hyperpolarizing Factors

Several EDHFs have thus far been demonstrated, including epoxyeicosatrienoic acids, K^+ ions, gap junctions, and hydrogen peroxide (H_2O_2).[13] Activation of these factors results in increased K^+ conductance through small-conductance K^+ channels, hyperpolarization, and vasodilation as with the NO-mediated pathway, described previously. EDHFs are believed to provide an alternative vasodilatory pathway in the setting of impaired NO-mediated responses.[14] Several studies support the finding that EDHFs have an important role in management of microvascular perfusion and have demonstrated a greater effect of EDHFs in smaller resistance vessels than in large arteries.[5,15] eNOS-derived reactive oxygen species, such as H_2O_2, are a source of EDHFs; however, there are several contributory enzymatic pathways for the production of superoxide anions and H_2O_2 in human and animal models.[10,16]

Adenosine Triphosphate-Sensitive Potassium Channel Activation and Vascular Smooth Muscle Hyperpolarization

Activation of K_{ATP} channels causes an efflux of intracellular K^+ ions, leading to hyperpolarization of the cell membrane, inactivation of voltage-gated Ca^{2+} channels, vasodilation, and improved regional blood flow.[17,18] K_{ATP} channels are activated by increases in intracellular lactate and hydrogen ions and decreases in cellular ATP, thereby coupling their function to cellular respiration. Excessive activation of K_{ATP} channels in vasodilatory shock is believed in part responsible for vascular smooth muscle vasopressor hyporeactivity. Additional activators of K_{ATP} channels include atrial natriuretic peptide, calcitonin gene-related peptide, and adenosine, which have all been identified in significantly elevated plasma levels in septic shock.[19–21] Despite promising animal studies,[22–24] the therapeutic use of K_{ATP} antagonists, such as the sulfonylurea glibenclamide, in humans with septic vasodilatory shock thus far has proved unsuccessful, improving neither arterial blood pressure nor vasopressor sensitivity.[2,25–27]

Vasoconstrictor Receptor Down-regulation and Hyposensitivity

With prolongation of the vasodilatory shocked state, vascular smooth muscle exhibits progressively impaired responses to circulating vasoconstrictors.[28] This is believed due to decreased vasoconstrictor receptor activity either through receptor down-regulation, uncoupling from intracellular second messengers, or both, in response to circulating inflammatory mediators.[28,29] As highlighted in a recent review by Burgdorff and colleagues,[3] down-regulation or decreased activity of several vasoconstrictor receptors has been demonstrated in vivo and in vitro in several human and animal models of vasodilatory shock due to sepsis. Decreased expression and/or function of angiotensin receptor type 1 and angiotensin receptor type 2, α_1-adrenergic receptors, and the V1 VP receptor subtype (V1R) have all been demonstrated in response to the activity of several cytokines, including IL-1β, TNF-α and INF-γ.[3,30–36] Despite good evidence supporting V1R down-regulation due to cytokine activity, there seems to be an exaggerated pressor effect of exogenously administered VP.[1,37,38] Furthermore, this occurs in the setting of relative deficiency of circulating endogenous VP in the established stages of vasodilatory shock, a major contributor to the pathologic vasodilation of this state.[39,40] The exact mechanism underlying this phenomenon is not clear; however, these findings have led to a focus on VP as a key element not only in the pathophysiology of vasodilatory shock but also potentially in its management.[40,41]

VASOPRESSIN

VP is a cyclic nonapeptide hormone also known as antidiuretic hormone. It plays an important role in the homeostatic mechanisms of the cardiovascular system, exhibiting multiple hormonal and osmoregulatory effects beyond its pressor activity.[40] Its significance in vasodilatory shock has been extensively investigated, and it has been identified as a primary protagonist in the acute vasoconstrictor response to both hemorrhagic and vasodilatory shock.[37–39,42–44] Equally important is the fall in VP levels identified in late-stage shock, which has raised the possibility of VP deficiency as a key factor in persistent vasodilatory shock as well as a possible target for therapeutic intervention.[37–39,44]

VP is synthesized in the magnocellular neurons of the paraventricular and supraoptic nuclei of the hypothalamus. It subsequently migrates as a prohormone bound to the axonal carrier protein, neurohypophysin, to the pars nervosa of the posterior pituitary via the supraoptic-hypophyseal tract. VP-containing storage granules in the posterior pituitary release VP from hypothalamic magnocellular neuron axonal terminals in response to depolarization.[40,45] Only 10% to 20% of the stored hormone can be rapidly released from the posterior pituitary, with the rate of release falling significantly thereafter, despite appropriate stimulation. This offers an explanation for the biphasic response observed in septic shock, with a late drop trough in VP levels.[46]

VP activity classically occurs through binding to the $G_{q/11}$ family of G-protein–coupled transmembrane receptors; however, G_s subtype binding has also been described.[40] Three receptor subtypes are responsible for the physiologic effects of VP: V1 (previously V1a), V2, and V3 (previously V1b). These are widely distributed through numerous tissues and organ systems (**Fig. 1**), resulting in widespread and varied effects when activated.

V1 Receptor

The V1R is responsible for most of the hemodynamic effects of VP. The gene encoding for V1R is found on the 12q14-15 region of chromosome 12.[47] This subtype is predominantly found in smooth muscle cells of the vasculature and in cardiac myocytes, although its distribution extends beyond this to multiple tissues and organ systems. Stimulation of vascular V1R causes receptor-coupled activation of intracellular phospholipase C (PLC) via $G_{q/11}$ binding, which in turn causes an increase in Ca^{2+}_i via the phosphatidyl-inositol pathway, resulting in vasoconstriction. G_s binding couples to the

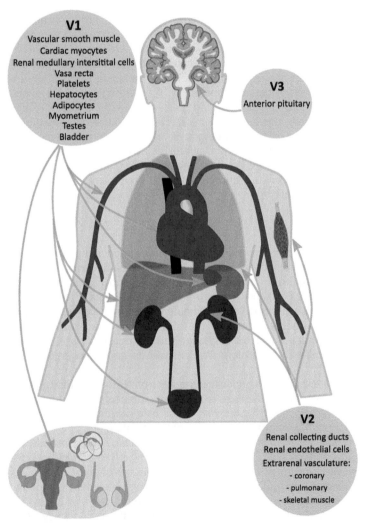

Fig. 1. Distribution of V1, V2, and V3 vasopressin receptor subtypes throughout the body.

cyclic AMP (cAMP) intracellular signaling cascade, activating multiple intracellular pathways.[48] In addition to activation of multiple second messenger signaling pathways, VP exhibits direct ion channel effects (**Fig. 2**), with dose-dependent blockade of K^+_{ATP} channels responsible for systemic vasodilation.[49] As described previously, these channels play a significant role in the regulation of arterial vascular tone. The inhibitory action of VP at this site may be an important aspect of the restoration of vascular tone—and therefore systemic blood pressure—in patients with vasodilatory shock, particularly due to endotoxemic sepsis.[22]

Renal expression of V1R can be seen in medullary interstitial cells and in the vasa recta. Medullary vascular V1R activation selectively decreases inner medullary blood flow without altering cortical blood flow, an effect that plays an important role in the kidney's ability to maximally concentrate urine in states of water deprivation.[50] The efferent glomerular artery and epithelial cells of the collecting duct also demonstrate V1R expression. Efferent arteriolar contraction in response to V1R stimulation produces an increase in glomerular filtration rate due to the lack of concurrent afferent arteriolar constriction, in contrast to catecholaminergic vasopressors.[48] This action likely accounts for the paradoxic increase in urine output seen with VP administration in vasodilatory shock, despite its typically antidiuretic effects.[51]

Platelet expression of V1R and the role of VP in platelet aggregation and hemostasis is an area of ongoing investigation. Stimulation of platelet V1R is known to result in increased Ca^{2+}_i, thereby facilitating thrombosis, although this may be an undesired

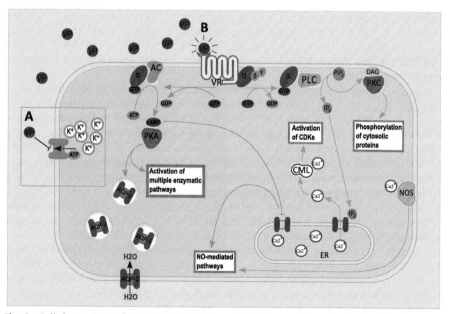

Fig. 2. Cellular actions of vasopressin. (*A*) Direct inhibition of K_{ATP} channels. (*B*) Indirect actions through vasopressin receptor-binding and activation of G-protein–coupled second messenger signaling pathways. AC, adenylyl cyclase; AQP-2, aquaporin-2 channel; CDKs, Ca^{2+}-dependent kinases; CML, calmodulin; DAG, diacylglycerol; ER, endoplasmic reticulum; GDP, guanosine diphosphate; GTP, guanosine triphosphate; IP₃, inositol 1,4,5-triphosphate; PIP_2, phosphatidylinositol 4.5-biphosphate; PKA, protein kinase A; PKC, protein kinase C; VR, VP receptor; α, G-protein alpha subunit; β, G-protein beta subunit; γ, G-protein gamma subunit.

effect in the setting of vasodilatory shock with microvascular dysfunction and the potential for microthrombus formation and worsened end organ perfusion.[52,53] There is, however, great variability in the aggregation response to VP of normal human platelets, and platelet V1R polymorphism has been proposed as a possible explanation for this observation.[48] It is, therefore, currently unknown whether V1R platelet activity is of any significance in the vasodilatory shock state. V1R has also been identified in the myometrium, bladder, spleen, testes, and on adipocytes and hepatocytes.[48] The exact action of V1R in all these regions remains to be characterized.

V2 Receptor

The V2 receptor subtype (V2R) is responsible for the antidiuretic and osmoregulatory effects of VP. Originally believed found exclusively in the collecting ducts and endothelial cells of the kidney, there is growing evidence to support the existence of extrarenal V2Rs in vascular and other tissues and with it an expansion in the significance of V2R beyond osmoregulation.[38,48,54] The chromosome Xq28 region carries the V2R gene, and V2R is structurally similar to V1R, differing only in the number of N-linked glycosylation sites. The 2 subtypes are, however, functionally distinct.[48]

The primary action of V2R in the kidney is to increase collecting duct permeability to water. This is achieved by interaction of VP-activated V2R with adenylyl cyclase, causing increased production of cAMP and activation of the protein kinase A enzymatic pathway (see **Fig. 2**). Aquaporin-2–containing vesicles subsequently fuse with the luminal membrane of the collecting duct, thereby increasing water permeability. Water is drawn down a concentration gradient from the collecting duct cells into the hyperosmolar renal interstitium, leaving behind more concentrated urine.[48,50] V2Rs also exist in the thick ascending limb of the loop of Henle, where they influence NaCl transport and the countercurrent multiplication mechanism.[54] V2R activation of a distinct urea transporter, further contributes to maintenance of the medullary concentrating gradient.[55,56]

Afferent arteriolar vasodilation is known to occur in response to V2R stimulation, although the underlying mechanism continues to be debated.[57] Vasodilation in response to VP activity has been demonstrated in several extrarenal vascular beds—including heart, lung, and skeletal muscle—and there is evidence to support V2 as the receptor subtype responsible in both human and animal models.[58] Endothelial V2R activation seems to increase cAMP, causing a decrease in Ca^{2+}_i and activation of NO-mediated mediated pathways (see **Fig. 2**), leading to vasodilation.[38,58] V2R expression has also been identified in splenic tissue and on human T cells, raising the possibility of an immunomodulatory role of VP via V2R. Moreover, pulmonary epithelial V2R activation has been found to cause a reduction in lipopolysaccharide-induced inflammation seen in a mouse model, as measured by a fall in IL-6 levels. V2R modulation of NF-κB signaling is believed the likely mechanism.[59] The significance of these findings, in particular their relevance in the widespread inflammatory response seen in vasodilatory shock, is unclear. It is possible that a combination of activation of NO-mediated pulmonary microvascular vasodilation and modulation of the inflammatory response may be of benefit in vasodilatory shock, although this remains unproved in large clinical trials.[60] Endothelial V2Rs also have an important role in hemostasis through stimulation of von Willebrand factor secretion in response to cAMP-mediated signaling.[61]

V3 Receptor

The V3 receptor subtype (V3R) is a distinct G-protein–coupled pituitary receptor that stimulates corticotropin secretion from the anterior pituitary in a dose-dependent manner when activated by VP. A variety of signaling pathways may be activated by V3R depending on its degree of expression, and over-expression is seen in corticotropin-hypersecretory tumors.[62] The gene encoding V3R is found on chromosome 1q32.[48]

Oxytocin Receptor

The oxytocin receptor (OTR) is present in myometrial and mammary myoepithelial smooth muscle cells, eliciting smooth muscle contraction through $G_{q/11}$-binding, activation of PLC signaling pathways, and increased Ca^{2+}_i.[38] It exhibits equal affinity for VP and oxytocin binding, and circulating VP, therefore, elicits full receptor activation. In addition to myometrial and mammary tissue, OTRs are also abundantly found in vascular endothelial cells where activation and increased Ca^{2+}_i stimulates increased eNOS activity and NO-mediated vasodilation. Furthermore, OTRs can be found in the heart, where they stimulate release of atrial natriuretic peptide, a hormone whose actions influence natriuresis, blood pressure control, and cardiomyocyte differentiation.[38,48] It is clear that there are conflicting actions of OTRs and the various VP receptor subtypes; however, the precise implications of these variable effects is at present unknown.

VASOPRESSIN AND VASODILATORY SHOCK

Under normal physiologic conditions, the effect of exogenous VP on arteriolar tone and systolic blood pressure is negligible.[40] In contrast, a key feature of vasodilatory shock states is marked hypersensitivity to exogenously administered VP in conjunction with the previously highlighted deficiency in plasma VP levels.[38,39]

Hypersensitivity to physiologic doses of VP has been demonstrated in multiple animal models of vasodilatory shock due to sepsis and in several small human studies.[38] The mechanisms behind this observation are thought to relate to effects of VP on the key pathophysiologic pathways of vasodilatory shock already described. Inhibition of iNOS by VP has been demonstrated both in vitro and in vivo; however, this has not been correlated with a change in serum nitrate/nitrite levels in patients with septic shock receiving exogenous VP.[63–65] In addition, there are several studies supporting the notion that excessive activation of K_{ATP} channels may be mitigated by VP activity. This may be through direct closure of the channel or through activation of calcineurin, a Ca^{2+}-dependent phosphatase important in regulating gene transcription that has been shown to inhibit K_{ATP} channel activity.[49,66,67] Furthermore, in the setting of adrenoceptor desensitization and adrenergic vasoconstrictor hyposensitivity, VP has been shown to exhibit exaggerated pressor effects as well as significant synergy with concurrently initiated adrenergic pressors, despite evidence of V1R desensitization.[3,29,33,37] Possible mechanisms proposed for this observation, in addition to those already discussed, include utilization of an alternate pathway for increasing Ca^{2+}_i; sensitization of the endothelial smooth muscle contractile apparatus to Ca^{2+} through inhibition of myosin light chain phosphatase; stimulation of production of the vasoconstrictor endothelin-1; and cross-regulation of adrenergic receptor cycling by nonreciprocal inhibition of β-adrenoceptor internalization through intracellular trafficking of β-arrestins.[38]

Several studies have characterized an early peak in VP levels in response to septic or hemorrhagic shock, with levels typically reaching 10-fold to 20-fold those seen in response to increased plasma osmolality. These subsequently fall away to basal levels as shock becomes established, which is believed to worsen vasoplegia due to inadequate VP levels for efficacy of the described pathways.[40] Proposed mechanisms underlying this biphasic response include a combination of depletion of neurohypophyseal stores,[68] decreased stimulation of VP release due to impaired autonomic reflexes or tonic inhibition of atrial stretch receptors,[69] and inhibition of release due to increased endothelial and pituitary NO[70–72] or high circulating levels of NE acting centrally.[45]

Deficiency of VP in this setting may have repercussions that go beyond impaired vascular reactivity. There has been much interest in the actions of VP outside of the well-established systemic arterial vasoconstrictor effects, particularly in the setting of septic shock. Of particular significance, several studies have demonstrated favorable pulmonary effects in septic shock with a decrease in pulmonary artery pressure under normoxic or hypoxic conditions and a possible decrease in the pulmonary inflammatory response.[40,59] Pulmonary vasodilation seems to be a V1R effect and is NO-mediated. It The immunomodulatory effects of VP are complex and as yet incompletely elucidated. VP expression has been demonstrated in multiple immune cells, including peripheral T cells, B cells, and monocyte/macrophage cells. It has also been found in human thymic epithelial cells and splenic B cells. Release of VP occurs in response to acute and chronic inflammatory stimuli, and its deficiency has been shown to increase natural killer cell activity in a rat model. Furthermore, VP seems to potentiate corticotropin release from peripheral monocytes, and it plays a role in T-cell activation and modulation of primary antibody production.[73] Moreover, there is evidence to support the effect of VP on astrocyte expression of TNF-α and IL-1β via V1R activity and on renal expression of Toll-like receptor 4 and NF-κB. The latter effect was associated with a decrease in downstream cytokine production; however, this also resulted in decreased bacterial clearance from the lower urinary tract, bringing into question the net benefit of the decreased inflammatory response.[73]

The widespread inflammatory response seen in vasodilatory shock inevitably results in increased endothelial permeability and capillary leak syndrome, a phenomenon that renders fluid resuscitation and maintenance of intravascular volume repletion problematic. Pulmonary edema inevitably ensues, exacerbating lung injury and worsening acute respiratory distress syndrome. Such edema is not confined solely to the lung, and numerous organs suffer from the resultant impaired oxygen extraction and delayed recovery of function.

In an ovine model of septic shock the use of terlipressin, a VP analog with relative V1R selectivity, demonstrated a decrease in positive fluid balance within 12 hours of onset of shock compared with VP treatment. This finding may point toward the role of V1R activation in limiting edema formation, potentially through decreased endothelial permeability.[74]

A major compounding factor contributing to the organ dysfunction seen in vasodilatory shock, particularly of septic etiology, is microcirculatory failure. Hemodynamic optimization is currently limited to guidance by macrocirculatory indices, such as mean arterial pressure, or surrogate markers of tissue perfusion, such as blood lactate levels. Optimization, however, of the macrocirculation is not necessarily accompanied by improved microcirculatory function.[75] As a potent vasoconstrictor, the potential for VP to exacerbate microcirculatory compromise, thereby leading to worsened outcomes, has been of particular concern. In numerous experimental studies, the use of VP in the setting of insufficient volume resuscitation, or when administered in high dose or by bolus dosing, was found to cause significant microcirculatory compromise in splanchnic, renal and cutaneous circulations.[76] This was somewhat ameliorated by the use a V1R-selective agent, despite the loss of vasodilatory effects of V2R activation, described previously. The use of the highly V1R-selective agent, selepressin, was found superior to either VP or NE in restoring microcirculatory function, although this was assessed by the surrogate measure of blood lactate levels.[77]

Clinical studies have emphasized the complexity of the interplay between the macro-circulation, microvascular function, and vasopressor use. Numerous studies have provided significantly variable results.[76] It seems that microcirculatory failure and the reversal thereof are perhaps determined more by factors other than the use of a specific vasopressor agent, such as adequacy of volume resuscitation, timing of therapy, and disease progression.[78] In comparison to adrenergic vasopressors, VP and its analogs demonstrated no increased risk of adverse outcomes.[79]

Despite the evidence demonstrating the potential benefits of VP receptor agonism in improving vascular tone, minimizing edemagenesis, and decreasing pulmonary inflammation and hypertension, clinical trials have thus far failed to deliver the expected improvements in outcomes.

Important Clinical Trials

The largest randomized controlled trial of VP use in septic shock to date is the multi-center Vasopressin and Septic Shock Trial (VASST) that compared the use of NE alone with that of NE and low-dose VP (0.01–0.03 U/min) in 778 patients with septic shock. The primary endpoint assessed was all-cause mortality at 28 days from the commencement of study infusion and was powered to detect a 10% absolute difference in mortality with an assumed 60% mortality rate in the NE group. No significant difference in the primary endpoint was found between the 2 groups, although analysis of an a priori defined subgroup of patients with less severe septic shock showed decreased mortality with VP treatment.[60] The observed mortality rates in both groups were significantly lower than predicted (39.3% and 35.4% in the NE and VP groups, respectively), likely having an impact on the power. Although not reaching statistical significance, a relative reduction in mortality of 10% was seen in the VP group. Stratified group analysis of patients receiving early VP ($\leq$12 h), demonstrated a trend toward higher mortality in the NE group (40.5% vs 33.2%; $P = .12$) that was not seen with later VP initiation (37.5% vs 37.7%; $P = .97$), suggesting the timing of VP initiation may be important. Furthermore, post hoc analysis of trial data indicated a trend toward both improved renal function with VP and a survival benefit when corticosteroids were coadministered.[80,81] Decreased serum creatinine, renal failure, use of renal replacement therapy (RRT), and mortality was found associated with VP use.[80] A multivariate logistic regression analysis of patients in the risk category of the risk, injury, failure, loss of function, and end-stage kidney disease (RIFLE) criteria for acute kidney failure showed a slight increase in mortality with increasing NE dose (odds ratio [OR] 1.03; 99% CI, 1.00–1.06; $P = .02$). The use of VP seemed protective (OR 0.33; 99% CI, 0.1–1.09; $P = .02$).

These findings led to the recent VANISH (Vasopressin versus Norepinephrine as Initial Therapy in Septic Shock) randomized clinical trial of 409 patients with septic shock. The use of early ($\leq$6 h of hypotension) VP versus NE, either with or without hydrocortisone, was assessed for any impact on the incidence of acute kidney injury, RRT, survival, or adverse events in the 28-day period postrandomization.[82] The number of kidney-failure free days was the primary outcome, measured as 2 summary measures: (1) the proportion of patients who never developed kidney failure and (2) the median number of days alive and free of kidney failure in those who died, experienced kidney failure, or both. Secondary outcome measures included rates of RRT, mortality, and serious adverse events. There was less use of RRT in the VP-treated group compared with the NE-treated group (24.5% vs 35.3%; difference −9.9%, 95% CI, −19.3 to −0.6%); however, there was no difference in the number of kidney-failure free days for those who died or experienced kidney failure (median 9 [interquartile range 1 to −24] days vs 13 [interquartile range 1 to −25] days; difference

−4 days; 95% CI, −11–5). There was once again no difference seen in either mortality or in the rate of serious adverse events, despite the early use of VP (median 3.5 hours after onset of shock) in significantly higher doses (up to 0.06 U/min) than those used in VASST. Both VASST and VANISH demonstrated a catecholamine-sparing effect of VP use, and, although no mortality benefit was seen in either study, it has been suggested that the early use of VP may help reduce the adrenergic burden associated with traditional vasoactive agents.[79] This may be important given the previously identified association of higher doses of catecholamines with increased mortality in septic patients,[83] and the lack of a significant effect in these studies may have been a question, certainly in VASST at least, of study power.

The relationship between VP and cortisol secretion is well established. As previously described, VP is known to stimulate corticotropin release through V3R binding. Furthermore, in septic shock, patients with low plasma cortisol levels or impaired responses to corticotropin were consistently found to have an increased VP level, at least in the early stages of shock.[84] These findings have led to the suggestion that there may be regulatory interdependence between VP and cortisol secretion, with VP release increasing to stimulate increased corticotropin production in the setting of relative adrenal insufficiency.[79] Moreover, post hoc analysis of the VASST cohort found that VP levels in patients who received hydrocortisone were significantly higher than those who did not at both 6 hours and 24 hours. The combination of low-dose VP and hydrocortisone administration was also associated with decreased mortality and organ dysfunction.[81] Study design of the VANISH trial incorporated assessment of the possible interaction of corticosteroids with VP in a 2 × 2 factorial design that included a group who received hydrocortisone in combination with early VP. No impact was found from the use of corticosteroids; however, fewer than half of all patients received the second study drug (hydrocortisone/placebo) and the investigators, therefore, acknowledge that the power might be lacking to draw any significant conclusions.[82] The interaction of corticosteroids and VP in the physiologic response to, and management of, vasodilatory shock remains controversial, and more evidence is required before any definitive conclusions can be made.

Selective VP receptor agonism may well be the key to delivering improved outcomes in the clinical setting. Terlipressin, a synthetic analog with relative V1:V2R selectivity of approximately 2:1, was shown to reduce catecholamine requirements more effectively than VP in the TERLIVAP (Continuous Terlipressin Versus Vasopressin Infusion in Septic Shock) pilot study.[85] Subsequent studies reported, however, several concerning adverse events related to microvascular ischemia and decreased cardiac output.[86–88] It is likely that the adverse events observed may relate to the differing pharmacokinetic properties of VP and terlipressin, with the latter having a much longer half-life (24 minutes vs 6 hours, respectively) and, therefore, less titratability. Furthermore, it seems that bolus dosing of terlipressin also contributed to the development of adverse events.[86] Selepressin, a short-acting VP analog with even greater V1R selectivity, is showing promise in experimental and early clinical trials as a potential option for efficacious management of vasoplegia in vasodilatory shock, while avoiding some undesirable V2R-mediated effects previously outlined, such as fluid retention, selective vasodilation, and potentially increased platelet aggregation.[77,89] The recently completed phase IIb/III SEPSIS-ACT (Selepressin Evaluation Programme for Sepsis-Induced Shock - Adaptive Clinical Trial) randomized, placebo-controlled, clinical trial (NCT02508649) will provide an increased understanding of the efficacy and safety of selepressin in this setting once final results are released.

SUMMARY

The vasoplegia seen in vasodilatory shock is the final common pathway for all advanced states of shock. A multitude of interrelated mechanisms clearly contribute to the pathophysiology of this state; however, these remain incompletely understood. As such, the availability of successful interventions to mitigate the disease burden of this ubiquitous condition continues to prove elusive. The myriad multisystem effects of VP through its receptor subtypes provide several promising opportunities for pharmacotherapeutic targeting. Finding the right balance of receptor subtype agonism/antagonism to simultaneously achieve optimal outcomes while avoiding harm will, however, require still more investigation. Selective V1R agonists may prove to be at least 1 piece of this puzzle, although this remains to be seen.

REFERENCES

1. Landry DW, Oliver JA. The pathogenesis of vasodilatory shock. N Engl J Med 2001;345:588–95.

2. Matsuda N, Hattori Y. Vascular biology in sepsis: pathophysiological and therapeutic significance of vascular dysfunction. J Smooth Muscle Res 2007;43(4): 117–37.

3. Burgdorff AM, Bucher M, Schumann J. Vasoplegia in patients with sepsis and septic shock: pathways and mechanisms. J Int Med Res 2018;46(4):1303–10.

4. Ochoa JB, Udekwu AO, Billiar TR, et al. Nitrogen oxide levels in patients after trauma and during sepsis. Ann Surg 1991;214(5):621–6.

5. Vo PA, Lad B, Tomlinson JAP, et al. Autoregulatory role of endothelium-derived nitric oxide (NO) on lipopolysaccharide-induced vascular inducible NO synthase expression and function. J Biol Chem 2005;280(8):7236–43.

6. Wort SJ, Evans TW. The role of the endothelium in modulating vascular control in sepsis and related conditions. Br Med Bull 1999;55(1):30–48.

7. Li X, Stark GR. NFκB-dependent signalling pathways. Exp Hematol 2002;30(4): 285–96.

8. Ignarro LJ. Endothelium-derived nitric oxide: pharmacology and relationship to the actions of organic nitrate esters. Pharm Res 1989;6(8):651–9.

9. Moncada S, Palmer RMJ, Higgs EA. The discovery of nitric oxide as the endogenous nitrovasodilator. Hypertension 1988;12(4):365–72.

10. Sharawy N. Vasoplegia in septic shock: do we really fight the right enemy? J Crit Care 2014;29(1):83–7.

11. Jaggar JH, Porter VA, Lederer WJ, et al. Calcium sparks in smooth muscle. Am J Physiol Cell Physiol 2000;278(2):C235–56.

12. Kilbourn RG, Gross SS, Jubran A, et al. NG-methyl-l-arginine inhibits tumor necrosis factor-induced hypotension: implications for the involvement of nitric oxide. Proc Natl Acad Sci U S A 1990;87(9):3629–32.

13. Ohashi J, Sawada A, Nakajima S, et al. Mechanisms for enhanced endothelium-derived hyperpolarizing factor-mediated responses in microvessels in mice. Circ J 2012;76(7):1768–79.

14. Cohen RA, Vanhoutte PM. Endothelium-dependent hyperpolarization: beyond nitric oxide and cyclic GMP. Circulation 1995;92(11):3337–49.

15. Urakami-Harasawa L, Shimokawa H, Nakashima M, et al. Importance of endothelium-derived hyperpolarizing factor in human arteries. J Clin Invest 1997;100(11):2793–9.

16. Matoba T, Shimokawa H, Nakashima M, et al. Hydrogen peroxide is an endothelium-derived hyperpolarizing factor in mice. J Clin Invest 2000;106(12): 1521–30.
17. Jackson WF. Ion channels and vascular tone. Hypertension 2000;35:173–8.
18. Quayle JM, Nelson MT, Standen NB. ATP-sensitive and inwardly rectifying potassium channels in smooth muscle. Physiol Rev 1997;77(4):1165–232.
19. Schneider F, Lutun P, Couchot A, et al. Plasma cyclic guanosine 3'–5' monophosphate concentrations and low vascular resistance in human septic shock. Intensive Care Med 1993;19(2):99–104.
20. Arnalich F, Sanchez JF, Martinez M, et al. Changes in plasma concentrations of vasoactive neuropeptides in patients with sepsis and septic shock. Life Sci 1995;56(2):75–81.
21. Martin C, Leone M, Viviand X, et al. High adenosine plasma concentration as a prognostic index for outcome in patients with septic shock. Crit Care Med 2000;28(9):3198–202.
22. Landry DW, Oliver JA. The ATP-sensitive K+ channel mediates hypotension in endotoxemia and hypoxic lactic acidosis in dog. J Clin Invest 1992;89(6):2071–4.
23. Geisen K, Végh A, Krause E, et al. Cardiovascular effects of conventional sulfonylureas and glimepiride. Horm Metab Res 1996;28(9):496–507.
24. Gardiner SM, Kemp PA, March JE, et al. Regional haemodynamic responses to infusion of lipopolysaccharide in conscious rats: effects of pre- or post-treatment with glibenclamide. Br J Pharmacol 1999;128(8):1772–8.
25. Warrillow S, Egi M, Bellomo R. Randomized, double-blind, placebo-controlled crossover pilot study of a potassium channel blocker in patients with septic shock. Crit Care Med 2006;34(4):980–5.
26. Morelli A, Lange M, Ertmer C, et al. Glibenclamide dose response in patients with septic shock: effects on norepinephrine requirements, cardiopulmonary performance, and global oxygen transport. Shock 2007;28(5):530–5.
27. Lange M, Morelli A, Westphal M. Inhibition of potassium channels in critical illness. Curr Opin Anaesthesiol 2008;21(2):105–10.
28. Rozenfeld V, Cheng JW. The role of vasopressin in the treatment of vasodilation in shock states. Ann Pharmacother 2000;34(2):250–4.
29. Levy B, Collin S, Sennoun N, et al. Vascular hyporesponsiveness to vasopressors in septic shock: from bench to bedside. Intensive Care Med 2010;36(12): 2019–29.
30. Bucher M, Ittner KP, Hobbhahn J, et al. Downregulation of angiotensin II type 1 receptors during sepsis. Hypertension 2001;38(2):177–82.
31. Bucher M, Hobbhahn J, Kurtz A. Nitric oxide-dependent down-regulation of angiotensin II type 2 receptors during experimental sepsis. Crit Care Med 2001;29(9):1750–5.
32. Schmidt C, Höcherl K, Kurt B, et al. Blockade of multiple but not single cytokines abrogates downregulation of angiotensin II type-I receptors and anticipates septic shock. Cytokine 2010;49(1):30–8.
33. Schmidt C, Kurt B, Höcherl K, et al. Inhibition of NF-κB activity prevents downregulation of α1-adrenergic receptors and circulatory failure during CLP-induced sepsis. Shock 2009;32(3):239–46.
34. Fadel F, André-Grégoire G, Gravez B, et al. Aldosterone and vascular mineralocorticoid receptors in murine endotoxic and human septic shock. Crit Care Med 2017;45(9):e954–62.
35. Holmes CL, Walley KR. Arginine vasopressin in the treatment of vasodilatory septic shock. Best Pract Res Clin Anaesthesiol 2008;22(2):275–86.

36. Schmidt C, Höcherl K, Kurt B, et al. Role of nuclear factor-KB-dependent induction of cytokines in the regulation of vasopressin V1A-receptors during cecal ligation and puncture-induced circulatory failure. Crit Care Med 2008;36(8):2363–72.

37. Morales D, Madigan J, Cullinane S, et al. Reversal by vasopressin of intractable hypotension in the late phase of hemorrhagic shock. Circulation 1999;100(3):226–9.

38. Barrett LK, Singer M, Clapp LH. Vasopressin: mechanisms of action on the vasculature in health and in septic shock. Crit Care Med 2007;35(1):33–40.

39. Landry DW, Levin HR, Gallant EM, et al. Vasopressin deficiency contributes to the vasodilation of septic shock. Circulation 1997;95(5):1122–5.

40. Holmes CL, Patel BM, Russell JA, et al. Physiology of vasopressin relevant to management of septic shock. Chest 2001;120(3):989–1002.

41. Holmes CL, Landry DW, Granton JT. Science review: vasopressin and the cardiovascular system part 2 – clinical physiology. Crit Care 2004;8(1):15–23.

42. Errington ML, Rocha e Silva M Jr. Vasopressin clearance and secretion during haemorrhage in normal dogs and in dogs with experimental diabetes insipidus. J Physiol 1972;227(2):395–418.

43. Zerbe RL, Feurstein G, Kopin IJ. Effect of captopril on cardiovascular, sympathetic and vasopressin responses to hemorrhage. Eur J Pharmacol 1981;72:391–5.

44. Arnauld E, Czernichow P, Fumoux F, et al. The effects of hypotension and hypovolaemia on the liberation of vasopressin during haemorrhage in the unanaesthetized monkey (macaca mulatta). Pflugers Arch 1977;371(3):193–200.

45. Leng G, Brown CH, Russell JA. Physiological pathways regulating the activity of magnocellular neurosecretory cells. Prog Neurobiol 1999;57(6):625–55.

46. Sklar AH, Schrier RW. Central nervous system mediators of vasopressin release. Physiol Rev 1983;63(4):1243–80.

47. Thibonnier M, Graves MK, Wagner MS, et al. Structure, sequence, expression, and chromosomal localization of the human v1avasopressin receptor gene. Genomics 1996;31(3):327–34.

48. Holmes CL, Landry DW, Granton JT. Science review: vasopressin and the cardiovascular system part 1 – receptor physiology. Crit Care 2003;7(6):427–34.

49. Wakatsuki T, Nakaya Y, Inoue I. Vasopressin modulates K(+)-channel activities of cultured smooth muscle cells from porcine coronary artery. Am J Physiol 1992;263(2 Pt 2):H491–6.

50. Franchini KG, Cowley AW. Renal cortical and medullary blood flow responses during water restriction: role of vasopressin. Am J Physiol 1996;270(6 Pt 2):R1257–64.

51. Holmes CL, Walley KR, Chittock DR, et al. The effects of vasopressin on hemodynamics and renal function in severe septic shock: a case series. Intensive Care Med 2001;27(8):1416–21.

52. Filep J, Rosenkranz B. Mechanism of vasopressin-induced platelet aggregation. Thromb Res 1987;45(1):7–15.

53. Launay JM, Vittet D, Vidaud M, et al. V1a-vasopressin specific receptors on human platelets: potentiation by ADP and epinephrine and evidence for homologous down-regulation. Thromb Res 1987;45(4):323–31.

54. Juul KV, Bichet DG, Nielsen S, et al. The physiological and pathophysiological functions of renal and extrarenal vasopressin V2 receptors. Am J Physiol Renal Physiol 2014;306(9):F931–40.

55. Bankir L. Antidiuretic action of vasopressin: quantitative aspects and interaction between V1a and V2 receptor-mediated effects. Cardiovasc Res 2001;51(3): 372–90.

56. Nielsen S, Knepper MA. Vasopressin activates collecting duct urea transporters and water channels by distinct physical processes. Am J Physiol 1993;265(2 Pt 2):F204–13.

57. Tamaki T, Kiyomoto K, He H, et al. Vasodilation induced by vasopressin V2 receptor stimulation in afferent arterioles. Kidney Int 1996;49(3):722–9.

58. Kaufmann JE, Iezzi M, Vischer UM. Desmopressin (DDAVP) induces no production in human endothelial cells via V2 receptor- and cAMP-mediated signaling. J Thromb Haemost 2003;1(4):821–8.

59. Boyd JH, Holmes CL, Wang Y, et al. Vasopressin decreases sepsis-induced pulmonary inflammation through the V2R. Resuscitation 2008;79(2):325–31.

60. Russell JA, Walley KR, Singer J, et al. Vasopressin versus norepinephrine infusion in patients with septic shock. N Engl J Med 2008;358(9):877–87.

61. Kaufmann JE, Oksche A, Wollheim CB, et al. Vasopressin-induced von Willebrand factor secretion from endothelial cells involves V2 receptors and cAMP. J Clin Invest 2000;106(1):107–16.

62. Thibonnier M, Preston JA, Dulin N, et al. The human V3 pituitary vasopressin receptor: ligand binding profile and density-dependent signalling pathways. Endocrinology 2018;138(10):4109–22.

63. Kusano E, Tian S, Umino T, et al. Arginine vasopressin inhibits interleukin-1 beta-stimulated nitric oxide and cyclic guanosine monophosphate production via the V1 receptor in cultured rat vascular smooth muscle cells. J Hypertens 1997; 15(6):627–32.

64. Moreau R. Terlipressin inhibits in vivo aortic iNOS expression induced by lipopolysaccharide in rats with biliary cirrhosis. Hepatology 2002;36(5):1070–8.

65. Dunser MW, Werner ER, Wenzel V, et al. Arginine vasopressin and serum nitrite/nitrate concentrations in advanced vasodilatory shock. Acta Anaesthesiol Scand 2004;48(7):814–9.

66. Tsuchiya M, Tsuchiya K, Maruyama R, et al. Vasopressin inhibits sarcolemmal ATP-sensitive K+ channels via V1 receptors activation in the Guinea pig heart. Circ J 2002;66(3):277–82.

67. Wilson AJ, Jabr RI, Clapp LH. Calcium modulation of vascular smooth muscle ATP-sensitive K+ channels: role of protein phosphatase-2B. Circ Res 2000; 87(11):1019–25.

68. Sharshar T, Carlier R, Blanchard A, et al. Depletion of neurohypophyseal content of vasopressin in septic shock. Crit Care Med 2002;30(3):497–500.

69. Sharshar T, Gray F, Lorin de la Grandmaison G, et al. Apoptosis of neurons in cardiovascular autonomic centres triggered by inducible nitric oxide synthase after death from septic shock. Lancet 2003;362(9398):1799–805.

70. Reid IA. Role of nitric oxide in the regulation of renin and vasopressin secretion. Front Neuroendocrinol 1994;15(4):351–83.

71. Giusti-Paiva A, De Castro M, Antunes-Rodrigues J, et al. Inducible nitric oxide synthase pathway in the central nervous system and vasopressin release during experimental septic shock. Crit Care Med 2002;30(6):1306–10.

72. Carnio EC, Stabile AM, Batalhão ME, et al. Vasopressin release during endotoxaemic shock in mice lacking inducible nitric oxide synthase. Pflugers Arch 2005; 450(6):390–4.

73. Russell JA, Walley KR. Vasopressin and its immune effects in septic shock. J Innate Immun 2010;2(5):446–60.

74. Rehberg S, Ertmer C, Köhler G, et al. Role of arginine vasopressin and terlipressin as first-line vasopressor agents in fulminant ovine septic shock. Intensive Care Med 2009;35(7):1286–96.
75. Dünser M, Hjortrup BP, Pettilä V. Vasopressors in shock: are we meeting our target and do we really understand what we are aiming at? Intensive Care Med 2016;42(7):1176–8.
76. Hessler M, Kampmeier TG, Rehberg S. Effect of non-adrenergic vasopressors on macro- and microvascular coupling in distributive shock. Best Pract Res Clin Anaesthesiol 2016;30(4):465–77.
77. He X, Su F, Taccone FS, et al. A selective V1A receptor agonist, selepressin, is superior to arginine vasopressin and to norepinephrine in ovine septic shock. Crit Care Med 2016;44(1):23–31.
78. Morelli A, Donati A, Ertmer C, et al. Effects of vasopressinergic receptor agonists on sublingual microcirculation in norepinephrine-dependent septic shock. Crit Care 2011;15(5):R217.
79. Schurr JW, Szumita PM, DeGrado JR. Neuroendocrine derangements in early septic shock: pharmacotherapy for relative adrenal and vasopressin insufficiency. Shock 2017;48(3):284–93.
80. Gordon AC, Russell JA, Walley KR, et al. The effects of vasopressin on acute kidney injury in septic shock. Intensive Care Med 2010;36(1):83–91.
81. Russell JA, Walley KR, Gordon AC, et al. Interaction of vasopressin infusion, corticosteroid treatment, and mortality of septic shock. Crit Care Med 2009;37(3):811–8.
82. Gordon AC, Mason AJ, Thirunavukkarasu N, et al. Effect of early vasopressin vs norepinephrine on kidney failure in patients with septic shock: the VANISH randomized clinical trial. JAMA 2016;316(5):509–18.
83. Dünser MW, Ruokonen E, Pettilä V, et al. Association of arterial blood pressure and vasopressor load with septic shock mortality: a post hoc analysis of a multicenter trial. Crit Care 2009;13(6):R181.
84. Sharshar T, Blanchard A, Paillard M, et al. Circulating vasopressin levels in septic shock. Crit Care Med 2003;31(6):1752–8.
85. Morelli A, Ertmer C, Rehberg S, et al. Continuous terlipressin versus vasopressin infusion in septic shock (TERLIVAP): a randomized, controlled pilot study. Crit Care 2009;13(4):R130.
86. Ishikawa K, Wan L, Calzavacca P, et al. The effects of terlipressin on regional hemodynamics and kidney function in experimental hyperdynamic sepsis. PLoS One 2012;7(2):e29693.
87. Lange M, Ertmer C, Westphal M. Vasopressin vs. terlipressin in the treatment of cardiovascular failure in sepsis. Intensive Care Med 2008;34(5):821–32.
88. Singer M. Arginine vasopressin vs. terlipressin in the treatment of shock states. Best Pract Res Clin Anaesthesiol 2008;22(2):359–68.
89. Russell JA, Vincent JL, Kjølbye AL, et al. Selepressin, a novel selective vasopressin V1A agonist, is an effective substitute for norepinephrine in a phase IIa randomized, placebo-controlled trial in septic shock patients. Crit Care 2017;21(1):213.

Hydrocortisone in Vasodilatory Shock

Balasubramanian Venkatesh, MD[a,b,c,*], Jeremy Cohen, PhD[a,d,e]

KEYWORDS

- Vasodilatory shock • Corticosteroids • Septic shock

KEY POINTS

- Vasodilatory shock is the most common type of circulatory shock seen in critically ill patients and sepsis is the predominant cause of vasodilatory shock.
- Corticosteroids as an adjunct therapy in septic shock act through 2 mechanisms: immune modulation and cardiovascular modulation.
- The results from the 2 recent randomized controlled trials of corticosteroids have strengthened the rationale for the use of hydrocortisone in critically ill patients with septic shock.
- The recommended dosage of intravenous hydrocortisone is 200 mg daily by bolus or infusion for 7 days.
- Future areas of work could be directed at elucidating mechanism of shock reversal, interaction of hydrocortisone with other therapeutic agents, identifying steroid responsiveness using biochemical or gene signatures, and clarifying the role of fludrocortisone.

Vasodilatory shock is the most common type of circulatory shock seen in critically ill patients and sepsis is the predominant cause of vasodilatory shock. Sepsis and septic shock are major health care problems affecting millions of people around the world each year and killing as many as 1 in 4 people.[1] Systemic vasodilatation and arterial hypotension are the hallmarks of septic shock. Treatment of vasodilatory shock often includes fluids and vasopressors. One of the most commonly used adjunctive

Funding source: Dr B. Venkatesh was funded by a Medical Research Future fund Practitioner Fellowship.

[a] Department of Intensive Care, The Wesley Hospital, Coronation Drive, QLD 4066, Australia; [b] Department of Intensive Care, Princess Alexandra Hospital, Ipswich Road, University of Queensland, QLD 4102, Australia; [c] Division of Critical Care, The George Institute for Global Health, University of New South Wales, King Street, NSW 2050, Australia; [d] Department of Intensive Care, The Royal Brisbane and Women's Hospital, University of Queensland, Herston Road, QLD 4066, Australia; [e] Division of Critical Care, The George Institute for Global Health, King Street, Sydney, NSW 2050, Australia
* Corresponding author. Department of Intensive Care, The Wesley Hospital, Coronation Drive, QLD 4066, Australia.
E-mail address: bvenkatesh@georgeinstitute.org.au

Crit Care Clin 35 (2019) 263–275
https://doi.org/10.1016/j.ccc.2018.11.005
0749-0704/19/© 2018 Elsevier Inc. All rights reserved.

therapies for septic shock is corticosteroids. This article describes the pathophysiology of septic shock and discusses the current evidence regarding the role of hydrocortisone in its management.

REGULATION OF VASCULAR SMOOTH MUSCLE TONE AND VASOPLEGIA OF SEPSIS

For optimal vasoconstriction, hormonal or neuronal ligands, such as noradrenaline and angiotensin II, bind to receptors on vascular smooth muscle, increase intracellular calcium through second messengers, and activate the myosin adenosine triphosphatase (ATPase), resulting in muscle contraction. Systemic hypotension occurs as a result of failure of the vascular smooth muscle to constrict. Pathologic vasodilatory shock (vasoplegia) is characterized not only by hypotension but also by reduced vasomotor responsiveness to vasopressor drugs such as noradrenaline and adrenaline.[2]

Initial research on the mechanisms of the vasoplegia of sepsis[2] focused on increased nitric oxide and prostacyclin synthesis triggered by the inflammatory response, elevated adrenomedullin[3] and activation of transient receptor potential vanilloid type 4 (TRPV4) channel.[4] However, studies investigating the role of nitric oxide synthase blockers[5] and prostaglandin inhibitors[6] have not reported any beneficial effects on clinically relevant outcomes. Data on adrenomedullin and TRPV4 activation are preliminary and there are no approved pharmacologic antagonists for these agents. If untreated, the hypotension associated with sepsis results in macrocirculatory and microcirculatory failure, leading to organ dysfunction and increased mortality. A substantial body of research in the last decade has focused on understanding the mechanisms for vasoplegia and developing new therapies to reverse circulatory failure.[2]

Role of Corticosteroids

Although glucocorticoids (GCs) have been studied as an adjunct therapy in the management of septic shock for more than 6 decades, it is only recently that their mechanisms of action have been clearly delineated. Cortisol is a hormone with multiple actions in regulating metabolism, the immune system, and vascular responsiveness to circulating catecholamines. GCs (mainly cortisol) exert their actions via an intracellular receptor, a 777 amino acid cytoplasmic protein found in nearly all nucleated cells. Cortisol passes through cell membranes to bind with this receptor, following which the steroid-receptor complex migrates to the nucleus and influences gene transcription.[7,8] However, once inside the cell there is a further level of control exerted on GCs by the actions of the 11β-hydroxysteroid dehydrogenase (11β-HSD) enzyme system, which modulates the intracellular concentrations of cortisol and cortisone (**Fig. 1**).

GCs play a pivotal role in the normal body metabolism and affect a wide variety of systems. It has been estimated that GCs affect 22% of the genome of mononuclear blood cells.[9] There is, in addition, accumulating evidence for nongenomic effects of cortisol, in which as yet unidentified membrane receptors may be implicated.[10] In the liver, cortisol stimulates glycogen deposition by increasing glycogen synthase and inhibiting the glycogen-mobilizing enzyme glycogen phosphorylase.[11] Hepatic gluconeogenesis is stimulated, leading to increased blood glucose levels. Concurrently, glucose uptake by peripheral tissues is inhibited.[12] Free fatty acid release into the circulation is increased and triglyceride levels rise.

In the circulatory system, cortisol increases blood pressure both by direct actions on smooth muscle and via renal mechanisms. The actions of pressor agents such as catecholamines are potentiated; whereas nitric oxide–mediated vasodilatation is reduced.[13,14] Renal effects include an increase in glomerular filtration rate, sodium

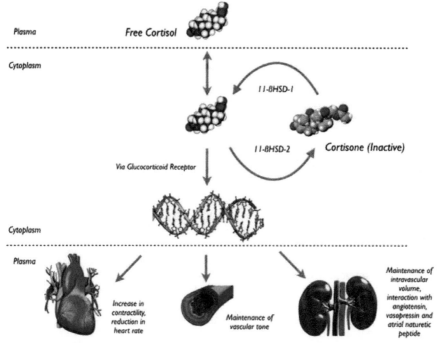

Fig. 1. Actions of cortisol in regulation of cardiovascular system. Free cortisol passes through the cell wall into the cytoplasm. The intracellular isoenzymes 11-beta-hydroxysteroid dehydrogenase (11β-HSD) 1 and 2 regulate the interconversion of cortisol and inactive cortisone. Cortisol binds to the GC receptor, which translocates to the nucleus where it binds to DNA to upregulate and downregulate specific gene activity, leading to tissue-specific effects.

transport in the proximal tubule, and sodium retention and potassium loss in the distal tubule.[15]

The primary effects of cortisol on the immune system are antiinflammatory and immunosuppressive. Lymphocyte cell counts decrease, whereas neutrophil counts increase.[15] Accumulation of immunologically active cells at inflammatory sites is decreased. The production of cytokines is inhibited, an effect that is mediated via nuclear factor (NF)-kβ. This occurs both by induction of NF-kβ inhibitor or by direct binding of cortisol to the NF-kβ molecule, thus preventing its translocation to the nucleus. Although the well-defined effects of cortisol on the immune system are primarily inhibitory, it is also suggested that normal host defense function requires some cortisol secretion.

Corticosteroids and Vascular Tone

Corticosteroids have a central role in the maintenance of blood pressure in health through a variety of mechanisms. These are thought to include the regulation of intravascular volume by generation of angiotensin, vasopressin, and atrial natriuretic peptide; control of fluid and electrolyte balance; and effects on vascular contractility.[16] The influence of corticosteroids on the heart and vascular wall is still incompletely understood. Topical application of corticosteroids causes vasoconstriction[17] and corticosteroids potentiate the contractile response to noradrenaline and angiotensin II. They also have direct effects on the heart, increasing cardiac contractility and reducing heart rate.

CLINICAL TRIALS OF HYDROCORTISONE IN SEPTIC SHOCK

Hydrocortisone was introduced into clinical practice by Philip Hench in 1950. Steroids were first used for the management of sepsis in patients with poststreptococcal infections in 1951.[18] Since then, corticosteroid therapy has undergone several transformations from steroid success in sepsis and malaria in the 1970s and early 1980s[19,20] to steroid excess (30 mg/Kg methylprednisolone) in severe sepsis in the mid to late 1980s.[21] The high-dose steroid approach resulted in excess morbidity and mortality in the steroid group, thus leading to total abandonment of its use in early 1990s. However, this phase was short-lived.

The renaissance in steroid use particularly in lower dosages (200–300 mg of hydrocortisone per day) was driven by trials in the late 1990s demonstrating improved hemodynamic status and vasopressor wean with the use of steroids,[22] as well as the possibility that there exists a state of adrenal suppression secondary to critical illness, termed relative adrenal insufficiency or critical illness–related corticosteroid insufficiency. This group of patients were identified by a blunted cortisol response (<250 nmol/L) to corticotropin and termed nonresponders.[23,24]

Two randomized controlled trials (RCTs) of low-dose corticosteroids in subjects with septic shock were conducted in the 2000s: the Ger-Inf-05 in 2002 and the CORTICUS (Corticosteroid Therapy of Septic Shock) trial in 2008. The Ger-Inf-05 trial ($n = 299$) evaluated the role of hydrocortisone 200 mg or fludrocortisone 50 µg per day compared with placebo. The key findings were: shock was reversed more rapidly in the steroid group and there was no difference in mortality between the groups in an intention to treat analysis; however, in subjects assigned to the intervention group there was an improved survival in the corticotropin nonresponders (63% vs 53%, CI 0.47–0.95, $P = .02$).[25] Of note, more than 75% of subjects in the trial were identified as nonresponders, a figure substantially higher than anticipated and nearly a quarter of the subjects received etomidate, a known adrenal suppressant.

The lack of convincing evidence of benefit of hydrocortisone in the Ger-Inf-05 study, coupled with its small sample size prompted the conduct of the CORTICUS study. This European multicenter study, initially designed to enroll 800 subjects, evaluated the role of 200 mg of hydrocortisone per day versus placebo in subjects with septic shock. The trial was stopped prematurely (after enrollment of 499 subjects) when lower than expected recruitment resulted in termination of funding and expiry of the study drug supply. This study also demonstrated reversal of shock; however, there was no beneficial effect of hydrocortisone on overall mortality (34% vs 31%, $P = .51$) or in the subgroups of corticotropin responders or nonresponders, and more episodes of superinfection in the subjects who received steroids were reported.[26] About 19% of subjects in the CORTICUS trial were exposed to etomidate. As in the Ger-Inf-05 trial, this trial was significantly underpowered to detect a clinically important treatment effect.

The results from these 2 trials and the plethora of systematic reviews that followed continued to generate substantial debate about the role of corticosteroids, resulting in global uncertainty and marked variation in clinical practice. Furthermore, how significant the effect of etomidate as a confounder was in both these trials remained unclear.

In 2018, 2 large parallel group RCTs of corticosteroids in septic shock were reported that have added substantially to the evidence base and provided much needed clarity to this question. The ADRENAL (Adjunctive Corticosteroid Treatment in Critically Ill Patients with Septic Shock) trial ($n = 3800$), which was powered adequately to detect a 5% point absolute risk reduction in mortality, evaluated the role of 200 mg of hydrocortisone administered as an intravenous infusion in etomidate-naïve mechanically ventilated subjects with septic shock. Although there was no difference in the primary outcome (90-day mortality) between the treatment groups, some secondary outcomes were better in the hydrocortisone group: faster reversal of shock, earlier time to liberation from mechanical ventilation, earlier time to intensive care unit (ICU) discharge, and a lower incidence of blood transfusion.[27]

The APROCCHSS study (n = 1241) commenced as a 2-by-2 factorial design trial, evaluating the effect of hydrocortisone combined with fludrocortisone, drotrecogin alfa, or their respective combinations or respective placebos on survival from septic shock. After withdrawal of activated protein C from the market in 2011, the trial continued as a parallel group design comparing hydrocortisone 200 mg in 4 divided doses or oral fludrocortisone 50 µg against placebo. In this study, the inclusion criteria required a higher inotropic or pressor support and an organ failure score; however, it did not mandate mechanical ventilatory support. Prior receipt of etomidate in the current hospital admission was not an exclusion. A corticotropin test was performed before randomization. The APROCCHSS (Activated protein C and corticosteroids for human septic shock) study demonstrated a survival benefit in the active treatment arm (43% vs 49.1%, P = .03). As in the ADRENAL trial, some secondary outcomes were also better in the steroid group: shorter time to weaning from mechanical ventilation and vasopressor therapy, and reaching a sequential organ failure assessment (SOFA) score below 6. In contrast to the original Ger-Inf-05 trial, there was no differential treatment effect in the group of corticotropin nonresponders.[28]

Following the publication of the 2 recent RCTs, the debate has continued about the role of hydrocortisone in septic shock and the reasons for the discordant results on mortality. Next, several questions in relation to these 2 trials specifically are addressed, as well as several other relevant issues related to the use of hydrocortisone in septic shock (**Table 1**).

Was the Mortality Benefit in APROCCHSS Because of a Different Trial Population?

As noted, the ADRENAL and APROCCHSS trials differed in their key finding on the role of the intervention on the primary outcome: 90-day mortality. The former demonstrated no treatment effect, whereas in the latter there was a 6% point absolute risk reduction in the intervention arm. Although the 2 trials had several design features in common (adequate power, predominantly medical sepsis, and similar bacteremia rates), there were key differences. In the ADRENAL trial the need for mechanical ventilation was an inclusion criterion and etomidate exposure in the current hospital admission was an exclusion. In the APROCCHSS trial, subjects were required to have a much higher vasopressor requirement (0.25 µg/kg/min of noradrenaline) at entry. At baseline, subjects in the APROCCHSS cohort had a higher lactate concentrations and a greater proportion of subjects were on renal replacement therapy. The question has been raised whether the difference in the treatment effect on the primary outcome was because the subjects in APROCCHSS trial were a sicker cohort. In addition, etomidate exposure was not an exclusion in the APROCCHSS trial and what proportion of subjects may have been exposed to it is not clearly specified in the published report. However, analysis of the primary outcome in the ADRENAL trial in the prespecified subgroups of greater sickness severity (Acute Physiology and Chronic Health Evaluation [APACHE] >25) and severe shock (noradrenaline dosage >15 µg/min, which corresponds to 0.22 µg/kg/min in a 70 kg individual) did not reveal a differential treatment effect on mortality.

Three meta-analyses following the publication of ADRENAL and APROCCHSS trials differ in the conclusion regarding the benefit of steroids on mortality, 2 reporting no

Table 1
Major randomized controlled trials of low-dose steroids in septic shock

	Ger-Inf-05	CORTICUS	ADRENAL	APROCCHSS
Sample size	299	499	3800	1241
Inclusion criteria	Septic shock	Septic shock	Septic shock + IPPV	Septic shock, SOFA score, and a pressor requirement (0.25 µg/kg/min of noradrenaline)
Predominantly medical sepsis cohort	Y	N	Y	Y
Proportion mechanically ventilated	90%	90%	100%	92%
Baseline plasma lactate (mmol/L)	4.4 ± 4.4	3.9 ± 3.6	3.8 ± 3.0	4.4 ± 4.9
Treatment				
Drugs	HC/FC	HC	HC	HC/FC
Dosage (mg/µg) per day	200/50	200	200	200/50
Duration (days)	7	11	7	7
Mode of administration of HC	Bolus	Bolus	Infusion	Bolus
Tapering	N	Y	N	N
Corticotropin test	Y	Y	Not performed	Y
Nonresponders (%)	77%	46%	N/A	54%
Etomidate usage	Y 24%	Y 19%	N	Unspecified
Mortality benefit with HC				
Intention to treat	—	—	—	—
In-hospital	N	N	N/A	Y
28 d	N	N	N	N
90 d	N	N/A	N	Y
6 mo	N/A	N/A	N	Y
Differential mortality effect in nonresponders to corticotropin	Y	N	N/A	N
Other outcomes				
Shock reversal	Y	Y	Y	Y
Weaning from mechanical ventilation	N/A	N/A	Y	Y
Length of ICU stay	N/A	N	Y	N
Length of hospital stay	N/A	N	N	N
Adverse effects with HC	N	Y (superinfections)	Y (metabolic)	Y (metabolic)

Abbreviations: FC, fludrocortisone; HC, hydrocortisone; IPPV, intermittent positive pressure ventilation; N/A, not applicable.

benefit and a third reporting a potential small benefit.[29–31] Additional post hoc analyses are likely to provide further insight into this important question.

Is Fludrocortisone Responsible for the Beneficial Effect on Mortality in the APROCCHSS Trial?

Of note, the trials that have reported a reduction in mortality with steroids in septic shock incorporated fludrocortisone in the intervention arm (Ger-inf-05 and APROCCHSS). In the former, the survival benefit was only in the subgroup of nonresponders. The rationale for including fludrocortisone is the suggestion that there may be primary adrenal insufficiency in sepsis, requiring both GC and mineralocorticoid supplementation, as well as downregulation of the mineralocorticoid receptor.[32] At dosages of 200 mg of hydrocortisone per day, there is sufficient plasma concentration to activate the mineralocorticoid receptor and produce the desired mineralocorticoid effects.[33] Fludrocortisone is normally recommended for primary adrenal insufficiency when subjects are on a maintenance dosage of GCs but not at the dosages of hydrocortisone used in septic shock. Pharmacokinetic considerations also argue against the potential role of fludrocortisone in reducing mortality. Studies have shown that oral absorption of fludrocortisone is limited in critically ill patients.[34] A previous RCT comparing hydrocortisone with hydrocortisone or fludrocortisone combination did not demonstrate a beneficial effect on mortality.[35] Although a beneficial effect of fludrocortisone cannot be excluded with certainty, additional pharmacokinetic-pharmacodynamic data will inform the debate.

Should Hydrocortisone Be Administered by Infusion or Bolus?

In the ADRENAL trial, the total daily dose of hydrocortisone was administered as an infusion, whereas it was administered as bolus doses in the APROCCHSS trial. Bolus administration is the widely used method; however, administration by infusion has been demonstrated to attenuate the inflammatory response and reverse shock.[36] It is the recommended mode in patients with Addisonian crisis[37] and practice guidelines for septic shock suggest that infusions may minimize metabolic side effects.[38,39]

There are limited data comparing these 2 delivery strategies. Of note, there was evidence of hemodynamic benefit in both trials. There are no head-to-head trials comparing bolus with infusion, and a recent meta-analysis did not demonstrate any effect from method of administration on outcome.[30] At present, there is no good evidence to recommend either delivery method over the other.

Is Corticotropin Testing Required Before Administration of Hydrocortisone?

The corticotropin test gained importance as an important predictor of steroid responsiveness after the Ger-Inf-05 trial demonstrated an improved outcome with corticosteroids in the subgroup of subjects who were nonresponders to corticotropin. However, these findings were not replicated in CORTICUS or the more recent APROCCHSS trial. The corticotropin test has limited utility in critically ill patients,[40] which is in accord with conclusions from a recent international task force meeting on adrenal insufficiency.[41]

What is the Optimal Duration of Hydrocortisone Therapy?

Of the 4 RCTs of corticosteroids in septic shock, 3 trials evaluated 7-day courses of corticosteroids without tapering. The CORTICUS trial in addition to the 7-day course incorporated a tapering regime over an additional 4 days. An analysis of the hemodynamic data from the ADRENAL trial suggests that the differences in mean arterial pressure and heart rate between the 2 groups seemed to narrow after day 7, corresponding with cessation of study drug treatment. It is possible that duration of therapy beyond 7 days may translate into a greater proportion of patients achieving resolution of shock. However, there is no robust evidence to recommend a duration of hydrocortisone beyond 7 days.

Is There Evidence to Support a Repeat Course of Hydrocortisone if There is a Relapse of Shock?

There are very limited published data evaluating the efficacy of a repeat course of hydrocortisone for a relapse of septic shock. Briegel and colleagues[42] demonstrated that a repeat administration of a hydrocortisone infusion in a small number of subjects with relapsed shock was associated with shock reversal. However, there are no large scale RCTs confirming this finding.

Does the Type of Vasopressor Influence Responsiveness to Hydrocortisone?

Although there are reports of absolute or relative deficiencies of endogenous vasoactive hormones, such as vasopressin and angiotensin II, in patients with shock states, there is no evidence to suggest that the beneficial effects of hydrocortisone are associated with a specific type of vasopressor. Early reports of synergy between vasopressin and hydrocortisone observed in a subgroup analysis of the VASST (Vasopressin versus Norepinephrine Infusion in Patients with Septic Shock) study[43] were not reproduced in the subsequent VANISH (The Vasopressin vs Norepinephrine as Initial Therapy in Septic Shock) trial.[44] Similarly, no evidence of a treatment interaction with hydrocortisone was observed in a trial comparing adrenaline with noradrenaline.[45]

Is a 300 mg Dose of Hydrocortisone Superior to 200 mg in Septic Shock?

Early work evaluating low-dose steroids era by Bollaert and colleagues[46] and Briegel and colleagues[22] used 300 mg of hydrocortisone per day in subjects with septic shock as the dosing regimen demonstrated reversal of shock in these subjects. However, the 4 RCTs of adjunctive hydrocortisone in septic shock used 200 mg of hydrocortisone. One study has performed a head-to-head comparison of 200 mg with 300 mg of hydrocortisone in subjects with septic shock. There were no differences in mortality or adverse events between the 2 dosing regimens but redosing of hydrocortisone due to shock relapse was more frequent in the 300 mg group.[47] There is no clear evidence to support the use of 300 mg of hydrocortisone per day.

Does Hydrocortisone Require the Presence of Ascorbic Acid and Thiamine to Be More Efficacious?

It has been suggested that the beneficial effects of hydrocortisone may be potentiated by the concomitant administration of ascorbic acid and thiamine based on the results of a retrospective before–after study.[48] This question is currently the subject of investigation in ongoing clinical trials.

Is Hydrocortisone Useful for the Prevention of Septic Shock?

Although several trials have consistently demonstrated the reversal of septic shock by hydrocortisone, an RCT ($n = 353$) investigating its use in subjects with severe sepsis did not demonstrate a reduction in the incidence of septic shock compared with placebo (21.2% vs 22.9%, $P = .70$).[49]

Are the Mechanisms for Variability in Vascular Responsiveness to Vasopressors in Septic Shock Clearly Understood?

It is unclear why certain patients demonstrate shock resolution and others do not. In the ADRENAL trial, more than 75% of the subjects demonstrated reversal of shock, which was significantly faster and of a greater magnitude in the hydrocortisone group. What is also unknown is why some patients respond to exogenous cortisol early, whereas others take a longer time to achieve shock resolution. There is evidence of a variability in tissue sensitivity to GCs reported in patients with septic shock, although the mechanisms underpinning this are unclear.[50] In septic shock, there is marked variability in plasma cortisol concentrations.[51] There is renewed interest in the role of angiotensin II in septic shock following the publication of a recent RCT.[52] In health, the actions of angiotensin, hydrocortisone, and aldosterone are linked through complementary and intersecting biological mechanisms. Studies have also reported the angiotensin-converting enzyme (ACE) gene, the angiotensin receptor gene, and GC receptor polymorphisms in isolation in sepsis associated with poor outcomes.[53–55] However, given that clinical trials have demonstrated evidence of benefit with all 3 agents on shock reversal, studies examining the interactions between these 3 agents, respective pathways, the activities of ACE 1 and 2, and the impact of the genetic polymorphisms associated with their receptor expressions on shock reversal are critical and lacking. An improved understanding of the mechanisms behind the biological basis of their therapeutic effects and possible synergy may facilitate a targeted approach to the administration of these agents.

PRACTICE RECOMMENDATIONS

Published evidence to date suggests that adjunctive corticosteroid therapy may be associated with either no or, at best, a small reduction in mortality. There is clear evidence of benefit seen in the patient-centered outcomes of time to withdrawal of ventilation and time in ICU, as well as a faster reversal of shock. This may translate into significant cost savings. These may be sufficient considerations for clinicians to prescribe corticosteroids more frequently, especially in the absence of evidence of harm.

The authors recommend the following practice guidelines for clinicians commencing adjunctive corticosteroid treatment of patients with septic shock:

1. Hydrocortisone should be prescribed in a dosage of 200 mg/d
2. The recommended duration is for 7 days and can be administered by either infusion or bolus
3. Hydrocortisone can be used in all patients with septic shock irrespective of which vasopressor is being used to maintain the blood pressure
4. There is no requirement for dose tapering
5. The role of repeat course of hydrocortisone in the case of a relapse of shock needs further evaluation and there is no robust evidence to support or argue against its use
6. There is no requirement to perform a corticotrophin test before commencing hydrocortisone
7. Additional fludrocortisone is not necessary
8. There is no robust evidence to support the use of ascorbic acid and thiamine as additional adjuvant therapies with hydrocortisone
9. There is no evidence to support the use of hydrocortisone in the prevention of septic shock.

SUMMARY AND FUTURE QUESTIONS

The new evidence provided by the ADRENAL and APROCCHSS trials has strengthened the rationale for the use of hydrocortisone in critically ill patients with septic shock. Although its role in reducing mortality remains unclear, there are significant beneficial effects on other important patient-centered outcomes that are likely to also translate into potentially significant cost savings.

Future areas of work could be directed at elucidating mechanism of shock reversal, interaction of hydrocortisone with other therapeutic agents, identifying steroid responsiveness using biochemical or gene signatures, and clarifying the role of fludrocortisone.

REFERENCES

1. Finfer S, Bellomo R, Lipman J, et al. Adult-population incidence of severe sepsis in Australian and New Zealand intensive care units. Intensive Care Med 2004;30: 589–96.
2. Levy B, Fritz C, Tahon E, et al. Vasoplegia treatments: the past, the present, and the future. Crit Care 2018;22:52.
3. Valenzuela-Sanchez F, Valenzuela-Mendez B, Rodriguez-Gutierrez JF, et al. New role of biomarkers: mid-regional pro-adrenomedullin, the biomarker of organ failure. Ann Transl Med 2016;4:329.
4. Dalsgaard T, Sonkusare SK, Teuscher C, et al. Pharmacological inhibitors of TRPV4 channels reduce cytokine production, restore endothelial function and increase survival in septic mice. Sci Rep 2016;6:33841.
5. Lopez A, Lorente JA, Steingrub J, et al. Multiple-center, randomized, placebo-controlled, double-blind study of the nitric oxide synthase inhibitor 546C88: effect on survival in patients with septic shock. Crit Care Med 2004;32:21–30.
6. Bernard GR, Wheeler AP, Russell JA, et al. The effects of ibuprofen on the physiology and survival of patients with sepsis. The Ibuprofen in Sepsis Study Group. N Engl J Med 1997;336:912–8.
7. Chrousos GP. The hypothalamic-pituitary-adrenal axis and immune-mediated inflammation. N Engl J Med 1995;332:1351–62.
8. Weinberger C, Hollenberg SM, Rosenfeld MG, et al. Domain structure of human glucocorticoid receptor and its relationship to the v-erb-A oncogene product. Nature 1985;318:670–2.
9. Galon J, Franchimont D, Hiroi N, et al. Gene profiling reveals unknown enhancing and suppressive actions of glucocorticoids on immune cells. FASEB J 2002;16: 61–71.
10. Iwasaki Y, Aoki Y, Katahira M, et al. Non-genomic mechanisms of glucocorticoid inhibition of adrenocorticotropin secretion: possible involvement of GTP-binding protein. Biochem Biophys Res Commun 1997;235:295–9.
11. Stalmans W, Laloux M. Glucocorticoids and hepatic glycogen metabolism. In: Baxter JD, Rousseau GG, editors. Glucocorticoid hormone action. New York: Springer-Verlag; 1979. p. 518–33.
12. Olefsky JM. Effect of dexamethasone on insulin binding, glucose transport, and glucose oxidation of isolated rat adipocytes. J Clin Invest 1975;56:1499–508.
13. Grunfeld JP, Eloy L. Glucocorticoids modulate vascular reactivity in the rat. Hypertension 1987;10:608–18.
14. Saruta T, Suzuki H, Handa M, et al. Multiple factors contribute to the pathogenesis of hypertension in Cushing's syndrome. J Clin Endocrinol Metab 1986;62:275–9.

15. Larsen P, Kronenburg H, Melmed S, et al. Williams textbook of endocrinology. Philadelphia: Saunders; 2003.
16. Hadoke PW, Iqbal J, Walker BR. Therapeutic manipulation of glucocorticoid metabolism in cardiovascular disease. Br J Pharmacol 2009;156:689–712.
17. Walker BR, Connacher AA, Webb DJ, et al. Glucocorticoids and blood pressure: a role for the cortisol/cortisone shuttle in the control of vascular tone in man. Clin Sci (Lond) 1992;83:171–8.
18. Hahn E, Houser H, Rammelkamp CJ, et al. Effect of cortisone on acute streptococcal infections and poststreptococcal complications. J Clin Invest 1951;30: 274–81.
19. Hoffman SL, Punjabi NH, Kumala S, et al. Reduction of mortality in chloramphenicol-treated severe typhoid fever by high-dose dexamethasone. N Engl J Med 1984;310:82–8.
20. Schumer W. Steroids in the treatment of clinical septic shock. Ann Surg 1976;184: 333–41.
21. Bone RC, Fisher CJ Jr, Clemmer TP, et al. A controlled clinical trial of high-dose methylprednisolone in the treatment of severe sepsis and septic shock. N Engl J Med 1987;317:653–8.
22. Briegel J, Forst H, Haller M, et al. Stress doses of hydrocortisone reverse hyperdynamic septic shock: a prospective, randomized, double-blind, single-center study. Crit Care Med 1999;27:723–32.
23. Annane D, Sebille V, Troche G, et al. A 3-level prognostic classification in septic shock based on cortisol levels and cortisol response to corticotropin. JAMA 2000; 283:1038–45.
24. Marik PE. Critical illness-related corticosteroid insufficiency. Chest 2009;135: 181–93.
25. Annane D, Sebille V, Charpentier C, et al. Effect of treatment with low doses of hydrocortisone and fludrocortisone on mortality in patients with septic shock. JAMA 2002;288:862–71.
26. Sprung CL, Annane D, Keh D, et al. Hydrocortisone therapy for patients with septic shock. N Engl J Med 2008;358:111–24.
27. Venkatesh B, Finfer S, Cohen J, et al. Adjunctive glucocorticoid therapy in patients with septic shock. N Engl J Med 2018;378:797–808.
28. Annane D, Renault A, Brun-Buisson C, et al. Hydrocortisone plus fludrocortisone for adults with septic shock. N Engl J Med 2018;378:809–18.
29. Rochwerg B, Oczkowski SJ, Siemieniuk RAC, et al. Corticosteroids in sepsis: an updated systematic review and meta-analysis. Crit Care Med 2018;46:1411–20.
30. Rygård SL, Butler E, Granholm A, et al. Low-dose corticosteroids for adult patients with septic shock: a systematic review with meta-analysis and trial sequential analysis. Intensive Care Med 2018;44:1003–16.
31. Zhu Y, Wen Y, Jiang Q, et al. The effectiveness and safety of corticosteroids therapy in adult critical III patients with septic shock: a meta-analysis of randomized controlled trials. Shock 2018. https://doi.org/10.1097/SHK.0000000000001202.
32. Fadel F, Andre-Gregoire G, Gravez B, et al. Aldosterone and vascular mineralocorticoid receptors in murine endotoxic and human septic shock. Crit Care Med 2017;45:e954–62.
33. Charmandari E, Kino T, Chrousos GP. Glucocorticoids. In: Yaffe SJ, Aranda JV, editors. Neonatal and pediatric pharmacology. 4th edition. Philadelphia: Lippincott Williams and Wilkins; 2010. p. 760–72.
34. Polito A, Hamitouche N, Ribot M, et al. Pharmacokinetics of oral fludrocortisone in septic shock. Br J Clin Pharmacol 2016;82:1509–16.

35. Investigators CS, Annane D, Cariou A, et al. Corticosteroid treatment and intensive insulin therapy for septic shock in adults: a randomized controlled trial. JAMA 2010;303:341–8.
36. Keh D, Boehnke T, Weber-Cartens S, et al. Immunologic and hemodynamic effects of "low-dose" hydrocortisone in septic shock: a double-blind, randomized, placebo-controlled, crossover study. Am J Respir Crit Care Med 2003;167: 512–20.
37. Arlt W. The approach to the adult with newly diagnosed adrenal insufficiency. J Clin Endocrinol Metab 2009;94:1059–67.
38. Loisa P, Parviainen I, Tenhunen J, et al. Effect of mode of hydrocortisone administration on glycemic control in patients with septic shock: a prospective randomized trial. Crit Care 2007;11:R21.
39. Rhodes A, Evans LE, Alhazzani W, et al. Surviving sepsis campaign: international guidelines for management of sepsis and septic shock: 2016. Intensive Care Med 2017;43:304–77.
40. Venkatesh B, Cohen J. The utility of the corticotropin test to diagnose adrenal insufficiency in critical illness: an update. Clin Endocrinol (Oxf) 2015;83(3): 289–97.
41. Annane D, Pastores SM, Rochwerg B, et al. Guidelines for the diagnosis and management of critical illness-related corticosteroid insufficiency (CIRCI) in critically ill patients (Part I): Society of Critical Care Medicine (SCCM) and European Society of Intensive Care Medicine (ESICM) 2017. Intensive Care Med 2017;43:1751–63.
42. Briegel J, Kellermann W, Forst H, et al. Low-dose hydrocortisone infusion attenuates the systemic inflammatory response syndrome. The Phospholipase A2 Study Group. Clin Investig 1994;72:782–7.
43. Russell JA, Walley KR, Singer J, et al. Vasopressin versus norepinephrine infusion in patients with septic shock. N Engl J Med 2008;358:877–87.
44. Gordon AC, Mason AJ, Thirunavukkarasu N, et al. Effect of early vasopressin vs norepinephrine on kidney failure in patients with septic shock: the VANISH randomized clinical trial. JAMA 2016;316:509–18.
45. Myburgh JA, Higgins A, Jovanovska A, et al. A comparison of epinephrine and norepinephrine in critically ill patients. Intensive Care Med 2008;34:2226–34.
46. Bollaert PE, Charpentier C, Levy B, et al. Reversal of late septic shock with supraphysiologic doses of hydrocortisone. Crit Care Med 1998;26:645–50.
47. Hyvernat H, Barel R, Gentilhomme A, et al. Effects of increasing hydrocortisone to 300 mg per day in the treatment of septic shock: a pilot study. Shock 2016;46: 498–505.
48. Marik PE, Khangoora V, Rivera R, et al. Hydrocortisone, vitamin C, and thiamine for the treatment of severe sepsis and septic shock: a retrospective before-after study. Chest 2017;151:1229–38.
49. Keh D, Trips E, Marx G, et al. Effect of hydrocortisone on development of shock among patients with severe sepsis: the HYPRESS randomized clinical trial. JAMA 2016;316:1775–85.
50. Cohen J, Pretorius CJ, Ungerer JPJ, et al. Glucocorticoid sensitivity is highly variable in critically ill patients with septic shock and is associated with disease severity. Crit Care Med 2016;44:1034–41.
51. Venkatesh B, Mortimer RH, Couchman B, et al. Evaluation of random plasma cortisol and the low dose corticotropin test as indicators of adrenal secretory capacity in critically ill patients: a prospective study. Anaesth Intensive Care 2005; 33:201–9.

52. Khanna A, English SW, Wang XS, et al. Angiotensin II for the treatment of vaso-dilatory shock. N Engl J Med 2017;377:419–30.
53. Cvijanovich NZ, Anas N, Allen GL, et al. Glucocorticoid receptor polymorphisms and outcomes in pediatric septic shock. Pediatr Crit Care Med 2017;18:299–303.
54. Dou XM, Cheng HJ, Meng L, et al. Correlations between ACE single nucleotide polymorphisms and prognosis of patients with septic shock. Biosci Rep 2017; 37 [pii:BSR20170145].
55. Nakada TA, Russell JA, Boyd JH, et al. Association of angiotensin II type 1 receptor-associated protein gene polymorphism with increased mortality in sep-tic shock. Crit Care Med 2011;39:1641–8.

Erythropoietin in Critical Illness and Trauma

Craig French, MBBS, FANZCA, FCICM[a,b,c,]*

KEYWORDS

- Erythropoietin • Critical illness • Trauma • Red blood cell transfusion

KEY POINTS

- Erythropoietin (EPO) is a 34kd hormone essential for red cell production.
- The results of high-quality clinical trials conducted in critically ill patients do not support the routine use of EPO as a red blood cell transfusion agent.
- Locally produced EPO plays a key role in the response to injury and inflammation via the inhibition of apoptosis.
- Although a substantial body of preclinical and clinical evidence exists and suggests that EPO improves the outcome of critically ill trauma patients, further research is required.

INTRODUCTION

Erythropoietin (EPO) is a pleiotropic cytokine essential for the production of red blood cells (RBC). Commercial preparations of EPO have the following Food and Drug Administration (FDA)-approved indications: treatment of anemia in patients with chronic renal failure; treatment of anemia in zidovudine-treated human immunodeficiency virus (HIV)-infected patients; treatment of anemia in patients with cancer on chemotherapy; and for the reduction of allogeneic blood transfusion in surgery patients. It is now recognized that EPO has nonhemopoietic functions including the response to tissue injury. This article provides and overviews the history and biochemistry of EPO, together with its potential applications in critical illness, including as a transfusion sparing agent and for tissue protection following severe trauma.

HISTORY OF ERYTHROPOIETIN

The story of EPO began in the late nineteenth century in France when Francois-Gilbert Viault, a histologist, observed an increase in the number of his own RBC following

Disclosure Statement: Nothing to disclose.
a Western Health, Footscray Hospital, Gordon Street Footscray, Melbourne, VIC 3011, Australia; b The University of Melbourne, Parkville, VIC 3010, Australia; c Monash University, School of Public Health and Preventive Medicine, 553 St Kilda Road, Melbourne, VIC 3004, Australia
* Department of Intensive Care, Footscray Hospital, Level 1 North Block, 160 Gordon Street, Footscray, Victoria 3011, Australia.
E-mail address: Craig.French@wh.org.au

3 weeks at altitude.[1] In the early twentieth century Carnot and DeFlandre hypothesized that red cell production was regulated by a substance they called *hemopoietin*.[2] They observed that the injection of plasma from rabbits who suffered hemorrhage into normal rabbits had led to an increase in red cell mass. The term "erythropoietin" was first used in 1948 by Finnish researchers Bonsdorrf and Jalavisto.[3] They demonstrated an increase in red cell precursors in the bone marrow of rabbits injected with plasma from rabbits exposed to hypoxia. Over the following decade further animal studies reproduced these results[4,5] and the principle site of production of EPO was identified as the kidneys.[6] However, it was not until 1977 that Miyake and colleagues[7] finally purified human EPO from the urine of patients with aplastic anemia. In 1985, 2 groups cloned the EPO gene: Lin and colleagues[8] in Chinese hamster ovary cells and Jacobs and colleagues[9] in African green monkey kidney cells. This allowed the development of human recombinant EPO (rHuEPO) for use as a drug. In 1988, the rHuEPO, epoetin alfa, received regulatory approval in the United States for human therapeutic use.

STRUCTURE OF ERYTHROPOIETIN AND MECHANISM OF ENHANCED ERYTHROPOIESIS

EPO comprises 165 amino acids and 4 carbohydrate side chains with a molecular mass of 34kD and a compact globular structure.[10] It is essential for normal red cell production and the dominant site of synthesis is the renal cortex. EPO production is increased in response to a decrease in tissue oxygen partial pressure.[11] Hypoxia-inducible factor-2 is now recognized as the primary transcription factor for expression of the EPO gene and hypoxia-inducible factor-alpha prolyl-hydroxylases the primary O_2 sensors in control of EPO production.[12] EPO binds to a specific receptor (EPOR) that is present on the surface of colony-forming unit–erythroids (CFU-Es).[13] Activation of EPOR inhibits apoptosis of CFU-Es leading to an increase in the number of normoblasts and subsequently reticulocytes and RBC.[11]

ANEMIA IN CRITICAL ILLNESS

Anemia and allogeneic blood transfusion are common in the critical illness and both are independently associated with poor outcome.[14–17] The World Health Organization (WHO) defines anemia as a hemoglobin concentration of less than 130 g/L in men and 120/g in women.[18] Two large cohort studies have demonstrated on admission to intensive care units (ICUs) that more than 60% of patients have a hemoglobin concentration less than 120 g/L and 25% less than 90 g/L.[14,15] Further it is demonstrated that hemoglobin concentration further declines rapidly (in patients not transfused) in the following 72 hours (up to 50 g/L from admission) and thereafter more slowly such that most of the overwhelming patients with an ICU length of stay of 1 week or more have a hemoglobin concentration of less than 90 g/L on at least one occasion.[16] The cause of anemia of critical illness is multifactorial and complex. Many of the etiologic factors are shared with the anemia of chronic disease; it is their relative contribution that differs.[19] Contributing factors include hemodilution; overt or occult blood loss, including iatrogenic secondary to phlebotomy; decreased red cell survival due to increased uptake by the reticuloendothelial system; and impaired erythropoiesis.

Although anemia is common, the effect of allogenic RBC transfusion in critically ill patients not actively bleeding is uncertain. RBC transfusion has been associated with increased mortality, ventilator associated pneumonia, nosocomial infection, acute respiratory distress syndrome, and multiple organ failure.[20] However, the data are inconsistent and any association time dependent. Rüttinger and colleagues[21] (2007) examined the relationship between RBC transfusion and mortality in 3037 patients admitted to a surgical ICU. This prospective cohort study demonstrated a significant association between RBC transfusion and ICU mortality when the analysis was adjusted for admission variables only. When adjustment was made for severity of illness and organ dysfunction throughout the ICU admission any association was lost. This may suggest that red cell transfusion is a surrogate marker for disease severity and is not causally related to mortality or adverse outcomes in critically ill patients. Accordingly, in the absence of strong evidence of benefit and possible adverse outcomes, restrictive RBC transfusion practices, including single unit transfusion, are advised.[22] As result there has been substantial focus on nontransfusion interventions, including EPO, for the treatment of anemia in the ICU.

ERYTHROPOIETIN AS A RED BLOOD CELL TRANSFUSION-SPARING AGENT IN CRITICAL ILLNESS

In healthy individuals the normal serum EPO concentration is 5 to 10 IU/L.[23] However, in patients who are critically ill endogenous EPO levels are inappropriately low.[24–26] After controlling for hemoglobin levels, EPO levels were reduced by approximately 75% compared with ambulatory patients with iron deficiency anemia.[26] As a consequence of these data it was postulated that the administration of rHuEPO would decrease the need for allogenic red cell transfusion in critical illness and potentially improve patient outcomes.

Howard Corwin's group, over a 15-year period, evaluated the effectiveness of EPO as a transfusion-sparing agent in critically ill patients.[27–29] In 1999, they reported the results of a 160-patient single-center pilot study (EPO-1).[27] In this study participants were randomized to receive 300unit/kg of rHuEPO or placebo administered by subcutaneous injection. Study treatment commenced 72 hours following ICU admission and continued daily for 5 days and then second daily until ICU discharge for up to 6 weeks to achieve a hematocrit (Hct) concentration of greater than 38%. In this pilot study the cumulative total number of RBC units transfused was significantly less in the rHuEPO group than the placebo group, with 166 units administered to the 80 patients randomized to EPO and 305 units administered in the placebo group. The final Hct concentration of the patients with rHuEPO was also significantly greater than the final Hct concentration of placebo patients (35.1 ± 5.6 vs 31.6 ± 4.1; $P<.01$, respectively). No adverse safety signals were observed.

The results of EPO-1 supported the evaluation of rHuEPO in a larger population. In 2002 the EPO-2 trial was published.[28] This randomized double-blind placebo-controlled trial was conducted in 65 Unites States medical centers between December 1998 and June 2001. The study enrolled 1302 participants. Eligible patients were those patients in the ICU for 48 hours with an expected length of stay of at least an additional 48 hours and an Hct of less than 38%. In contrast to EPO-1, patients received a single subcutaneous injection of 40,000 units of epoetin alfa (or placebo) on day 3 and then weekly after for a maximum of 3 doses. Study drug was also withheld if the Hct was 38%. This study demonstrated a 19% reduction in the total number of RBC units transfused in the rHuEPO group (1963 units, placebo vs 1590 units, rHuEPO). No difference in mortality was observed between the 2 groups (14% in rHuEPO vs 15% in placebo) and the incidence of reported serious adverse events was comparable.

In 1999, a landmark study of allogeneic RBC administration to critically ill patients was published.[30] The Transfusion Requirements in Critical Care trial evaluated the effect of a restrictive (70–90 g/L) versus liberal (100–120 g/L) RBC transfusion strategy in critically ill patients. It is highly likely that clinical transfusion practice will influence any evaluation of EPO as a transfusion-sparing agent. It was possible therefore that the reduction in the number of red cell transfusions observed in EPO-1 and EPO-2 may be less or even disappear with a restrictive transfusion strategy. As a consequence, EPO-3 was conducted in 115 medical centers between December 2003 and June 2006.[29] This trial enrolled 1460 participants. Inclusion and exclusion criteria were similar to EPO-2: study drug was withheld when the hemoglobin concentration was greater than 120 g/L rather than a Hct of 38%. Study treatment was 40,000 units of epoetin alfa administered subcutaneously on study day 1 and weekly thereafter to a maximum of 3 doses.

In contrast to EPO-1 and EPO-2, no significant difference in the percentage of patients who received an RBC transfusion was observed (46.0% in the epoetin alfa group vs 48.3% in the placebo group; relative risk, 0.95; 95% confidence interval [CI], 0.85–1.06; $P = .34$), no difference in the median units transfused per patient and no difference in the total number of units transfused (1525 vs 1530). Interestingly, mortality at day 29 (a secondary endpoint) was lower in the epoetin alfa group than the placebo group (8.5% vs 11.4% $P = .02$). Although lower mortality in the study population was observed, there was an increase in the incidence of clinical thrombotic events (16.5% vs 11.5% $P = .008$), including pulmonary embolism, deep venous thrombosis, stroke, myocardial infarction, and cardiac arrest.

The meta-analysis commissioned by National Blood Authority of Australia evaluates the effect of EPO when used as a transfusion-sparing agent on blood transfusion.[22] The results are stratified by prevailing transfusion practice (restrictive or liberal) at the time the study was conducted. Although overall a reduction in RBC transfusion is observed, the effect is not significant where a restrictive transfusion strategy is used (3 trials; 43.7%; risk ratio [RR] 0.68; 95% CI 0.43, 1.07). No effect on mortality was observed (11 trials; 14% vs 16%; RR 0.90; 95% CI 0.77, 1.05) and no significant difference deep vein thrombosis (7 trials; 5% vs 4%; RR 1.06; 95% CI 0.69, 1.64), stroke (3 trials; 2% vs 3%; RR 0.76; 95% CI 0.41, 1.41), or myocardial infarction (2 trials; 2% vs 1%; RR 0.80; 95% CI 0.05, 13.82). Given the lack of clear effect on RBC transfusion and no effect on patient-centered outcomes, a high-level recommendation was made against the routine use of erythropoiesis stimulating agents in critically ill anemic patients.[22]

ERYTHROPOIETIN—MORE THAN JUST ERYTHROPOIESIS

As detailed previously, EPO is produced in response to hypoxia and increases red cell mass via the inhibition of apoptosis of red cell precursors. In this role EPO acts as a circulating hormone. Over the last 2 decades a greater understanding of EPO's potential nonhemopoietic functions has emerged.[31] It is now generally accepted that EPO can be produced outside the renal cortex and that EPORs are expressed in a wide variety of tissues, not just erythroid progenitor cells.[32] Further not all EPORs are the same with distinct isoforms now recognized.[33] When produced outside the renal cortex EPO has a paracrine/autocrine function rather than the hormonal role it occupies in erythropoiesis.

ENDOGENOUS ERYTHROPOIETIN HAS PROTECTIVE EFFECTS FOLLOWING TISSUE INJURY

Although the inflammatory response is adaptive and essential for clearing tissue debris following injury, the authors now appreciate the key protective role that endogenous EPO production plays critically limiting further tissue damage. A delicate balance exists between EPO and proinflammatory cytokines, such as tumor necrosis factor alpha (**Fig. 1**).

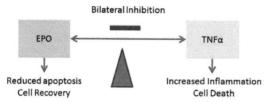

Fig. 1. Balance existing between EPO and proinflammatory cytokines, such as tumor necrosis factor alpha.

The basic science rationale for EPO-mediated tissue protection following trauma is extremely strong:

1. EPO production is increased in response to trauma and inflammation: an endogenous self-defense mechanism driven by hypoxia-inducible transcription factor.[34]
2. EPO binds to a specific tissue protective receptor (EPOR-βcR), whose expression is increased in response to trauma and inflammation, triggering key protective responses in injured tissues/organs **(Fig. 2)**.[35,36]
3. EPOR-βcR complex expression has been identified in a wide variety of tissues and body areas, including the central and peripheral nervous system,[37] heart,[38] kidney,[39] endothelium,[40] and skeletal muscle,[41] all of which are vulnerable in critically ill multitrauma patients.
4. The whole tissue protective effects of EPO compounds have been demonstrated in multiple animal models focusing on these tissues/body areas, including focal cerebral ischemia,[42] embolic stroke,[43] traumatic brain injury,[44] myocardial ischemia,[39] acute kidney injury,[45] limb ischemia,[46] and wound healing.[47]
5. Increased levels of EPO are required to trigger this tissue protective effect compared with the traditional erythropoietic response, making it an ideal pharmacologic target.[48] The EPOR-βcR complex (also known as the innate repair receptor [IRR]) is essential for these tissue protective effects. In a murine model, no tissue protective effect of EPO was observed in its absence.[45]
6. EPO administration may be delayed for some hours after injury with effects qualitatively similar to its immediate administration. Exogenous EPO's or its derivatives tissue's protective effects are still observed where administration has been delayed for up to 48 hours.[49]

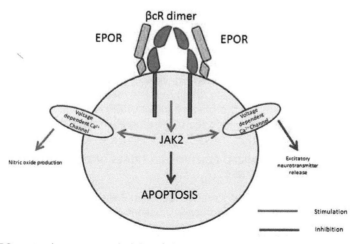

Fig. 2. EPO protective responses in injured tissues/organs.

EPO is therefore a highly plausible and attractive pharmaceutical candidate to reduce secondary tissue and organ damage. It has the potential to prevent deaths and reduce severe disability in critically ill trauma patients.

EXOGENOUS ERYTHROPOIETIN MAY IMPROVE SURVIVAL AND REDUCES SEVERE DISABILITY IN TRAUMA PATIENTS

Trauma is a global public health issue. The WHO estimates that more than 5 million people die each year from traumatic injuries worldwide.[50] These represent 9% of all deaths and are 1.7 times the number of fatalities that result from HIV/AIDS, tuberculosis, and malaria combined. More than 1.3 million of these deaths are a result of road trauma: by 2020 this is projected to increase to more than 2 million.[51] Traumatic injury has significant social and economic impact: globally the estimated annual cost of road trauma alone is estimated to be in excess of US $500 billion.[52] As outlined earlier, initial clinical interventional studies in the critically ill evaluated the use of EPO as a possible RBC transfusion-sparing agent.[27–29] These studies provided the first signal in humans that EPO administration may improve patient outcome in critically ill trauma patients when a striking protective effect was observed in the trauma subgroups of these trials.[53]

In the EPO-2 study,[28] 1620 of the 1302 enrolled patients (47.7%) had a trauma diagnosis. EPO significantly reduced day 28 mortality: EPO 15/314 (4.8%) versus Control 33/316 (10.4%); $P = .009$. In the EPO-3 study,[29] 793 (54.3%) of the 1460 patients had a trauma diagnosis. EPO reduced day 29 mortality: EPO 14/402 (3.5%) versus 26/391 (6.6%); $P = .04$. These studies targeted general populations and did not determine the burden of disability. In 2015, a 606-patient randomized controlled trial of EPO in critically ill patients with severe and moderate traumatic brain injury (EPO-TBI) was published.[54] EPO again lowered mortality in critically ill trauma patients (adjusted odds ratio 0.58, 95% CI, 0.34–0.99; $P = .04$; adjusted hazard ratio 0.62, 95% CI, 0.39–0.97). Thus, EPO has reduced the mortality of critically ill trauma patients in 3 double-blind randomized controlled trials.

In contrast to earlier studies, EPO-TBI study reported the pattern (region involved) and severity (focal vs diffuse brain injury and associated multitrauma) of injury and assessed the burden of disability with functional assessment at 6 months. Post hoc analyses of the EPO-TBI trial were conducted to identify any differential effect in patient subgroups.[55,56] These analyses suggested that EPO had a particularly striking protective effect on those patients with traumatic brain injury (TBI) with coexisting multiple trauma: its administration significantly decreased mortality (HR 0.42, 95% CI 0.20–0.87; $P = .02$) and was associated with an 18% relative increase in the number of patients surviving at 6 months without severe disability (48.8% to 57.6%, $P = .17$). Further, in another follow-up study EPO significantly increased Quality Adjusted Life Years ($P<.001$) at 6 months.[57] Taken together these results provide strong evidence of a potentially clinically relevant protective effect of EPO on critically ill trauma patients. This evidence is further supported by a comprehensive recent meta-analysis.

META-ANALYSIS OF RANDOMIZED CONTROLLED TRIALS OF ERYTHROPOIETIN IN CRITICALLY ILL TRAUMA PATIENTS

A recent systematic review of the literature identified 9 eligible randomized controlled trials that randomly assigned 2607 critically ill patients following trauma to EPO.[58] An update performed in January 2018 identified one further eligible randomized controlled trial with an additional 151 patients.[59]

EPO therapy is associated with a highly significant and substantial 36% relative risk reduction in the latest reported mortality. Importantly, the exclusion of lower-quality studies had no substantive impact on the results, no statistical heterogeneity exists (RR 0.62, 95% CI 0.48–0.81, P = .0004; I2 = 0%), and the benefit remained significant after trial sequential analysis adjustment to account for the multiple hypothesis testing inherent in meta-analytic techniques. Three trials reported functional outcome and disability using the GOSE.[54,59,60] A 22% improvement in the number of patients with severe disability (RR 1.22 95% CI 0.82–1.81; P = .33 I2 = 84%) was observed.

Although there is strong evidence for benefit, uncertainty remains regarding EPO's effectiveness. All previously conducted randomized controlled trials have limitations: in some, trauma patients were retrospectively or prospectively defined subgroups; in others, outcomes of interest were a secondary endpoint; and some were of low quality and did not assess functional outcome. Accordingly, the large body of clinical evidence is insufficient to justify recommending the routine administration of EPO or its incorporation into practice guidelines.

ERYTHROPOIETIN—THE MOST PROTECTIVE DOSE, ROUTE, AND FREQUENCY OF ADMINISTRATION IN THE CRITICALLY ILL

Of the patients included in the abovementioned meta-analysis, the majority (2193/2607) were enrolled in trials using a weekly dose of 40,000 units. Four clinical studies administered EPO subcutaneously (n = 2067).[28,29,54,61] A sensitivity analysis performed as part of the meta-analysis did not demonstrate any differential effect of the route of administration on mortality. Four studies administered multiple doses of EPO—usually weekly.[28,29,54,61] Although a weekly dose of 40,000 units was originally developed as a transfusion-sparing regimen, it has been repeatedly associated with improved patient outcome in critically ill trauma patients. Further there is evidence from the preclinical literature that these relatively large doses are necessary to activate tissue protective receptors and essential for EPO's protective effects.[45] Furthermore, a detailed post hoc analysis of the EPO-TBI study demonstrated maximum benefit accrued with 2 doses of 40,000 units of EPO (separated by 7 days).[62]

ERYTHROPOIETIN—IS IT SAFE IN CRITICALLY ILL TRAUMA PATIENTS?

Some early clinical trials, mainly in patients with cancer, suggested an increased rate of thrombosis with EPO prompting a US FDA Black Box warning in 2007. However, detection of thrombosis was based on clinical evaluation. In the EPO-TBI study, there was no difference in the rate of objectively assessed (ultrasound examination) deep venous thrombosis with EPO (15.7%) compared with placebo (18.1%) or in a composite thromboembolic endpoint (EPO 20.3% vs placebo 22.8%).[54] In a post hoc analysis, no association between EPO use and venous thromboembolic events was demonstrated.[63] Thromboembolic events related to EPO administration in the critically ill have also be subject to meta-analysis and no adverse safety findings were demonstrated.[58] These findings support the relative safety of exogenous EPO to critically ill trauma patients (**Table 1**).

NONERYTHROPOIETIN LIGANDS OF THE INNATE REPAIR RECEPTOR

Data suggest that the locally produced EPO that binds to the IRR differs from the EPO produced by the renal cortex.[64] In particular, locally produced EPO lacks the 4 carbohydrate moieties terminated with sialic acids. It has therefore been termed hyposialated EPO (hsEPO). The removal of these carbohydrate moieties dramatically

Table 1
Thromboembolic adverse events reported in randomized controlled trials

Outcome	Studies	Participants	No. of Events	Risk Ratio (95% CI)	P Value
Deep Venous Thrombosis (lower limb)	6	2491	162	0.97 (0.72, 1.29)	.81
Pulmonary Embolism	3	991	34	1.10 (0.57, 2.14)	.78
Cardiac Arrest	4	2225	45	0.83 (0.42, 1.65)	.59

reduces the half-life of hsEPO compared with EPO (1.4 minute vs 4–6 hours). This is consistent with its paracrine/autocrine role. Novel molecules are being developed, which are specific ligands for the IRR and that do activate EPOR. These may result in the inhibition of inflammation, apoptosis, and activation of repair without the concern of increased thromboembolic events that exist with exogenous rHuEPO administration.[35] The potential application of such molecules is limited not only to severe trauma but also in chronic diseases such as diabetes and chronic pain.[65]

SUMMARY

Eugene Goldwasser described his 3 decades of identifying, isolating, and purifying EPO as a "bloody long journey."[66] Determining any role in critical illness is taking even longer! What is clear is that in the modern era of restrictive red cell transfusion practice EPO's routine use as a transfusion-sparing agent cannot be recommended—no reliable effect on the incidence of transfusion or other patient centered outcome has been demonstrated. EPOs (or non-EPO IRR ligands) role in tissue repair, modulation of inflammation, and prevention of apoptosis remains uncertain. Although there exists a large body of preclinical and clinical evidence that suggests a role for exogenous rHuEPO in the most severely ill trauma patients, it is insufficient to guide practice. The uncertainty will only be addressed by the conduct of definitive well-designed clinical trials.

REFERENCES

1. Viault F. Sur l'augmentation considerable du nombre des globules rouge dans le sang chez les inhabitants des hauts plateaux de l'Amerique du Sud. C R Acad Sci Paris 1890;111:917–8.
2. Camot P, Deflandre C. Sur l'activite hemopoietique du serum au cours de la regeneration du sang. C R Acad Sci Paris 1906;143:384–6.
3. Bonsdorff E, Jalavisto E. A humoral mechanism in anoxic erythrocytosis. Acta Physiol Scand 1948;16:150–70.
4. Reissmann KR. Studies on the mechanism of erythropoietic stimulation in parabiotic rats during hypoxia. Blood 1950;5:372–80.
5. Erslev AJ. Humoral regulation of red cell production. Blood 1953;8:349–57.
6. Jacobson LO, Goldwasser E, Fried W, et al. Role of the kidney in erythropoiesis. Nature 1957;179:633–4.
7. Miyake T, Kung CK, Goldwasser E. Purification of human erythropoietin. J Biol Chem 1977;252(15):5558–64.
8. Lin FK, Suggs S, Lin CH, et al. Cloning and expression of the human erythropoietin gene. Proc Natl Acad Sci U S A 1985;82(22):7580–4.
9. Jacobs K, Shoemaker C, Rudersdorf R, et al. Isolation and characterization of genomic and cDNA clones of human erythropoietin. Nature 1995;313(6005):806–10.

10. Jelkmann W. Erythropoietin. J Endocrinol Invest 2003;26(9):832–7.
11. Jelkmann W. Regulation of erythropoietin production. J Physiol 2011;589(Pt 6): 1251–8.
12. Warnecke C, Zaborowska Z, Kurreck J, et al. Differentiating the functional role of hypoxia-inducible factor (HIF)-1α and HIF-2α (EPAS-1) by the use of RNA interference:erythropoietin is a HIF-2α target gene in Hep3B and Kelly cells. FASEB J 2004;18:1462–4.
13. Broudy VC, Lin N, Brice M, et al. Erythropoietin receptor characteristics on primary human erythroid cells. Blood 1991;77(12):2583–2V590.
14. Vincent JL, Baron J-F, Reinhart K, et al. Anemia and blood transfusion in critically ill patients. JAMA 2002;288(12):1499–507.
15. Corwin HL, Gettinger A, Pearl RG, et al. The CRIT Study: anemia and blood transfusion in the critically ill–current clinical practice in the United States. Crit Care Med 2004;32(1):39–52.
16. Nguyen BV, Bota DP, Melot C, et al. Time course of hemoglobin concentrations in nonbleeding intensive care unit patients. Crit Care Med 2003;31(2):406–10.
17. Rodriguez RM, Corwin HL, Gettinger A, et al. Nutritional deficiencies and blunted erythropoietin response as causes of the anemia of critical illness. J Crit Care 2001;16(1):36–41.
18. Blanc B, Finch CA, Hallberg L, et al. Nutritional anaemias. Report of a WHO Scientific Group. World Health Organ Tech Rep Ser 1968;405:1–40.
19. Eckardt K-U. Anaemia of critical illness– implications for understanding and treating rHuEPO resistance. Nephrol Dial Transplant 2002;17(Suppl 5):48–55.
20. Marik PE, Corwin HL. Efficacy of red blood cell transfusion in the critically ill: a systematic review of the literature. Crit Care Med 2008;36(9):2667–74.
21. Rüttinger D, Wolf H, Kuchenhoff H, et al. Red cell transfusion: an essential factor for patient prognosis in surgical critical illness? Shock 2007;28(2):165–71.
22. National Blood Authority of Australia. Patient blood management guidelines module 4- critical care. National Blood Authority; 2012. ISBN 978-0-9872519-9-2.
23. Cazzola M. How and when to use erythropoietin. Curr Opin Hematol 1998;5(2): 103–8.
24. Krafte-Jacobs B. Anemia of critical illness and erythropoietin deficiency. Intensive Care Med 1997;23(2):137–8.
25. Krafte-Jacobs B, Levetown ML, Bray GL, et al. Erythropoietin response to critical illness. Crit Care Med 1994;22(5):821–6.
26. Rogiers P, Zhang H, Leeman M, et al. Erythropoietin response is blunted in critically ill patients. Intensive Care Med 1997;23(2):159–62.
27. Corwin HL, Gettinger A, Rodriguez RM, et al. Efficacy of recombinant human erythropoietin in the critically ill patient: a randomized, double-blind, placebo-controlled trial. Crit Care Med 1999;27(11):2346–50.
28. Corwin HL, Gettinger A, Pearl RG, et al. Efficacy of recombinant human erythropoietin in critically ill patients: a randomized controlled trial. JAMA 2002;288(22): 2827–35.
29. Corwin HL, Gettinger A, Fabian TC, et al. Efficacy and safety of epoetin alfa in critically ill patients. N Engl J Med 2007;357:965–76.
30. Hebert PC, Wells G, Blajchman MA, et al. A multicenter, randomized, controlled clinical trial of transfusion requirements in critical care. Transfusion Requirements in Critical Care Investigators, Canadian Critical Care Trials Group. N Engl J Med 1999;340(6):409–17.
31. Nekoui A, Blaise G. Erythropoietin and nonhematopoietic effects. Am J Med Sci 2017;353(1):76–81.

32. Brines M, Cerami A. The receptor that tames the innate immune response. Mol Med 2012;18:486–96.
33. Leist M, Ghezzi P, Grasso G, et al. Derivatives of erythropoietin that are tissue protective but not erythropoietic. Science 2004;305:239–42.
34. Shein NA, Horowitz M, Alexandrovich AG, et al. Heat acclimation increases hypoxia-inducible factor 1alpha and erythropoietin receptor expression. J Cereb Blood Flow Metab 2005;25(11):1456–65.
35. Collino M, Thiemermann C, Cerami A, et al. Flipping the molecular switch for innate protection and repair of tissues: long-lasting effects of a non-erythropoietic small peptide engineered from erythropoietin. Pharmacol Ther 2015;151:32–40.
36. Bohr S, Patel SJ, Vasko R, et al. Modulation of cellular stress response via the erythropoietin/CD131 heteroreceptor complex in mouse mesenchymal-derived cells. J Mol Med (Berl) 2015;93(2):199–210.
37. Brines M, Grasso G, Fiordaliso F, et al. Erythropoietin mediates tissue protection through an erythropoietin and common beta-subunit heteroreceptor. Proc Natl Acad Sci U S A 2004;101(41):14907–12.
38. Xu X, Cao Z, Cao B, et al. Carbamylated erythropoietin protects the myocardium from acute ischemia/reperfusion injury through a PI3K/Akt-dependent mechanism. Surgery 2009;146(3):506–14.
39. Kitamura H, Isaka Y, Takabatake Y, et al. Nonerythropoietic derivative of erythropoietin protects against tubulointerstitial injury in a unilateral ureteral obstruction model. Nephrol Dial Transplant 2008;23(5):1521–8.
40. Su KH, Shyue SK, Kou YR, et al. β common receptor integrates the erythropoietin signaling in activation of endothelial nitricoxide synthase. J Cell Physiol 2011;226(12):3330–9.
41. Collino M, Benetti E, Rogazzo M, et al. A nonerythropoietic peptide derivative of erythropoietin decreases susceptibility to diet-induced insulin resistance in mice. Br J Pharmacol 2014;171(24):5802–15.
42. Kilic E, Kilic U, Soliz J, et al. Brain-derived erythropoietin protects from focal cerebral ischemia by dual activation of ERK-1/-2 and Akt pathways. FASEB J 2005;19(14):2026–8.
43. Lapchak PA. Erythropoietin molecules to treat acute ischemic stroke: a translational dilemma! Expert Opin Investig Drugs 2010;19(10):1179–86.
44. Blixt J, Gunnarson E, Wanecek M. Erythropoietin attenuates the brain edema response after experimental traumatic brain injury. J Neurotrauma 2018;35(4):671–80.
45. Coldewey SM, Khan AI, Kapoor A, et al. Erythropoietin attenuates acute kidney dysfunction in murine experimental sepsis by activation of the beta-common receptor. Kidney Int 2013;84(3):482–90.
46. Nakano M, Satoh K, Fukumoto Y, et al. Important role of erythropoietin receptor to promote VEGF expression and angiogenesis in peripheral ischemia in mice. Circ Res 2007;100(5):662–9.
47. Haroon ZA, Amin K, Jiang X, et al. A novel role for erythropoietin during fibrin-induced wound-healing response. Am J Pathol 2003;163(3):993–1000, 5802–5815.
48. Brines M, Cerami A. Erythropoietin-mediated tissue protection: reducing collateral damage from the primary injury response. J Intern Med 2008;264:405–32.
49. Meng Y, Xiong Y, Mahmood A, et al. Dose-dependent neurorestorative effects of delayed treatment of traumatic brain injury with recombinant human erythropoietin in rats. J Neurosurg 2011;115(3):550–60.

50. Injuries and violence: the facts 2014. World Health Organization; 2014. ISBN 978 924150801 8.
51. Mathers CD, Loncar D. Projections of global mortality and burden of disease from 2002 to 2030. PLoS Med 2006;3:e442.
52. The global burden of disease. Geneva (Switzerland): World Health Organisation; 2012.
53. Napolitano LM, Fabian TC, Kelly KM, et al. Improved survival of critically ill trauma patients treated with recombinant human erythropoietin. J Trauma 2008;65(2): 285–9.
54. Nichol A, French C, Little L, et al. Erythropoietin in traumatic brain injury (EPO-TBI): a double-blind randomised controlled trial. Lancet 2015;386:2499–506.
55. Skrifvars MB, Bailey M, French C, et al. Erythropoietin in patients with traumatic brain injury and extracranial injury-A post hoc analysis of the erythropoietin traumatic brain injury trial. J Trauma Acute Care Surg 2017;83(3):449–56.
56. Skrifvars MB, French C, Bailey M, et al. Cause and timing of death and sub-group differential effects of erythropoietin in the EPO-TBI study. J Neurotrauma 2018; 35(2):333–40.
57. Knott RJ, Harris A, Higgins A, et al. Cost-effectiveness of erythropoietin in traumatic brain injury (EPO-TBI): a multinational trial based economic analysis, in press.
58. French CJ, Glassford NJ, Gantner D, et al. Erythropoiesis-stimulating agents in critically ill trauma patients: a systematic review and meta-analysis. Ann Surg 2017;265:54–62.
59. Li ZM, Xiao YL, Zhu JX, et al. Recombinant human erythropoietin improves functional recovery in patients with severe traumatic brain injury: a randomized, double blind and controlled clinical trial. Clin Neurol Neurosurg 2016;150:80–3.
60. Robertson CS, Hannay HJ, Yamal JM, et al. Effect of erythropoietin and transfusion threshold on neurological recovery after traumatic brain injury: a randomized clinical trial. JAMA 2014;312:36–47.
61. Nirula R, Diaz-Arrastia R, Brasel K, et al. Safety and efficacy of erythropoietin in traumatic brain injury patients: a pilot randomized trial. Crit Care Res Pract 2010; 2010 [pii:209848].
62. Gantner D, Bailey M, Presneill J, et al. Erythropoietin to reduce mortality in traumatic brain injury-a post-hoc dose-effect analysis. Ann Surg 2018;267:585–9.
63. Skrifvars MB, Bailey M, Presneill J, et al. Venous thromboembolic events in critically ill traumatic brain injury patients. Intensive Care Med 2017;43(3):419–28.
64. Erbayraktar S, Grasso G, Sfacteria A, et al. Asialoerythropoietin is a nonerythropoietic cytokine with broad neuroprotective activity in vivo. Proc Natl Acad Sci U S A 2003;100(11):6741–6.
65. Niesters M, Swartjes M, Heij L, et al. The erythropoietin-analogue ARA 290 for treatment of sarcoidosis-induced chronic neuropathic pain. Exp Opin Orphan Drugs 2013;1:77–87.
66. Goldwasser E. A bloody long journey: erythropoietin (Epo) and the person who isolated. Bloomington (IN): Xlibiris; 2011.

Hemoglobin A1c and Permissive Hyperglycemia in Patients in the Intensive Care Unit with Diabetes

Anca Balintescu, MD[a], Johan Mårtensson, MD, PhD[b,c,]*

KEYWORDS

- Diabetes • HbA1c • Critical care • Hyperglycemia • Hypoglycemia
- Glucose variability

KEY POINTS

- Quantification of glycated hemoglobin A1c, a measure of the average blood glucose level over the prior 2 to 3 months, can identify intensive care unit patients with deranged chronic glycemic control.
- Hyperglycemia and glucose fluctuations are better tolerated by patients with elevated glycated hemoglobin A1c than by patients with normal or near normal glycated hemoglobin A1c.
- Iatrogenic hypoglycemia, a potentially fatal complication, is common and is associated with greater risks among critically ill patients with elevated glycated hemoglobin A1c.
- Permissive hyperglycemia (blood glucose target 10–14 mmol/L) effectively decreases the incidence of hypoglycemia among critically ill patients with elevated glycated hemoglobin A1c.

INTRODUCTION

There are nearly half a billion adults with diabetes mellitus worldwide.[1] But about one-half of them are still unaware of their disease. For that reason, the prevalence of diabetes among critically ill patients admitted to the intensive care unit (ICU) has

Disclosure Statement: The authors declare that they have no conflicts of interest.
[a] Department of Clinical Science and Education Södersjukhuset, Section of Anaesthesia and Intensive Care, Karolinska Institutet, Södersjukhuset, Sjukhusbacken 10, Stockholm 118 83, Sweden; [b] Department of Physiology and Pharmacology, Section of Anaesthesia and Intensive Care, Karolinska Institutet, Solnavägen 9, Stockholm, 171 65 Solna, Sweden; [c] Function Perioperative Medicine and Intensive Care, Karolinska University Hospital, Stockholm 171 76, Sweden
* Corresponding author. Function Perioperative Medicine and Intensive care, Karolinska University Hospital, Stockholm 171 76, Sweden.
E-mail address: johan.martensson@sll.se

Crit Care Clin 35 (2019) 289–300
https://doi.org/10.1016/j.ccc.2018.11.010
0749-0704/19/© 2018 Elsevier Inc. All rights reserved.

been difficult to estimate. After the introduction of glycated hemoglobin A1c (HbA1c) measurement, which quantifies chronic glycemic control, it seems that the diabetes prevalence has been grossly underestimated among ICU patients.[2,3]

Quantification of the level of chronic glycemia in the critically ill provides important clinical information. In those patients with premorbid chronic hyperglycemia (elevated HbA1c), the clinician should expect more severe critical illness-associated dysglycemia and a different response to standard glucose control in the ICU than in patients with chronic normoglycemia (HbA1c in the normal range).

Since the Normoglycemia in Intensive Care Evaluation Survival Using Glucose Algorithm Regulation (NICE-SUGAR) trial,[4] which showed increased risk of hypoglycemia and higher mortality with target glucose of 4.5 to 6.0 mmol/L as compared with 8 to 10 mmol/L, a more liberal glucose control strategy is recommended for ICU patients with or without diabetes.[5–7] However, the question is whether such liberal control is liberal enough for those patients with diabetes, who are adapted to chronic hyperglycemia. Novel evidence from observational studies suggests that such patients may benefit from even more liberal targets. However, definitive answers from randomized trials are needed.

In this narrative review, we discuss the impact of the premorbid chronic glucose control on key domains of glycemic control in the ICU (hyperglycemia, hypoglycemia, and glucose variability) and the interaction between premorbid glycemic control and the association between glucose regulation and clinical outcomes. Additionally, we summarize the existing evidence surrounding a more liberal glucose control strategy in critically ill patients with diabetes.

ASSESSING CHRONIC GLYCEMIA IN CRITICALLY ILL PATIENTS

The diagnosis of diabetes can be established by a blood glucose of 11.1 mmol/L or greater after a 75-g oral glucose load, a fasting blood glucose of 7.0 mmol/L or greater, a random glucose of 11.1 mmol/L or greater, or by an HbA1c of 6.5% or greater (Diabetes Control and Complications Trial unit) or 48 mmol/mol or greater (International Federation of Clinical Chemistry unit).[8] Acute illness precludes the use of blood glucose for establishing the diagnosis owing to a high incidence of stress-induced hyperglycemia. In contrast, because HbA1c is not affected by critical illness per se, it is a more appropriate measure of ICU patients' chronic glycemic state (**Fig. 1**).[9] Notably, HbA1c should be interpreted with caution in patients receiving blood transfusions, in those with hemoglobinopathies, during hemolysis, and in the setting of chronic alcohol consumption.[10]

The concentration of HbA1c in whole blood reflects the average blood glucose level over the prior 2 to 3 months and is widely used to monitor long-term glycemic control in people with diabetes. The average glucose concentration can be estimated (estimated average glucose [eAG]) from HbA1c and the following equation[11]:

$$eAG \ (mmol/L) = 1.59 \times HbA1c \ (\%) - 2.59$$

GLYCATED HEMOGLOBIN A1C, ACUTE HYPERGLYCEMIA, AND OUTCOME

Observational studies reliably show an independent association between hyperglycemia in the ICU and increased mortality in patients without diabetes.[12–17] Whether this is also true for patients with diabetes is controversial. In a study of almost 260,000 ICU admissions, Falciglia and colleagues[13] demonstrated progressively greater mortality risk with increasing mean glucose of greater than 6.1 mmol/L. Although still significant, the relationship was markedly attenuated among the 77,850 patients with diabetes. Similarly, in an analysis of more than 160,000 patients from the eICU Collaborative

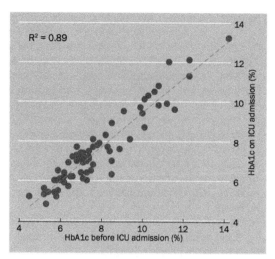

Fig. 1. Correlation between hemoglobin A1c (HbA1c) measured within 30 days before intensive care unit (ICU) admission and HbA1c measured on ICU admission. (*Data from* Luethi N, Cioccari L, Tanaka A, et al. Glycated hemoglobin A1c levels are not affected by critical illness. Crit Care Med 2016;44(9):1692–4.)

Research Database (16.7% had diabetes) a blood glucose level of greater than 10 mmol/L at any time in the ICU was independently associated with greater mortality and ICU length of stay.[17] Again, these associations were less pronounced among patients with diabetes than among those without diabetes. In contrast, hyperglycemia was not associated with mortality[12,14,16] or was associated with lower mortality[15] in other cohorts of critically ill patients with diabetes (**Table 1**).

Table 1
Association between hyperglycemia in intensive care unit and mortality in critically ill patients with diabetes

First Author, Year	Diabetes (n)	Blood Glucose, mmol/L		Association Between Hyperglycemia (vs Comparator) and Mortality
		Hyperglycemia	Comparator	
Whitcomb et al,[12] 2005[a]	574	>11.1	3.3–11.1	No significant association
Falciglia et al,[13] 2009[b]	77,850	>6.1	3.9–6.1	Hyperglycemia associated with higher mortality
Stegenga et al,[14] 2010[a]	188	>11.1	≤11.1	No significant association
Krinsley et al,[15] 2013[b]	12,880	>6.1	4.4–6.1	Hyperglycemia associated with lower mortality
Krinsley et al,[16] 2017[b]	1873	≥10	7.8–9.9	No significant association
Cichosz and Schaarup,[17] 2017[c]	27,458	>10	≤10	Hyperglycemia associated with higher mortality

[a] Study assessing blood glucose on intensive care unit admission.
[b] Study assessing mean glucose during the entire intensive care unit stay.
[c] Study assessing peak glucose during the entire intensive care unit stay.

The fact that the patients' premorbid level of glycemia was not considered in these studies may contribute to such contradictory findings. Indeed, emerging evidence suggest that premorbid glycemia (ie, HbA1c) modifies the relationship between hyperglycemia in ICU and mortality. Among 415 critically ill diabetes patients, an HbA1c of greater than 7% (vs ≤7%) was associated with progressively lower mortality if the mean glucose in ICU was greater than 10 mmol/L and greater mortality if mean glucose was less than 9 mmol/L (**Fig. 2**).[18] Additionally, Plummer and colleagues[19] demonstrated a 20% higher mortality risk for every 1 mmol/L increase in blood glucose above normoglycemia in patients without diabetes or in those with diabetes and an HbA1c of less than 7%. However, in patients with an HbA1c of 7% or greater, no association between any degree of acute hyperglycemia and mortality was found.[2] Finally, among patients with an HbA1c of greater than 8.5% in another study, no association between peak glucose and mortality was observed, not even when peak glucose reached 30 mmol/L.

These studies provide preliminary evidence that a level of hyperglycemia that is considered harmful in ICU patients without diabetes may be safe or even beneficial in ICU patients adapted to chronic hyperglycemia.

GLYCATED HEMOGLOBIN A1C, HYPOGLYCEMIA, AND OUTCOME

A decrease in blood glucose below normal levels (hypoglycemia) is associated with adverse clinical outcomes. Cardiac arrhythmias, myocardial infarction, seizures, stroke, and death have been associated with hypoglycemia in hospitalized and ambulant patients with diabetes.[20–23] In ICU patients, even moderate hypoglycemia (between 2.3 and 3.9 mmol/L) was independently associated with greater 90-day mortality, both in patients with and in those without diabetes.[24]

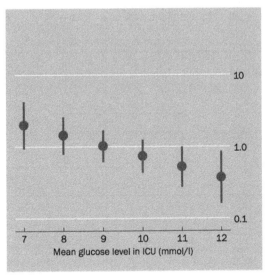

Fig. 2. Association between a high (>7%) versus low (≤7%) glycated hemoglobin A1c (HbA1c) and hospital mortality according to the average glucose level in intensive care unit (ICU) among 415 patients with diabetes. Values are adjusted odds ratios for hospital mortality. (*Data from* Egi M, Bellomo R, Stachowski E, et al. The interaction of chronic and acute glycemia with mortality in critically ill patients with diabetes. Crit Care Med 2011;39(1):105–11.)

Hypoglycemia triggers a myriad of neurohormonal counterregulatory responses such as a decrease in the secretion of insulin and an increase in the release of endogenous adrenaline, noradrenaline, cortisol, growth hormone, and glucagon. This hormonal defense mechanism increases blood glucose via accelerated hepatic glucose production with the immediate aim to restore glucose supply to the brain.

Hypoglycemia-induced counterregulation is impaired in patients with beta-cell failure (established type 1 diabetes or advanced type 2 diabetes). Because circulating insulin levels depend entirely on the absorption and clearance of administered insulin in such patients, their plasma insulin concentration will not decrease in response to hypoglycemia. Attenuated counterregulatory release of glucagon (owing to alpha-cell failure) and adrenaline is another feature in patients with beta-cell failure.[25] In response to such counterregulatory deficiency, patients with beta-cell failure are at significantly greater risk of iatrogenic hypoglycemia than those with preserved beta-cell function.

The critical level at which hypoglycemia-induced counterregulation occurs depends on the level of chronic glycemia. In patients without diabetes, counterregulatory responses occur just below the lower limit of normal blood glucose, that is, at 3.9 mmol/L or less,[26] a threshold that is typically used to define hypoglycemia. However, patients with poorly controlled diabetes are adapted to chronic hyperglycemia. In such patients, counterregulatory activation may occur already when blood glucose decreases to levels within the physiologic blood glucose concentration range,[26–31] so-called relative hypoglycemia.[32]

In addition to tight glycemic control,[24] greater HbA1c is independently associated with a greater risk of developing hypoglycemia.[33] For example, in a recent multicenter study of more than 3000 critically ill patients exposed to conventional glucose control (target blood glucose of 6–10 mmol/L), hypoglycemia (blood glucose of <3.9 mmol/L) occurred in 5% of those with an HbA1c of less than 6.5% whereas 1 in 5 patients with an HbA1c of 8% or greater developed hypoglycemia.[34] Importantly, patients with an HbA1c of 8% or greater also had a higher adjusted risk of death than patients with lower HbA1c at the same level of hypoglycemia (**Fig. 3**).

Several factors may explain why hypoglycemia is more dangerous among those patients who are exposed to chronic hyperglycemia before ICU admission. First, the distance between their eAG and the hypoglycemic threshold of 3.9 mmol/L (glycemic distance = eAG − 3.9) is greater than in patients with chronic normoglycemia. This glycemic distance would, for example, be 6 mmol/L in a patient with an HbA1c of 8% (eAG of 10 mmol/L) but only 3 mmol/L in a patient with an HbA1c of 6.0% (eAG of 7 mmol/L). A greater distance does indeed lead to a greater hypoglycemia-induced stress response.[27]

Second, as discussed elsewhere in this article, the release of stress hormones may occur already when the level of normoglycemia is reached in patients with chronic hyperglycemia. Hence, as blood glucose continues to decrease below 3.9 mmol/L, the stress response duration will be prolonged in such patients.[27]

Finally, patients with chronic hyperglycemia are likely have more advanced diabetes, more pronounced beta-cell failure, and an impaired counterregulatory defense against hypoglycemia. Their ability to accelerate endogenous glucose production is therefore impaired, which increases the risk that blood glucose continues to decrease before hypoglycemia is detected and treated.

Since the publication of NICE-SUGAR, the implementation of more liberal glucose control has decreased the incidence of hypoglycemia in the ICU.[4] The incidence remains, however, unacceptably high among patients with elevated HbA1c.[34] Future trials need to assess whether the use of continuous glucose monitoring[35] and/or

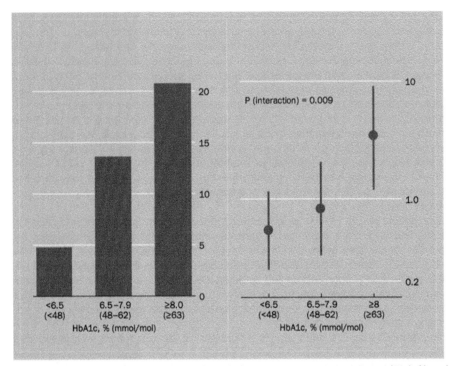

Fig. 3. Prevalence (%) of hypoglycemia (blood glucose concentration <3.9 mmol/L; *left*) and association adjusted odds ratio between hypoglycemia and hospital mortality (*right*) according to preadmission glycated hemoglobin A1c (HbA1c) level among 3084 critically ill patients. (*Data from* Egi M, Krinsley JS, Maurer P, et al. Pre-morbid glycemic control modifies the interaction between acute hypoglycemia and mortality. Intensive Care Med 2016;42(4):562–71.)

permissive hyperglycemia above 10 mmol/L can further decrease hypoglycemia incidence and whether such strategies will improve patient outcomes.

GLYCATED HEMOGLOBIN A1C, GLUCOSE VARIABILITY, AND OUTCOME

In addition to hyperglycemia and hypoglycemia, acute fluctuation in blood glucose (glucose variability) is a major feature of critical illness-associated dysglycemia. Emerging experimental and clinical evidence suggest harmful effects of glucose fluctuations independent of other glucose metrics.

In a study of 21 ambulant patients with type 2 diabetes, Monnier and colleagues[36] used continuous glucose monitoring to assess the contribution of mean glucose over 24 hours and glucose variability to oxidative stress (urinary excretion of 8-iso prostaglandin F2α [8-iso PGF2α]). In their multivariable linear regression analysis they found that glucose variability but not mean glucose was independently associated with greater excretion of urinary 8-iso PGF2α.

In a subsequent experimental study, Ceriello and colleagues[37] studied the effect of glucose variability compared with stable hyperglycemia on oxidative stress (plasma nitrotyrosine and urinary 8-iso PGF2α) and endothelial function (flow-mediated dilation of the brachial artery) in 12 healthy subject and 15 ambulant patients with diabetes (mean HbA1c of 7.7%) over 48 hours. Compared with stable hyperglycemia at 10 and

15 mmol/L, glucose fluctuations between 5 and 15 mmol/L resulted in greater endothelial dysfunction and oxidative stress in patients with or without diabetes. This effect was, however, more pronounced in the nondiabetic cohort.

In 2006, Egi and coworkers[38] demonstrated that, among 7000 patients from 4 ICUs, the standard deviation of blood glucose concentrations was associated with greater ICU mortality independent of illness severity and mean and peak glucose level (adjusted odds ratio, 1.28; 95% confidence interval, 1.14–1.44).

Additionally, Ali and coworkers[39] found an association between higher glycemic lability index, another measure of glucose variability, and hospital mortality among 1200 septic patients after adjusting for hypoglycemia, diabetes, insulin therapy, and number of organ failures. However, this association was only significant among patients with an average glucose level of less than 7.4 mmol/L.

Finally, Krinsley and coworkers[40] found that a standard deviation of glucose of greater than 27.7 mmol/L was independently associated with increased mortality, even after excluding patients with severe hypoglycemia. In all, these studies suggest that the average glucose level or the occurrence of hyperglycemia or hypoglycemia is not responsible for the relationship between glucose variability and mortality.

Despite evidence suggesting an independent association between glucose variability and oxidative stress in ambulant patients, critically ill patients with diabetes seem to be somewhat protected against the harmful effects of large glucose fluctuations. In fact, multiple studies have shown that the independent association between glucose variability and mortality is lost or at least markedly attenuated when diabetes patients are studied separately.[15,16,19,41] Furthermore, Plummer and coworkers[19] demonstrated a significant interaction between premorbid glycemic control (HbA1c) and the association between glucose variability and hospital mortality. Specifically, they found that this association was only evident among those patients with an HbA1c of 8.5% or greater,[19] further supporting the view that patients with insufficient chronic glycemic control may be adapted to and tolerate large glucose swings.

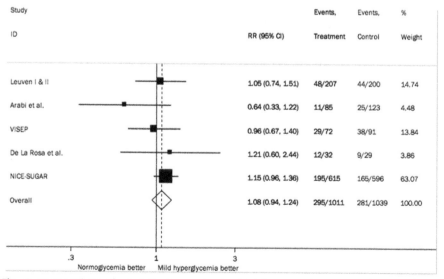

Fig. 4. Metaanalysis of mortality in randomized trials comparing normoglycemia (treatment) with mild hyperglycemia (control) in the subgroup of critically ill patients with diabetes.

Table 2
Before-and-after studies comparing liberal and conventional glucose targets in patients with diabetes

First Author, Year	n	HbA1c, %	Glucose Target, mmol/l		Main Findings
			Conventional	Liberal	
Kar et al,[46] 2016	83	≥7	6–10	10–14	Decreased risk of hypoglycemia (RR, 0.47; P = .09) and glucose variability (CV, 23.8% vs 33.2%; P<.01) with liberal control
Di Muzio et al,[32] 2016	80	All	6–10	10–14	Reduced incidence of relative hypoglycemia (22.5% vs 50.0%; P = .01) with liberal control
Luethi et al,[47] 2018	700	All	6–10	10–14	Reduced glucose variability (GLI, 59 vs 66 [mmol/l]²/h/wk; P = .02) with liberal control
Luethi et al,[47] 2018	314	≥7	6–10	10–14	Decreased incidence or hypoglycemia (4.1% vs 9.5%; P = .05) with liberal control

Abbreviations: CV, coefficient of variation; GLI, glucose lability index; HbA1c, glycated hemoglobin A1c; RR, relative risk.

PERMISSIVE HYPERGLYCEMIA

The diabetes prevalence was low (<20%) in previous randomized ICU trials comparing normoglycemia with mild hyperglycemia. Although the outcome effect did not reach statistical significance in any of the diabetic cohorts of the 5 trials,[4,42–45] the pooled relative risk (relative risk, 1.08; 95% confidence interval, 0.94–1.24) favors mild hyperglycemia (**Fig. 4**).

Since 2016, 3 before-and-after studies have compared liberal (blood glucose target 10–14 mmol/L) with conventional (blood glucose target 6–10 mmol/L) glucose control in ICU patients with diabetes (**Table 2**). Di Muzio and coworkers[32] found that such liberal control significantly decreased insulin requirements and the incidence of relative hypoglycemia (defined as a >30% decrease in blood glucose relative the premorbid eAG level). Additionally, Kar and coworkers[46] found that liberal control decreased the occurrence of hypoglycemia (relative risk, 0.47; $P = .09$) and attenuated glucose variability in 83 patients with an HbA1c of 7% or greater.

Finally, in a before-and-after study including 700 ICU patients with diabetes, Luethi and coworkers[47] assessed the effect of liberal control on various glucose metrics and exploratory clinical outcomes. Overall, they observed no significant effect on hypoglycemia incidence. However, among patients with an HbA1c of 7% or greater, the implementation of liberal control decreased the incidence of hypoglycemia from 9.5% to 4.1% ($P = .05$). The glycemic lability index was also lower during the liberal control period. Finally, the authors found no independent association between liberal control and mortality, duration of mechanical ventilation, ICU-free days to day 30, changes in serum creatinine, or white cell count.

In their aggregate, these studies provide preliminary evidence that more liberal glucose targets between 10 and 14 mmol/L attenuates both glucose variability and the risk of hypoglycemia in patients with an HbA1c of greater than 7%. In addition, they suggest that exposure to such liberal control may be safe in critically ill patients with diabetes.

However, these observational studies do not provide sufficient high-quality evidence to recommend a practice change. Therefore, the feasibility, safety, and potential clinical efficacy of liberal glucose control must be confirmed or refuted by adequately powered randomized controlled trials. Until the results of such trials have been published, we suggest that blood glucose be frequently monitored and that blood glucose be kept in the upper target blood glucose range of 6 to 10 mmol/L to minimize the risk of hypoglycemia in patients with elevated HbA1c.

SUMMARY

A significant proportion of patients with diabetes who are admitted to the ICU have elevated HbA1c indicating that they are adapted to a chronic hyperglycemic state. Compared with patients without diabetes and those with well-controlled diabetes, patients with poor diabetic control respond differently to critical illness-associated dysglycemia. Although they seem to tolerate hyperglycemia and fluctuating blood glucose concentrations, the risks associated with hypoglycemia are markedly greater among patients with an elevated HbA1c. Novel observational evidence suggests that permissive hyperglycemia (blood glucose target of 10–14 mmol/L) is safe and reduces the risk of hypoglycemia among critically ill patients with an HbA1c of greater than 7%. The safety and clinical benefits, if any, of permissive hyperglycemia must be further assessed in randomized controlled trials.

REFERENCES

1. Cho NH, Shaw JE, Karuranga S, et al. IDF diabetes atlas: global estimates of diabetes prevalence for 2017 and projections for 2045. Diabetes Res Clin Pract 2018;138:271–81.
2. Plummer MP, Bellomo R, Cousins CE, et al. Dysglycaemia in the critically ill and the interaction of chronic and acute glycaemia with mortality. Intensive Care Med 2014;40(7):973–80.
3. Carpenter DL, Gregg SR, Xu K, et al. Prevalence and impact of unknown diabetes in the ICU. Crit Care Med 2015;43(12):e541–50.
4. Finfer S, Chittock DR, Su SY, et al. Intensive versus conventional glucose control in critically ill patients. N Engl J Med 2009;360(13):1283–97.
5. Rhodes A, Evans LE, Alhazzani W, et al. Surviving Sepsis Campaign: international guidelines for management of sepsis and septic shock: 2016. Intensive Care Med 2017;43(3):304–77.
6. Moghissi ES, Korytkowski MT, DiNardo M, et al. American Association of Clinical Endocrinologists and American Diabetes Association consensus statement on inpatient glycemic control. Endocr Pract 2009;15(4):353–69.
7. Nolan JP, Soar J, Cariou A, et al. European Resuscitation Council and European Society of Intensive Care Medicine Guidelines for post-resuscitation care 2015: section 5 of the European Resuscitation Council Guidelines for Resuscitation 2015. Resuscitation 2015;95:202–22.
8. American Diabetes Association. 2. Classification and diagnosis of diabetes: standards of medical care in diabetes-2018. Diabetes Care 2018;41(Suppl 1): S13–27.
9. Luethi N, Cioccari L, Tanaka A, et al. Glycated hemoglobin A1c levels are not affected by critical illness. Crit Care Med 2016;44(9):1692–4.
10. Gallagher EJ, Le Roith D, Bloomgarden Z. Review of hemoglobin A(1c) in the management of diabetes. J Diabetes 2009;1(1):9–17.
11. Nathan DM, Kuenen J, Borg R, et al. Translating the A1C assay into estimated average glucose values. Diabetes Care 2008;31(8):1473–8.
12. Whitcomb BW, Pradhan EK, Pittas AG, et al. Impact of admission hyperglycemia on hospital mortality in various intensive care unit populations. Crit Care Med 2005;33(12):2772–7.
13. Falciglia M, Freyberg RW, Almenoff PL, et al. Hyperglycemia-related mortality in critically ill patients varies with admission diagnosis. Crit Care Med 2009;37(12): 3001–9.
14. Stegenga ME, Vincent JL, Vail GM, et al. Diabetes does not alter mortality or hemostatic and inflammatory responses in patients with severe sepsis. Crit Care Med 2010;38(2):539–45.
15. Krinsley JS, Egi M, Kiss A, et al. Diabetic status and the relation of the three domains of glycemic control to mortality in critically ill patients: an international multicenter cohort study. Crit Care 2013;17(2):R37.
16. Krinsley JS, Maurer P, Holewinski S, et al. Glucose control, diabetes status, and mortality in critically ill patients: the continuum from intensive care unit admission to hospital discharge. Mayo Clin Proc 2017;92(7):1019–29.
17. Cichosz SL, Schaarup C. Hyperglycemia as a predictor for adverse outcome in ICU patients with and without diabetes. J Diabetes Sci Technol 2017;11(6):1272–3.
18. Egi M, Bellomo R, Stachowski E, et al. The interaction of chronic and acute glycemia with mortality in critically ill patients with diabetes. Crit Care Med 2011; 39(1):105–11.

19. Plummer MP, Finnis ME, Horsfall M, et al. Prior exposure to hyperglycaemia attenuates the relationship between glycaemic variability during critical illness and mortality. Crit Care Resusc 2016;18(3):189–97.

20. Turchin A, Matheny ME, Shubina M, et al. Hypoglycemia and clinical outcomes in patients with diabetes hospitalized in the general ward. Diabetes Care 2009; 32(7):1153–7.

21. Hsu PF, Sung SH, Cheng HM, et al. Association of clinical symptomatic hypoglycemia with cardiovascular events and total mortality in type 2 diabetes: a nationwide population-based study. Diabetes Care 2013;36(4):894–900.

22. Chow E, Bernjak A, Williams S, et al. Risk of cardiac arrhythmias during hypoglycemia in patients with type 2 diabetes and cardiovascular risk. Diabetes 2014; 63(5):1738–47.

23. Goto A, Arah OA, Goto M, et al. Severe hypoglycaemia and cardiovascular disease: systematic review and meta-analysis with bias analysis. BMJ 2013;347: f4533.

24. Finfer S, Liu B, Chittock DR, et al. Hypoglycemia and risk of death in critically ill patients. N Engl J Med 2012;367(12):1108–18.

25. Cryer PE. Mechanisms of hypoglycemia-associated autonomic failure in diabetes. N Engl J Med 2013;369(4):362–72.

26. Schwartz NS, Clutter WE, Shah SD, et al. Glycemic thresholds for activation of glucose counterregulatory systems are higher than the threshold for symptoms. J Clin Invest 1987;79(3):777–81.

27. Korzon-Burakowska A, Hopkins D, Matyka K, et al. Effects of glycemic control on protective responses against hypoglycemia in type 2 diabetes. Diabetes Care 1998;21(2):283–90.

28. Amiel SA, Sherwin RS, Simonson DC, et al. Effect of intensive insulin therapy on glycemic thresholds for counterregulatory hormone release. Diabetes 1988;37(7): 901–7.

29. Boyle PJ, Schwartz NS, Shah SD, et al. Plasma glucose concentrations at the onset of hypoglycemic symptoms in patients with poorly controlled diabetes and in nondiabetics. N Engl J Med 1988;318(23):1487–92.

30. Levy CJ, Kinsley BT, Bajaj M, et al. Effect of glycemic control on glucose counterregulation during hypoglycemia in NIDDM. Diabetes Care 1998;21(8):1330–8.

31. Spyer G, Hattersley AT, MacDonald IA, et al. Hypoglycaemic counter-regulation at normal blood glucose concentrations in patients with well controlled type-2 diabetes. Lancet 2000;356(9246):1970–4.

32. Di Muzio F, Presello B, Glassford NJ, et al. Liberal versus conventional glucose targets in critically ill diabetic patients: an exploratory safety cohort assessment. Crit Care Med 2016;44(9):1683–91.

33. Mahmoodpoor A, Hamishehkar H, Beigmohammadi M, et al. Predisposing factors for hypoglycemia and its relation with mortality in critically ill patients undergoing insulin therapy in an intensive care unit. Anesth Pain Med 2016;6(1): e33849.

34. Egi M, Krinsley JS, Maurer P, et al. Pre-morbid glycemic control modifies the interaction between acute hypoglycemia and mortality. Intensive Care Med 2016; 42(4):562–71.

35. Ancona P, Eastwood G, Lucchetta L, et al. The performance of flash glucose monitoring in critically ill patients with diabetes. Crit Care Resusc 2017;19:167–74.

36. Monnier L, Mas E, Ginet C, et al. Activation of oxidative stress by acute glucose fluctuations compared with sustained chronic hyperglycemia in patients with type 2 diabetes. JAMA 2006;295(14):1681–7.

37. Ceriello A, Esposito K, Piconi L, et al. Oscillating glucose is more deleterious to endothelial function and oxidative stress than mean glucose in normal and type 2 diabetic patients. Diabetes 2008;57(5):1349–54.

38. Egi M, Bellomo R, Stachowski E, et al. Variability of blood glucose concentration and short-term mortality in critically ill patients. Anesthesiology 2006;105(2): 244–52.

39. Ali NA, O'Brien JM Jr, Dungan K, et al. Glucose variability and mortality in patients with sepsis. Crit Care Med 2008;36(8):2316–21.

40. Krinsley JS. Glycemic variability: a strong independent predictor of mortality in critically ill patients. Crit Care Med 2008;36(11):3008–13.

41. Donati A, Damiani E, Domizi R, et al. Glycaemic variability, infections and mortality in a medical-surgical intensive care unit. Crit Care Resusc 2014;16(1):13–23.

42. Van den Berghe G, Wilmer A, Milants I, et al. Intensive insulin therapy in mixed medical/surgical intensive care units: benefit versus harm. Diabetes 2006; 55(11):3151–9.

43. Arabi YM, Dabbagh OC, Tamim HM, et al. Intensive versus conventional insulin therapy: a randomized controlled trial in medical and surgical critically ill patients. Crit Care Med 2008;36(12):3190–7.

44. Brunkhorst FM, Engel C, Bloos F, et al. Intensive insulin therapy and pentastarch resuscitation in severe sepsis. N Engl J Med 2008;358(2):125–39.

45. De La Rosa Gdel C, Donado JH, Restrepo AH, et al. Strict glycaemic control in patients hospitalised in a mixed medical and surgical intensive care unit: a randomised clinical trial. Crit Care 2008;12(5):R120.

46. Kar P, Plummer MP, Bellomo R, et al. Liberal glycemic control in critically ill patients with type 2 diabetes: an exploratory study. Crit Care Med 2016;44(9): 1695–703.

47. Luethi N, Cioccari L, Biesenbach P, et al. Liberal glucose control in ICU patients with diabetes: a before-and-after study. Crit Care Med 2018;46(6):935–42.

Osteoporosis and the Critically Ill Patient

Neil R. Orford, MBBS, FCICM, PhD[a,b,c,*], Julie A. Pasco, DipEd, PhD, MEpi[a,c,d,e], Mark A. Kotowicz, MBBS, FRACP[a,c,e]

KEYWORDS

- Critical illness • Long-term outcomes • Osteoporosis • Fracture • Bone loss
- Bone mineral density

KEY POINTS

- Improved survival after critical illness has led to recognition of impaired recovery following critical illness as a major public health problem.
- A consistent association between critical illness and accelerated bone loss has been described, including changes in bone turnover markers, bone mineral density, and fragility fracture rate.
- The exact role of biochemical changes to bone; changes to osteoclast and osteoblast number, maturation, and activity; and relative contributions of humoral and cytokine pathways remains unresolved.
- Assessment of the effect of antifracture agents on fracture rate and mortality in the high-risk population of postmenopausal women with prolonged ventilation is warranted.

INTRODUCTION

Incomplete recovery following critical illness is a major public health problem. Each year approximately 150,000 Australians are admitted to the intensive care unit (ICU)[1] and, as mortality from critical illness has declined, the consequences of delayed and compromised functional recovery over subsequent months to years has become apparent.[2] Globally, quality of survival has been identified as among the largest health challenges for critically ill patients.[3]

Disclosure Statement: Authors have nothing to disclose.
[a] University Hospital Geelong, Barwon Health, Bellerine St, Geelong, VIC 3220, Australia; [b] Australian and New Zealand Intensive Care Research Centre (ANZIC-RC), Department of Epidemiology and Preventive Medicine (DEPM), Monash University, 553 St Kilda Rd, Melbourne, VIC 3004, Australia; [c] School of Medicine, Deakin University, 75 Pigdons Rd, Geelong, VIC 3216, Australia; [d] Department of Epidemiology and Preventive Medicine (DEPM), Monash University, Wellington Rd, Clayton, VIC 3800, Australia; [e] Department of Medicine, Melbourne Medical School-Western Campus, The University of Melbourne, McKechnie St, St Albans, VIC 3021, Australia
* Corresponding author. University Hospital Geelong, Barwon Health, Bellerine St, Geelong, VIC 3220, Australia.
E-mail address: neilo@barwonhealth.org.au

Crit Care Clin 35 (2019) 301–313
https://doi.org/10.1016/j.ccc.2018.11.006   criticalcare.theclinics.com

Osteoporosis is a chronic progressive disease and major public health issue, characterized by low bone mass, microarchitectural bone disruption, and skeletal fragility leading to fracture.[4] The lifetime risk of osteoporotic spine, hip, or wrist fracture is 30% to 40% in developed countries, and the lifetime risk of hip fracture is 1 in 6 in white females, with significant associated health burden of mortality, morbidity, and cost.[5-8] With 50% to 95% of those affected by osteoporosis not investigated or treated[5] and an annual cost of fractures exceeding 3.8 billion AUD in Australia,[6] 37 billion EUR in Europe, and 19 billion USD in the United States[7] in 2017, osteoporosis remains an important underdiagnosed and undertreated public health burden.[4]

Over the last decade a consistent association between critical illness and accelerated bone loss has been described, including changes in bone turnover markers (BTMs), bone mineral density (BMD), and fragility fracture rate.[8-10] In addition, an association between bone loss and increased mortality has been described in this population, as it has in the general population with and without fractures.[9-11] This article summarizes the current evidence for critical illness–associated bone loss, subsequent fracture and mortality, and future directions for research.

Bone Turnover Markers and Critical Illness

Bone is continually being remodeled to adapt to altered mechanical loading, repair microdamage, and meet requirements of mineral homeostasis, with a cycle of formation and resorption that is closely regulated and influenced by mechanical and biochemical factors.[11] Over the last 2 decades, the ability to measure the rate and direction of bone metabolic activity has become possible through the development of commercially available BTM tests.[12] These tests are divided into 2 categories, measures of bone resorption and measures of bone formation, providing a method to predict the rate of bone loss, subsequent fracture risk, and treatment response in clinical trials.[3,4]

Uncoupling of bone resorption and formation occurs in numerous conditions, including menopause, myeloma, rheumatoid arthritis, bone metastases, suppression of sex hormones (androgen deprivation therapy for prostate cancer in men and hormonal therapies for breast cancer in women), and in the presence of proinflammatory cytokines (interleukin [IL]-1, tumor necrosis factor [TNF]).[13] Estrogen deficiency increases the rate of remodeling and the volume of bone resorption by prolonging the lifespan of osteoclasts and decreasing the lifespan of osteoblasts. This leads to trabecular thinning, loss of connectivity between trabeculae, cortical thinning, and increased cortical porosity. As a result, bone fragility is more common in women than men, partly because the production of sex hormones does not decrease rapidly in men, with no subsequent increase in remodeling rate.

A systematic review in 2014[10] identified 10 studies[14-23] that described BTMs as an outcome in critically ill adults ventilated for greater than 24 hours.[10] Overall, these studies consistently reported an association between critical illness and BTMs consistent with uncoupling of bone formation and resorption. This includes an increase in osteoclastic bone resorption markers consistent with an increase in immature osteoblast number and activity, and reduced activity of mature osteoblasts. The relationship between duration of critical illness, sepsis, inflammation, loss of hypothalamic-pituitary axis pulsatility, and increase in BTMs has been explored. However, these relationships are only partially understood, with the confounding effects of premorbid disease, organ failure, and medications incompletely addressed.

Several studies have since added to the evidence of association between critical illness and change in BTMs. A prospective observational study of critically ill adults described an increase in the bone resorption marker serum collagen type 1 cross-linked c-telopeptide (CTX) during ICU admission, with median levels greater than the upper quartile normal range, returning to normal by 1 year. In contrast, the bone formation marker procollagen type 1 N-terminal propeptide (P1NP), was within normal limits during ICU admission and at 1 year, although median levels significantly increased during this time.[8] The Correction of Vitamin D Deficiency in Critically Ill Patients (VITdAL-ICU) study,[24] an interventional vitamin D3 randomized controlled trial in critically ill adults, reported increased CTX levels from day 1 of enrollment in ICU to day 28, normalizing by 6-months. Levels of osteocalcin (OC), a bone formation marker, were decreased during days 1 to 28, and normalized by 6 months. A prospective observational study of 28 adults with prolonged critical illness reported elevated CTX levels in 45% of subjects at admission, increasing to more than 80% of subjects in week 1 and 2, and more than 50% of subjects at week 5. In contrast, P1NP levels were reduced in 55% of subjects at admission to ICU and 10% of subjects by week 5.[25] A randomized controlled trial of ibandronate compared with placebo in 20 post-menopausal women with an ICU length of stay of greater than 5 days, reported increased serum CTX levels and reduced OC levels at entry into the study.[26] Finally, a prospective observational study reported serum sclerostin levels at admission and at 1 week, in 264 critically ill adults admitted to a medical ICU.[27] Sclerostin is a protein produced exclusively in the skeleton by osteocytes and a key negative regulator of bone formation. It acts through inhibition of the Wnt pathway, inhibiting terminal differentiation of osteoblasts and promoting apoptosis.[12] Overall serum sclerostin levels were increased on admission to ICU compared with controls and increased further over the following week. Levels varied with severity of illness, with significantly higher levels in patient with an Acute Physiology and Chronic Health Evaluation (APACHE) II score greater than 20 compared with less than 20. Increased levels were associated with the presence of liver cirrhosis and endstage renal disease.

There are several questions remaining about the use and understanding of BTMs in critically ill populations. First, the limitations to measurement and interpretation of BTMs in the critical care setting are unresolved. These include the effect of preanalytic variation due to nutrition delivery, body fluid compartment changes, organ dysfunction, circadian rhythm, and changes to protein binding.[12] Second, the relationship between elevated BTMs and subsequent fracture risk[12] and mortality,[9,10,28] described in noncritically ill patients, has not been established in critical illness.

In summary, the pattern of BTMs observed during and after critical illness is consistent with uncoupling of bone formation and resorption. This is characterized by accelerated bone loss beginning early in critical illness, persisting for weeks to months, and normalizing over the following year. In contrast, bone formation remains within normal limits. Although there are associations with duration of critical illness, sepsis, and inflammation, more data are required to understand the magnitude and duration of change, effect of confounding factors, and effect of critical illness on synthesis and clearance of markers independent of effects on bone formation and resorption.

Preclinical Studies

Over the last 5 years, animal and in vitro studies have begun to explore the mechanistic model of critical care–associated bone loss. A human in vitro model described several critical illness related osteoclast and angiogenic abnormalities.[20] The investigators reported an increase in peripheral blood mononuclear cells (PMNCs) primed to differentiate into mature osteoclasts in the blood of critically ill patients. The activity of mature osteoclasts depended on the presence of the circulating humoral factors receptor activator of nuclear factor kappa-B ligand (RANKL) and macrophage colony-stimulating factor (M-CSF). This activity was not suppressed by anticytokine (IL-6 and TNF-α) antibodies but was suppressed through blocking the low affinity IgG Fc receptor (FcɣRIII),

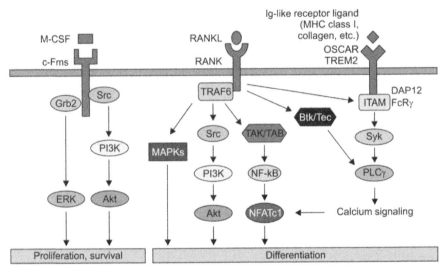

Fig. 1. Osteoclast differentiation pathways. c-Fms, M-CSF receptor; DAP12, nDNAX associated protein 12kD size; ERK, extracellular signal-regulated kinase; FcRγ: Fc Receptor; ITAM, immunoreceptor tyrosine-based activation motif; MAPK, mitogen-activated protein kinase; M-CSF, macrophage colony-stimulating factor; MHC, major histocompatibility complex; NFATc1, nuclear factor of activated T cells; NF-KB, nuclear factor-kB; OSCAR, osteoclast-associated receptor; PI3K, phosphatidylinositol 3-kinase; PLCγ, Phospholipase Cγ; RANK, receptor activator of nuclear factor-κ; RANKL: receptor activator of nuclear factor-κB ligand; TAK/TAB, TGF-B-activated kinase/TAK-1-binding protein; TRAF6, TNF receptor-associated factor 6; TREM2, triggering receptor expressed on myeloid cells 2. (*From* Kim JH, Kim N. Signaling pathways in osteoclast differentiation. Chonnam Med J 2016;52(1):12–6; with permission.)

an immunomodulatory tyrosine-based activation motif (ITAM) receptor (**Fig. 1**).[20,29] This suggests immunomodulatory factors may have an important role in critical illness osteoclast differentiation through noncanonical pathways. Finally, in a murine bone model, critical illness was associated with reduced angiogenesis factor expression, reduced mature bone formation, and reduced new vasculature formation.

The same investigators reported the effects of a rabbit burn model of critical illness on bone biochemistry and histomorphometry.[30] Critical illness was associated with a reduction in OC, decreased bone formation, and decreased trabecular tibial bone content and density. Surprisingly, there was no difference in the number and activity of osteoclasts compared with healthy controls. There was a decrease in early and late markers of osteoblast differentiation, and decreased expression of angiogenesis markers. Assessment of osteoclastogenesis found significant decrease in gene expression in the canonical pathway of RANKL, a trend to decreased osteoprotegerin (OPG) gene expression, with an unchanged OPG to RANKL ratio. In addition, gene expression of the noncanonical ITAM signaling pathway FcΥRIII and DAP12 (DNAX associated protein) receptors was significantly increased. This supports the hypothesis that FcΥRIII-positive monocytes, driven by circulating humoral factors and/or IgG antibodies through noncanonical ITAM signaling pathways, are an important pathway for osteoclastogenesis in critical illness, rather than canonical RANKL-OPG pathways.

A final animal model of critical illness bone loss study reported the mechanical, micro–computed tomography (CT), and bone histomorphometry effects in a rat model of sepsis at 24 and 96 hours.[31] Bone mechanical testing revealed no difference in femoral shaft strength, with a significantly decreased femoral neck fracture load. A rapid decrease on collagen elastic modulus occurred and slower decrease in mineral elastic modulus was observed. Interestingly, bone architecture and BMD were unchanged, as was morphometry. These findings suggest an early increase in bone fragility due to altered bone material properties, rather than osteoclast-driven bone turnover.

Overall, these studies provide improve evidence of the pathway for differentiation of PMNCs into mature active osteoclasts, and the relative role and interaction of canonical pathways, requiring the presence of RANKL or M-CSF, and noncanonical immunomodulatory ITAM pathways. They provide evidence of impaired angiogenesis and bone vascularization, and varied observations of reduced bone strength and mass during critical illness. The exact role of biochemical changes to bone; changes to osteoclast and osteoblast number, maturation, and activity; and relative contributions of humoral and cytokine pathways remains unresolved.

Bone Mineral Density and Critical Illness

The measurement of BMD by dual-energy X-ray absorptiometry (DXA) at the proximal femur and lumbar spine forms the basis of assessment and treatment of osteoporosis, with change in BMD estimated to account for 60% to 80% of variance in bone strength, and the central component of internationally agreed definitions of osteoporosis.[32] BMD values in individuals are expressed as an absolute value (grams per square centimeter), and in relation to a reference young adult population in standard deviation units, the T-score,[33] the basis of the World Health Organization (WHO) operational definition[34] of osteoporosis (T-score <–2.5), and osteopenia (T-score −2.5 to −1.0). In addition, BMD is used to assess response to treatment and as an outcome in antifracture trials.

Over the last 5 years, several studies have reported BMD measurements in critically ill patients. A prospective longitudinal cohort study described BMD trajectory for 1 and 2 years after critical illness.[8,35] In the year after critical illness, a significantly greater annual decrease in BMD was observed in subjects ventilated for greater than 24 hours who survived to ICU discharge compared with age-matched and sex-matched population controls[8] (**Table 1**). At ICU discharge, 45% of all subjects were osteopenic or osteoporotic, increasing to 55% at 1 year, with an increased proportion in women

Table 1
Annualized percent change in bone mineral density after critical illness compared with matched Geelong Osteoporosis Study controls

Variable	ICU	GOS	Difference (95% CI)	P Value
All	n = 66	n = 256	—	—
AP spine	−1.48 (4.37)	0.11 (1.12)	−1.59 (−2.18, −1.01)	<.001
Femur	−1.72 (3.43)	−0.53 (1.07)	−1.20 (−1.69, −0.70)	<.001
Women	n = 31	n = 120	—	—
AP spine	−2.85 (4.05)	−0.18 (1.08)	−2.67 (−3.49, −1.86)	<.001
Femur	−1.96 (4.03)	−0.65 (0.98)	−1.31 (−2.10, −0.51)	.001
Men	n = 35	n = 136	—	—
AP spine	−0.28 (4.34)	0.36 (1.10)	−0.64 (−1.45, 0.17)	.12
Femur	−1.52 (2.85)	−0.42 (1.13)	−1.10 (−1.7, −0.49)	<.001

Data are shown as mean plus standard deviation unless otherwise indicated.
Abbreviations: AP, anteroposterior; GOS, Geelong Osteoporosis Study.
From Orford NR, Lane SE, Bailey M, et al. Changes in bone mineral density in the year after critical illness. Am J Respir Crit Care Med 2016;193(7):736–44; Reprinted with permission of the American Thoracic Society. Copyright © 2018 American Thoracic Society. The American Journal of Respiratory and Critical Care Medicine is an official journal of the American Thoracic Society.

(ICU discharge 57%, 1 year 67%). The only other study to report T-score classification, the VITdAL-ICU study,[24] found 55% of all subjects were osteoporotic or osteopenic at a 6-month follow-up.

In the same cohort, participants not receiving antifracture treatment who completed 2-year post-ICU follow-up experienced ongoing loss of bone mass. In women, this was less in year 2 than in year 1 at both sites (femur year 1 at 2.8% ± 1.3% vs year 2 at 1.9% ± 0.7%, P = .6; spine year 1 at 4.8% ± 1.4% vs year 2 at 1.3% ± 1.8%, P = .08). In men, the annual decrease in femur BMD was significantly greater in year 2 than year 1 (femur year 1 at 1.9% ± 0.7% vs year 2 at 3.2% ± 0.7%, P = .03), with no difference in annual spine BMD change between year 1 and year 2 (spine year 1 at 0.0% ± 1.2% vs year 2 at 0.9% ± 1.5%, P = .6).[35]

No significant change in calcaneal BMD over a 10-day period was reported in a prospective study of critically ill subjects expected to be ventilated for greater than 48 hours. However, a significant decrease in BMD was observed in subjects with severe lung injury compared with ventilated control subjects (−2.81% vs +2.40%, P = .03).[36] Finally, a large retrospective cohort study of critically ill subjects with an ICU length of stay greater than 24 hours reported an overall 113% (± 19%) decrease in BMD per week.[37]

Overall, these studies describe accelerated loss of bone mass during and after critical illness, with the effect persisting for up to 2 years. In addition, a high proportion of patients are osteopenic or osteoporotic after ICU, suggesting a disease burden that may contribute to long-term morbidity and mortality. The factors that influence the trajectory of bone mass before and after critical illness have are not identified, partly due to the inherent difficulty performing long-term research in critically ill populations.

Critical Illness–Associated Fragility Fracture

The major consequence of accelerated bone loss is increased risk of fragility fracture and this has been described in critically ill patients.[9,38] An increased risk of fragility fracture was described in survivors of critical illness compared with age-matched and gender-matched population controls from a large population-based fracture study, the Geelong Osteoporosis Study (GOS).[9] The radiological databases of adult patients ventilated for greater than 24 hours who survived to ICU discharge were assessed for evidence of fragility fracture using the same ascertainment period as GOS. In the ICU survivor cohort, followed for a median of 3.7 years, 36 women (14.2%) sustained a fracture during the post-ICU time period, and an incident fracture rate of 3.84 (ICU survivors) and 2.41 (GOS controls) per 100 patient-years, respectively. In older women who survived ICU a significant increase in fracture rate and decreased time to fracture were observed compared with controls (hazard ratio 1.65, 95% CI 1.08–2.52) (P = .02).

A retrospective study of subjects admitted to ICU with a length of stay greater than 7 days, followed 178 matched to 2-year follow-up, and age-matched and gender-matched noncritically ill patients undergoing operations.[38] At 2 years the clinical fracture rate was 5% in the ICU group compared with 3.4% in the control group, with all fractures associated with falls. The risk of new fracture was 50% higher in the ICU cohort, although this was not significant (odds ratio 1.53, 95% CI 0.62–3.77, P = .35). The major limitation was the fracture ascertainment method, which involved a telephone call to the subject's local medical officer, with no subject interview, or radiological ascertainment of morphologic vertebral or clinical fractures.

In 2013, an analysis of annual osteoporosis and fracture rates was published in *Osteoporosis Australia*.[6] In the Australian community, 71% of women aged 50 years or older were osteopenic or osteoporotic, with an annual total fracture rate of 2.7%, vertebral fracture rate of 0.5%, and hip fracture rate of 0.4%. The GOS ICU longitudinal BMD and fracture studies revealed that 80% of women aged 50 years or older were osteopenic or osteoporotic in the year after ICU, with a total fracture rate of 6.0%, vertebral fracture rate of 3.2%, and hip fracture rate of 0.9% (**Table 2**).

In summary, the evidence regarding fragility fracture rates after critical illness, is limited, although there is higher quality evidence of increased rates of fragility fracture, particularly in the highest risk group of older women. Confirmation of postcritical illness fracture rates through larger database linkages is needed.

Mortality Associated with Accelerated Bone Loss

Osteoporosis is associated with increased mortality, with evidence that the common pathways shared by osteoporosis and atherosclerosis are associated with altered regulation of inflammation; innate immunity, apoptosis, and blocking of maturation and activity of osteoclast precursors; and increased all-cause and cardiovascular mortality.[28,39–42] The association between elevated BTMs, bone loss, and mortality has been reported in varied populations, including patients with cancer,[28] older ambulatory women,[43] and patients undergoing coronary angiogram.[41,42] Also, fragility fractures are associated with increased mortality. Age-adjusted mortality rates were increased for men and women for all ages, and all fractures except for minor fractures, for which increased mortality was only apparent for those older than 75 years. Increased mortality persisted for 5 years for all fractures and up to 10 years for hip fractures. In women, the increases in absolute mortality were higher than expected, with levels ranging from 1.32 to 13.2 per 100 person-years.[44]

This association is strengthened by evidence of reduced mortality associated with antifracture therapy. A meta-analysis of randomized controlled trials investigating antifracture agents for prevention of vertebral and nonvertebral fractures found treatment was associated with an 11% reduction in mortality in more than 1400 deaths in approximately 40,000 subjects.[45] In studies with higher baseline mortality (>10 per 1000 patient-years), a 17% risk reduction was observed. This effect seemed to be similar across the different classes of agents in the study. In addition, a prospective cohort study reported a reduction in mortality rates in community-based women and men receiving bisphosphonates in propensity score–adjusted analyses.[46]

Table 2
Comparison of bone health and therapy in women aged 50 years or older after critical illness to Australian population

Variable	Post-ICU Year 1	Australia Annual Rate
T-score		
Osteoporosis	36%	23%
Osteopenia	44%	48%
Normal	20%	29%
Cumulative annual fracture rate		
Hip	0.9%	0.4%
Vertebral	3.2%	0.5%
Wrist	0%	0.5%
Other	1.9%	1.2%
Total	6%	2.7%

From Refs.[6,8,9]

Currently there is no evidence of an association between abnormal BTMs, reduced bone mass, or fragility fracture and increased mortality following critical illness. There is limited evidence describing an association between antifracture therapy and reduced mortality (see later discussion).[37,47] The intersection of inflammatory and immune disturbance, high baseline mortality, and retrospective evidence of mortality benefit in antifracture agent users, suggest accelerated bone turnover may be associated with increased mortality following critical illness.

Antifracture Therapies and Critical Illness

The use of antifracture therapy after critical illness is very uncommon, with only 4% of ICU survivors treated at 1 year and 16% at 2 years, despite the treating physician's awareness of bone density results.[29] This combination of high prevalence and low treatment rates, suggests critically ill postmenopausal women are underdiagnosed, undertreated, and may benefit from antifracture therapy.

Three studies have reported the effects on bone turnover from treating vitamin D deficiency in critically ill patients. A comparison of parenteral vitamin D 200 IU with 500 IU daily in long-term surgical ICU patients receiving parenteral nutrition, found higher dose vitamin D was associated with a relatively small increase in serum OC and a decrease in serum CTX; however, this did not affect other BTMs. In addition, the decrease in inflammatory markers IL-6 and C-reactive protein over time was more pronounced with the higher dose vitamin D.[22] However, in a cohort of 55 ventilator-dependent chronic critically ill patients, treating vitamin D deficiency with calcitriol did not lead to a reduction in bone resorption markers.[16] Finally, post hoc analysis of the VITdAL-ICU study[24] reported no effect of high-dose vitamin D3 (540,000 IU) compared with placebo on 6-month serum OC, sclerostin, or CTX in 289 adult critically ill patients. It is important to consider potential safety issues of high-dose vitamin D, with an increase in falls and fractures observed in community-dwelling older women at risk of fractures[48]

Bisphosphonates bind to bone and suppress bone resorption by entering osteoclasts and inhibiting the enzyme farnesyl pyrophosphate synthase, resulting in disruption of osteoclast attachment to bone surface.[30] This class of agents is effective at reducing bone loss and vertebral and nonvertebral fractures associated with reduced mortality, and are recommended as first-line agents in treatment of osteoporosis.[31-33] A retrospective survey described a significant reduction in urine N-terminal telopeptide over an 18-day period in ventilator-dependent chronic critically ill patients when oral pamidronate was added to calcitriol alone.[16] A prospective trial that randomized 20 postmenopausal women requiring greater than 5 days of mechanical ventilation to a single dose of intravenous ibandronate versus placebo reported a significant decrease in bone resorption. However, this was transient, with serum CTX levels returning to baseline by day 11. There was no difference in serum OC levels between the ibandronate and placebo groups at day 11, although levels increased in both groups during the study. This suggests a lack of effect of ibandronate on bone formation and a gradual increase in osteoblast activity in both groups.[26]

Two studies have described an association between bisphosphonate use and mortality in critically ill subjects. A retrospective case series of 148 subjects with chronic critical illness compared outcomes of subjects who received pamidronate ($n = 118$) to those who did not ($n = 30$).[47] A lower ICU (0% vs 19%, $P = .008$) and 1-year mortality (20% vs 56%, $P = .004$) was reported with pamidronate, and this remained significant after adjustment for renal function and calcium levels. However, this study was limited by a single-center, unblinded, retrospective design, and lack of information about confounders, including preexisting risk factors, ICU severity illness, and ICU interventions.

A retrospective propensity-matched cohort study described outcomes in 245 subjects who had received bisphosphonates in the 5 years before an ICU admission of greater than 24 hours compared with ICU subjects who did not receive bisphosphonates. After matching for age, sex, comorbid disease, principal diagnosis, and year of admission, bisphosphonate use was associated with a significant decrease in hospital mortality rate ratio of 0.39 (95% CI 0.22–0.67, $P<.01$). In addition, a subgroup analysis of 37 subjects from the bisphosphonate group who underwent serial CT scans was compared with 74 matched subjects not using bisphosphonates. The bisphosphonate users had lower baseline bone density, with a significant attenuation of rate of vertebral bone loss compared with controls ($-3\% \pm 13\%$ vs $-15\% \pm 14\%$ per week, $P<.01$).[37]

Finally, an association between antifracture medications and bone loss in the 2 years after critical illness was reported.[35] Over a 2-year period after critical illness, 11% of participants were prescribed antifracture therapies, including alendronate, denosumab, strontium ranelate, and risedronate. In women, the use of antifracture therapy was associated with a significant difference in post-ICU annual change of BMD, with an increase in BMD in participants who received antifracture medication compared with a decrease in those that did not. In men, no association between antifracture therapy use and annual change in BMD was observed.

Overall, there is limited evidence suggesting benefit from bisphosphonates and other antifracture agents in terms of attenuated bone loss and mortality. Due to methodological limitations, the overall benefit, as well as specific risk and benefit related to agent, dose, duration, timing, subgroups, and duration, remain unclear.

Next Steps

There is increasing evidence that survivors of critical illness are at increased risk of accelerated bone loss, fragility fracture, and associated mortality. Currently, there is no routine intervention provided to prevent this and limited evidence that antifracture agents may have benefit. The 2 antifracture agents best suited to investigate for administration in critical illness are zoledronic acid and denosumab (see previous discussion of the class effects of zoledronic acid, a bisphosphonate). Denosumab, a fully human monoclonal antibody directed against RANKL, is the first biologic therapy approved to treat osteoporosis. Administered subcutaneously every 6 months, it is metabolized by organ-independent intracellular mechanisms, is a potent inhibitor of osteoclast activity, and is effective at reducing bone loss and fragility fractures.[31,32] The indications for use include prevention of bone loss and fractures in osteoporosis, bone metastases from solid tumors, men with prostate cancer and androgen deprivation, and women with breast cancer receiving aromatase inhibitors.[31–34] The RANKL antagonist effects of denosumab may result in inflammatory, cardiovascular, and cancer benefits, with associated reduction in mortality[35,36] and disease-free survival.[36]

Both denosumab and zoledronic acid are potential target interventions to study in critical illness. Both agents are likely to be effective at reducing bone resorption and preventing fragility fracture, and both agents show potential for extraskeletal benefit, including reduced mortality. The fracture reduction effect is likely to maximally benefit postmenopausal critically ill women owing to the high baseline risk. The immune, cardiovascular, and mortality effects, if present, may benefit all critically ill patients, although there is currently insufficient evidence to justify administration for this purpose.

A research program, including pilot assessment of safety and efficacy, as well as, if indicated, assessment of the effect of antifracture agents on vertebral or clinical fracture rate in the high-risk population of postmenopausal women with prolonged ventilation, may be warranted. In addition to fracture outcomes, assessment of the effect on mortality is important because a reduction of the magnitude reported in previous antifracture trails would have a significant impact on critically ill women.

SUMMARY

More is understood about critical illness–associated bone loss than was did a decade ago. There is increasing and consistent evidence of abnormal bone metabolism during critical illness, with a pattern of early increased bone resorption and suppression of bone formation that persists for up to a month, and changes to normal bone resorption and increased formation over the subsequent year. There is evidence of skeletal impact from the increased bone turnover associated with critical illness, with loss of BMD and increased fracture risk in subsequent years. There is preliminary evidence that antifracture interventions may be effective at attenuating bone loss and reducing mortality after critical illness.

There are important gaps in the knowledge and questions that need answers. The first is the contribution of precritical illness factors, critical illness factors, and recovery factors, to postcritical illness bone health, which remains unclear. Separating out the major influences on critical illness–related bone health will require larger participant cohorts, preferably with prospectively collected precritical illness data, which is a major challenge for critical care research in general. This is important because identification of the time and magnitude of skeletal insults may provide opportunities to intervene.

The second is understanding of biological pathways involved in bone loss, the interaction of cytokine pathways with bone turnover, and the nonskeletal effects of activation of bone metabolism, which are only beginning to be understood. Further investigation of these mechanisms, in both animal and human settings, may provide crucial information to guide interventions that alter both bone and inflammatory outcomes.

Finally, the prospect of reducing bone loss, fractures, and possibly mortality, in critically ill adults through ICU-based antifracture interventions is an intriguing area to investigate in future phase II and phase III randomized controlled trials. With careful design, these trials may also provide answers to the first 2 questions.

ACKNOWLEDGMENTS

Research contributing to this paper was supported by an unrestricted grant from the Intensive Care Foundation https://www.intensivecarefoundation.org.au.

REFERENCES

1. Kaukonen K-M, Bailey M, Suzuki S, et al. Mortality related to severe sepsis and septic shock among critically ill patients in Australia and New Zealand, 2000-2012. JAMA 2014;311(13):1308–16.
2. Hodgson CL, Udy AA, Bailey M, et al. The impact of disability in survivors of critical illness. Intensive Care Med 2017;43(7):992–1001.
3. Iwashyna TJ. Survivorship will be the defining challenge of critical care in the 21st century. Ann Intern Med 2010;153(3):204–5.
4. Nguyen TV, Center JR, Eisman JA. Osteoporosis: underrated, underdiagnosed and undertreated. Med J Aust 2004;180(5 Suppl):S18–22.
5. Kanis JA, Svedbom A, Harvey N, et al. The osteoporosis treatment gap. J Bone Miner Res 2014;29(9):1926–8.
6. Watts JJ, Abimanyi-Ochom J, Sanders K M. Osteoporosis costing all Australians. A new burden of disease analysis. Melbourne (VIC): Osteoporosis Australia; 2013. p. 1–80.

7. The global burden of osteoporosis: a factsheet. Available at: https://www. iofbonehealth.org/sites/default/files/media/PDFs/Fact%20Sheets/2014-factsheet-osteoporosis-A4.pdf.

8. Orford NR, Lane SE, Bailey M, et al. Changes in bone mineral density in the year after critical illness. Am J Respir Crit Care Med 2016;193(7):736–44.

9. Orford NR, Saunders K, Merriman E, et al. Skeletal morbidity among survivors of critical illness. Crit Care Med 2011;39(6):1295–300.

10. Orford N, Cattigan C, Brennan SL, et al. The association between critical illness and changes in bone turnover in adults: a systematic review. Osteoporos Int 2014;25(10):2335–46.

11. NIH consensus development panel on osteoporosis prevention, diagnosis, and therapy. Osteoporosis prevention, diagnosis, and therapy. JAMA 2001;285: 785–95.

12. Cavalier E, Bergmann P, Bruyère O, et al. The role of biochemical of bone turnover markers in osteoporosis and metabolic bone disease: a consensus paper of the Belgian Bone Club. Osteoporos Int 2016;27(7):2181–95.

13. Boyce BF, Li P, Yao Z, et al. TNFa and pathologic bone resorption. Keio J Med 2005;54(3):127–31.

14. Nierman DM, Mechanick JI. Bone hyperresorption is prevalent in chronically critically ill patients. Chest 1998;114(4):1122–8.

15. Lind L, Carlstedt F, Rastad J, et al. Hypocalcemia and parathyroid hormone secretion in critically ill patients. Crit Care Med 2000;28(1):93–9.

16. Nierman DM, Mechanick JI. Biochemical response to treatment of bone hyperresorption in chronically critically ill patients. Chest 2000;118(3):761–6.

17. Van den Berghe G, Baxter RC, Weekers F, et al. The combined administration of GH-releasing peptide-2 (GHRP-2), TRH and GnRH to men with prolonged critical illness evokes superior endocrine and metabolic effects compared to treatment with GHRP-2 alone. Clin Endocrinol (Oxf) 2002;56(5):655–69.

18. Van den Berghe G, Weekers F, Baxter RC, et al. Five-day pulsatile gonadotropin-releasing hormone administration unveils combined hypothalamic-pituitary-gonadal defects underlying profound hypoandrogenism in men with prolonged critical illness. J Clin Endocrinol Metab 2001;86(7):3217–26.

19. Van den Berghe G, Wouters P, Weekers F, et al. Reactivation of pituitary hormone release and metabolic improvement by infusion of growth hormone- releasing peptide and thyrotropin-releasing hormone in patients with protracted critical illness. J Clin Endocrinol Metab 1999;84:1311–23.

20. Owen HC, Vanhees I, Solie L, et al. Critical illness-related bone loss is associated with osteoclastic and angiogenic abnormalities. J Bone Miner Res 2012;27(7):1541–52.

21. Shapses SA, Weissman C, Seibel MJ, et al. Urinary pyridinium cross-link excretion is increased in critically ill surgical patients. Crit Care Med 1997;25(1):85–90.

22. Van den Berghe G. Bone turnover in prolonged critical illness: effect of vitamin D. J Clin Endocrinol Metab 2003;88(10):4623–32.

23. Smith LM, Cuthbertson B, Harvie J, et al. Increased bone resorption in the critically ill: association with sepsis and increased nitric oxide production. Crit Care Med 2002;30(4):837–40.

24. Schwetz V, Schnedl C, Urbanic-Purkart T, et al. Effect of vitamin D3 on bone turnover markers in critical illness: post hoc analysis from the VITdAL-ICU study. Osteoporos Int 2017;28(12):3347–54.

25. Gavala A, Makris K, Korompeli A, et al. Evaluation of bone metabolism in critically ill patients using CTx and PINP. Biomed Res Int 2016;2016(4):1–9.

26. Via MA, Potenza MV, Hollander J, et al. Intravenous ibandronate acutely reduces bone hyperresorption in chronic critical illness. J Intensive Care Med 2012;27(5): 312–8.

27. Koch A, Weiskirchen R, Ludwig S, et al. Relevance of serum sclerostin concentrations in critically ill patients. J Crit Care 2017;37(C):38–44.

28. Barnadas A, Manso L, la Piedra de C, et al. Bone turnover markers as predictive indicators of outcome in patients with breast cancer and bone metastases treated with bisphosphonates: results from a 2-year multicentre observational study (ZOMAR study). Bone 2014;68(C):32–40.

29. Kim JH, Kim N. Signaling pathways in osteoclast differentiation. Chonnam Med J 2016;52(1):12–6.

30. Vanhees I, Gunst J, Janssens T, et al. Enhanced immunoreceptor tyrosine-based activation motif signaling is related to pathological bone resorption during critical illness. Horm Metab Res 2013;45(12):862–9.

31. Puthucheary ZA, Sun Y, Zeng K, et al. Sepsis reduces bone strength before morphologic changes are identifiable. Crit Care Med 2017;45(12):e1254–61.

32. Kanis JA. Diagnosis of osteoporosis and assessment of fracture risk. Lancet 2002;359:1929–36.

33. Henry MJ, Pasco JA, Pocock NA, et al. Reference ranges for bone densitometers adopted Australia-wide: Geelong osteoporosis study. Australas Radiol 2004; 48(4):473–5.

34. Kanis JA. Assessment of fracture risk and its application to screening for post-menopausal osteoporosis: synopsis of a WHO report. Osteoporos Int 1994; 4(6):368–81.

35. Orford NR, Bailey M, Bellomo R, et al. The association of time and medications with changes in bone mineral density in the 2 years after critical illness. Crit Care 2017;21(1):69.

36. Rawal J, McPhail MJ, Ratnayake G, et al. A pilot study of change in fracture risk in patients with acute respiratory distress syndrome. Crit Care 2015;19(1):165.

37. Lee P, Ng C, Slattery A, et al. Preadmission bisphosphonate and mortality in critically ill patients. J Clin Endocrinol Metab 2016;101(5):1945–53.

38. Rousseau A-F, Cavalier E, Reginster J-Y, et al. Occurrence of clinical bone fracture following a prolonged stay in intensive care unit: a retrospective controlled study. Calcif Tissue Int 2017;1–8. https://doi.org/10.1007/s00223-017-0300-5.

39. Sambrook PN, Chen CJ, March L, et al. High bone turnover is an independent predictor of mortality in the frail elderly. J Bone Miner Res 2006;21(4):549–55.

40. Kanis JA, Oden A, Johnell O, et al. The components of excess mortality after hip fracture. Bone 2003;32(5):468–73.

41. Lerchbaum E, Schwetz V, Pilz S, et al. Association of bone turnover markers with mortality in women referred to coronary angiography: the Ludwigshafen Risk and Cardiovascular Health (LURIC) study. Osteoporos Int 2013;25(2):455–65.

42. Lerchbaum E, Schwetz V, Pilz S, et al. Association of bone turnover markers with mortality in men referred to coronary angiography. Osteoporos Int 2012;24(4): 1321–32.

43. Browner WS, Pressman AR, Nevitt MC, et al. Mortality following fractures in older women. The study of osteoporotic fractures. Arch Intern Med 1996;156(14): 1521–5.

44. Bliuc D, Nguyen ND, Milch VE, et al. Mortality risk associated with low-trauma osteoporotic fracture and subsequent fracture in men and women. JAMA 2009; 301(5):513–21.

45. Bolland MJ, Grey AB, Gamble GD, et al. Effect of osteoporosis treatment on mortality: a meta-analysis. J Clin Endocrinol Metab 2010;95(3):1174–81.

46. Center JR, Bliuc D, Nguyen ND, et al. Osteoporosis medication and reduced mortality risk in elderly women and men. J Clin Endocrinol Metab 2011;96(4): 1006–14.

47. Schulman RC, Moshier EL, Rho L, et al. Intravenous pamidronate is associated with reduced mortality in patients with chronic critical illness. Endocr Pract 2016;22(7):799–808.

48. Sanders KM, Stuart AL, Williamson EJ, et al. Annual high-dose oral vitamin D and falls and fractures in older women: a randomized controlled trial. JAMA 2010; 303(18):1815–22.

New Agents for the Treatment of Type 2 Diabetes

Renata Libianto, MBBS, BMedSci[a], Elif I. Ekinci, MBBS, FRACP, PhD[a,b],*

KEYWORDS

- Diabetes • New treatment • SGLT-2 inhibitors • GLP-1 agonists • DPP-4 inhibitors

KEY POINTS

- The US Food and Drug Administration mandated that all new agents for type 2 diabetes demonstrate cardiovascular safety.
- Within the last decade, the number of treatment options for type 2 diabetes have increased dramatically.
- Many of these newer agents have beneficial effects on cardiovascular and renal endpoints as well as benefits on weight.
- The benefits of new therapeutic options for type 2 diabetes need to be balanced against their potential adverse effects.

INTRODUCTION

Diabetes mellitus is highly prevalent. The World Health Organization estimates that its prevalence has nearly doubled since 1980, rising from 4.7% to 8.5% in the adult population.[1] It is now the eighth leading cause of death, and a significant proportion of deaths attributable to hyperglycemia occur prematurely, before the age of 70 years.[1] There is no cure at present for diabetes but treatment options have evolved considerably over the years. Banting and Best first extracted insulin in the 1920s, and sulfonylureas were discovered in the 1940s.[2] Metformin was first described in 1922 and its glucose-lowering action was discovered in animals in 1929.[3] However, it was not until 1994 that metformin was approved by the US Food and Drug Administration (FDA).[3] Meanwhile, thiazolidinediones, which were introduced in the late 1990s, are used less frequently now due to concerns regarding edema and worsening of heart failure.[4]

In the last decade, there has been a Renaissance of diabetes therapies. The development of continuous subcutaneous insulin infusion (insulin pump) and continuous

Disclosure: E.I. Ekinci has received grant funding from Viertel, RACP, Sir Edward 'Weary' Dunlop Medical Research Foundation, and the Diabetes Australia Research Program.
[a] Department of Medicine, The University of Melbourne, Austin Health, 300 Waterdale Road, Heidelberg West, Melbourne, Victoria 3081, Australia; [b] Department of Endocrinology, Austin Health, 300 Waterdale Road, Heidelberg West, Melbourne, Victoria 3081, Australia
* Corresponding author. Department of Endocrinology, Austin Health, 300 Waterdale Road, Heidelberg West, Melbourne, Victoria 3081, Australia.
E-mail address: elif.ekinci@unimelb.edu.au

Crit Care Clin 35 (2019) 315–328
https://doi.org/10.1016/j.ccc.2018.11.007
0749-0704/19/© 2018 Elsevier Inc. All rights reserved.

glucose monitoring systems are changing the treatment paradigm for people with type 1 diabetes. Meanwhile, noninsulin based agents are being manufactured and marketed at rapid succession for the treatment of type 2 diabetes. In the last decade, three newer classes of glucose-lowering medications that have been used are the sodium-glucose cotransporter (SGLT)-2 inhibitors, dipeptidyl peptidase (DPP)-4 inhibitors or gliptins, and glucagon-like peptide (GLP)-1 agonists.

In 2008, the FDA issued a *Guidance for Industry* requiring all new medications developed for diabetes treatment to demonstrate cardiovascular safety. This was based on the retraction of rosiglitazone, which was found to be associated with increased risk of cardiovascular death in a meta-analysis of 42 trials.[5] Since then, the FDA mandated that all sponsors for new treatment agents for type 2 diabetes to show that the therapy "will not result in an unacceptable increase in cardiovascular risk" (ie, noninferiority).[6] There is now evidence that both SGLT-2 inhibitors and GLP-1 agonists are associated with not just noninferiority but with superiority, with lower all-cause and cardiovascular mortality.[7]

This article will describe the mechanism of actions of each of the new classes of diabetes medications; their effects on cardiovascular, glycemic, and renal outcomes; and important safety considerations related to each class of medication (**Table 1**).

SODIUM-GLUCOSE COTRANSPORTER-2 INHIBITORS
Mechanism of Action

In healthy individuals, the proximal tubules of the kidneys are able to transport approximately 500 g of glucose per day, resulting in virtually complete reabsorption of the filtered glucose load.[8] Glucosuria is observed when the plasma glucose concentration exceeds 10 to 11.1 mmol/L. Several transport proteins are responsible for reabsorbing glucose in the proximal renal tubule. On the basolateral membrane, the sodium-potassium adenosine triphosphatase (Na+/K+ ATPase) transporter actively drives sodium from the tubular cells into the circulation. This creates a sodium gradient, which allows the SGLTs to transport glucose from the lumen into the cells by passively following this sodium gradient. SGLT-2 is the predominant transporter in the kidney, responsible for approximately 97% of the transport across the luminal membrane, whereas SGLT-1 is responsible for approximately 3% of the transport.[8] The glucose transporter (GLUT)-2 located on the basolateral membrane then transports glucose from the tubular cells into the circulation (**Fig. 1**).

The importance of SGLT-2 in glycemic regulation was demonstrated in animal studies. Zucker obese rats (a model of type 2 diabetes) had an increase in messenger RNA (mRNA) expression of SGLT-2 by 4.8-fold compared with lean controls,[9] perhaps as a coping mechanism to deal with the increased filtered glucose load in diabetes. However, this coping mechanism may worsen hyperglycemia and potentially enhance glucotoxicity in proximal tubular cells.[8] Meanwhile, induction of diabetes with streptozotocin in SGLT-2 knockout mice resulted in lesser increase of blood glucose level compared with wild-type mice ($\sim$16 mmol/L vs 26 mmol/L).[10] These studies demonstrate the importance of SGLT-2 in glucose homeostasis. Several SGLT-2 inhibitors are available in the market, including dapagliflozin, empagliflozin, ertugliflozin, canagliflozin, and sotagliflozin.

Effect on Cardiovascular Outcomes

Many of the initial cardiovascular endpoint trials demonstrated cardiovascular safety but did not demonstrate cardiovascular outcome superiority. Empagliflozin, in the well-known Empagliflozin Cardiovascular Outcome Event Trial in Type 2 Diabetes

Table 1
Summary of new treatment options for type 2 diabetes

Class	Drug Names and Dosages	Mechanism of Action	Cardiovascular Outcome	Glycemic Outcome	Weight Effect	Renal Outcome	Main Safety Considerations	Cost
SGLT-2 inhibitors	Dapagliflozin (5 or 10 mg, oral, daily) Empagliflozin (10 or 25 mg, oral, daily) Canagliflozin (100 or 300 mg, oral, daily) Ertugliflozin (5 or 15 mg, oral, daily)	Blocks SGLT-2 in the kidneys, thereby inducing glycosuria	Superior to placebo in reducing cardiovascular endpoint, in particular hospitalization for heart failure	Modest reduction in HbA1c of approximately 0.5%	Weight reduction of 2.5%	Reduce progression of nephropathy	• Genitourinary infection • Acute kidney injury • Euglycaemic ketoacidosis • Toe amputation (canagliflozin)	$$
GLP-1 agonists	Exenatide immediate-release (5–10 μg), subcutaneous, twice daily Exenatide extended-release (2 mg, subcutaneous, once weekly) Liraglutide (0.6–3 mg, subcutaneous, daily) Dulaglutide (0.75–1.5 mg, subcutaneous, weekly) Semaglutide (0.25–1 mg, subcutaneous, weekly) Lixisenatide (10–20 μg, subcutaneous, daily) Albiglutide (30–50 mg, subcutaneous, weekly)	Stimulates insulin release from the pancreas	Beneficial or neutral effect on cardiovascular outcome	Reduction in HbA1c of approximately 1%	Weight reduction by ~5%	Possible beneficial effect in reducing progression of nephropathy	• Gastrointestinal side effects • Possible pancreatitis • Worsening of diabetic retinopathy (semaglutide)	$$$

(continued on next page)

Table 1
(continued)

Class	Drug Names and Dosages	Mechanism of Action	Cardiovascular Outcome	Glycemic Outcome	Weight Effect	Renal Outcome	Main Safety Considerations	Cost
DPP-4 inhibitors	Sitagliptin (100 mg, oral, daily) Linagliptin (5 mg, oral, daily) Saxagliptin (2.5–5 mg, oral, daily) Alogliptin (25 mg, oral, daily) Vildagliptin (50 mg, oral, once or twice daily)	Inhibits DPP-4, the enzyme that deactivates GLP-1	Noninferior compared with placebo	Modest reduction in HbA1c of approximately 0.5%	Weight neutral	Possible beneficial effect in reducing progression of nephropathy.	• Gastrointestinal side effects • ?Pancreatitis • Hypersensitive reactions	$$

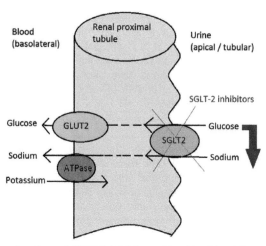

Fig. 1. Mechanism of action of SGLT-2 inhibitors. The Na+/K+ ATPase creates a sodium gradient across the basolateral membrane of the proximal renal tubule. The SGLT-2 channels cotransport sodium and glucose from the apical membrane into the tubule, and glucose is then transported into the circulation by the GLUT-2 channels. With inhibition of SGLT-2 channels, glucose is unable to be reabsorbed into the circulation and is excreted through the urine, thereby lowering plasma glucose concentration.

Mellitus Patients (EMPA-REG OUTCOME) trial,[11] exceeded this expectation by demonstrating a superior cardiovascular outcome and mortality. In this trial, more than 7000 subjects with diabetes and established cardiovascular disease were randomized to empagliflozin (at a dosage of 10 mg or 25 mg) or placebo daily. The primary outcome, which was a composite of cardiovascular death, nonfatal myocardial infarction, or nonfatal stroke, occurred in 10.5% in the empagliflozin group and 12.1% in the placebo group (hazard ratio [HR] 0.86, $P = .04$ for superiority) at 3.1 years of follow-up. The difference in mortality became apparent very early on in the trial, suggesting that the mechanism of the cardiovascular benefit was unlikely to be related to improvements in metabolic control. Furthermore, there was a significant reduction in cardiovascular mortality and heart failure hospitalization, without significant difference in the rates of myocardial infarction, unstable angina, or stroke as individual variables. Therefore, it is thought that the mechanisms that contribute to the reduction of cardiovascular mortality were likely to be driven by hemodynamic changes such as reduction in blood pressure, reduction in extracellular volume, and perhaps a reduction in sympathetic tone.[12] Another potential explanation is the so-called thrifty substrate hypothesis, which postulated that a shift toward utilization of beta-hydroxybutyrate as fuel source during treatment with SGLT-2 inhibitors (which is associated with mild hyperketonemia) results in a more efficient delivery and usage of oxygen.[13] Both empagliflozin dosages (10 and 25 mg) had similar effect on outcome measures without a dose-response relationship.

The Canagliflozin Cardiovascular Assessment Study (CANVAS) trial,[14] which similarly recruited patients with type 2 diabetes and high cardiovascular risk ($n >10,000$), also showed a reduction in the primary composite outcome of cardiovascular death, nonfatal myocardial infarction, and nonfatal stroke (HR 0.86, $P = .02$ for superiority) after a mean follow-up of 3.6 years. The rate of hospitalization for heart failure was, again, lower in the canagliflozin group; however, the reductions in the occurrence of each individual component of the composite outcome did not reach statistical significance. Nevertheless, these findings confirmed a class effect benefit of SGLT-2 inhibitors on cardiovascular outcomes. It is important to note that both the EMPA-REG OUTCOME and CANVAS trials involved high-risk patients with established cardiovascular disease at baseline. The cardiovascular benefits of SGLT-2 inhibitors compared with other glucose-lowering medications have been further validated in real-world, based on data collected across 6 countries of more than 300,000 patients (half of whom were taking SGLT-2 inhibitors).[15]

Effect on Glycemic Outcomes

SGLT-2 inhibitors modestly improve hemoglobin A1c (HbA1c) in patients with type 2 diabetes. In the cardiovascular outcome trials, the mean differences in HbA1c with empagliflozin and canagliflozin compared with placebo were −0.54% and −0.58%, respectively.[11,14] However, the benefits of using SGLT-2 inhibitors extend beyond improvement in HbA1c because they also have weight loss and blood pressure-lowering effects.[11,16,17] In a trial comparing canagliflozin and the DPP-4 inhibitor sitagliptin, the use of canagliflozin was associated with a 2.5% weight reduction (compared with 0.3% with sitagliptin) and a reduction in systolic blood pressure by 5.1 mm Hg (compared with 0.99 mm Hg with sitagliptin).[18] Another advantage of SGLT-2 inhibitors is the lower risk of hypoglycemia compared with agents such as sulfonylureas or insulin. In a study that compared the addition of dapagliflozin or glipizide to metformin in subjects with type 2 diabetes who have inadequate glycemic control, hypoglycemia occurred in 3.5% in the dapagliflozin group, compared with 40.8% in the glipizide group.[19]

Effect on Renal Outcomes

In the EMPA-REG OUTCOME trial previously described, the long-term renal effect of empagliflozin was a prespecified secondary outcome.[20] In this trial, incident or worsening nephropathy (defined as progression to macroalbuminuria, doubling of serum creatinine level, initiation of renal-replacement therapy, or death from renal disease) occurred less frequently in the empagliflozin group compared with placebo (HR 0.61, 95% CI 0.53–0.70). In the CANVAS trial, renal outcome comprised progression of albuminuria, reduction in estimated glomerular filtration rate, the need for renal-replacement therapy, and death from renal causes. The data suggested a possible benefit of canagliflozin in these measures,[14] although the trial was not designed to primarily assess renal outcome.

Safety Considerations

Due to its mechanism of action by causing glycosuria, SGLT-2 inhibitors could cause genital infections.[11,14] There have also been postmarketing reports of acute kidney injury, likely secondary to intravascular volume depletion.[21] Despite these postmarketing reports, the large cardiovascular outcome trials (EMPA-REG OUTCOME and CANVAS) did not report any excess incidence of acute kidney injury in their original studies.[11,14] Given the current available data, the FDA recommends assessment and monitoring of kidney function in patients with risk factors for kidney injury, such as those with preexisting chronic kidney disease, congestive heart failure, or taking medications such as diuretics or antihypertensive.[21]

A safety concern that has arisen is related to SGLT-2 inhibitors potentially increasing the risk of euglycemic diabetic ketoacidosis (DKA).[22] The incidence rate of DKA was approximately 0.5 per 1000 patient-years in people taking SGLT-2 inhibitors compared with 0.2 per 1000 patient-years in people taking other agents,[23] although in the original EMPA-REG OUTCOME and CANVAS trials there was no excess incidence of DKA reported. The ketoacidosis may be difficult to diagnose due to the absence of substantial hyperglycemia. The mechanism is not clearly understood, but potentially include reduced insulin production due to glycosuria, promotion of glucagon secretion by pancreatic alpha-cells that express SGLT-2, and reduction in renal clearance of ketone bodies.[24,25] For this reason, off-label use of SGLT-2 inhibitors in people with type 1 diabetes is discouraged. However, the evidence in type 2 diabetes is controversial, with a recent meta-analysis reporting no increase in risk of DKA among people with type 2 diabetes.[26] Nevertheless, patients who become ill while taking SGLT-2 inhibitors should have their serum ketones checked. It may be prudent to withhold SGLT-2 inhibitors in the perioperative period.[27] The current recommendations are to withhold SGLT-2 inhibitors for at least 3 days preoperatively, consider postponing nonurgent surgery if SGLT-2 inhibitors have not been ceased before surgery and blood ketones are greater than 0.6 mmol/L, routinely check blood glucose and ketone levels in the perioperative period, perform venous blood gas to measure pH if blood ketone is greater than 0.6 mmol/L in patients who have been on SGLT-2 inhibitor, and SGLT-2 inhibitor should be restarted when patient is eating and drinking and is close to being discharged.[28]

In the canagliflozin (CANVAS) trial, there was an excess risk of amputation, predominantly at the level of the toe or metatarsal, compared with placebo.[14] The underlying pathophysiology is not well-elucidated. One theory is that canagliflozin may cause volume depletion resulting in tissue underperfusion in people who already have compromised vasculature.[14] However, real-world data suggest that the risk of amputation is probably not a class-effect because empagliflozin and dapagliflozin were not associated with excess rate of amputation compared with nonusers of SGLT-2 inhibitors in patients with established diabetic foot wounds.[29]

GLUCAGON-LIKE PEPTIDE-1 AGONISTS
Mechanism of Action: The Incretin Effect

GLP-1 is an incretin hormone released by intestinal L cells in response to food intake. It simulates the release of insulin from pancreatic beta-cells in a glucose-dependent manner[30] (**Fig. 2**). It also slows gastric emptying, increases satiety, and reduces plasma glucagon. The release of GLP-1 is accentuated by oral administration of glucose, more so compared with intravenous administration. Incretin hormones are responsible for 70% of the total insulin secretion following oral glucose administration, and GLP-1 is the most potent of the incretins.[30] People with type 2 diabetes demonstrate impaired GLP-1 secretion postprandially, which may explain the inappropriate insulin response.[31] The other incretin is glucose-dependent insulinotropic peptide (GIP). In type 2 diabetes, plasma concentrations of GIP are normal or increased but the insulinotropic effect is deficient, possibly as a result of downregulation of GIP receptor expression due to hyperglycaemia.[32]

Synthetic GLP-1 receptor agonists are administered subcutaneously and are resistant to degradation by the enzyme DPP-4, making them suitable for clinical use. The GLP-1 agonists that are available on the market include exenatide, exenatide extended-release, liraglutide, dulaglutide, semaglutide, albiglutide, and lixisenatide. Most of these agents require daily or twice daily administration, with the exception of exenatide extended-release, dulaglutide, and semaglutide, which are administered weekly.

Effect on Cardiovascular Outcomes

Trials have demonstrated either beneficial or neutral effect of GLP-1 agonists on cardiovascular outcomes. In the Liraglutide Effect and Action in Diabetes: Evaluation of

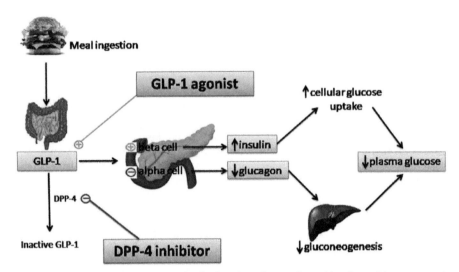

Fig. 2. The incretin effect. Incretins (including GLP-1) are released by the gut in response to oral glucose ingestion. They stimulate pancreatic beta-cells to release insulin and inhibit glucagon production by alpha-cells, which result in lowering of plasma glucose concentration. GLP-1 is inactivated by the enzyme DPP-4; inhibition of DPP-4, therefore, leads to glucose lowering.

Cardiovascular Outcome Results (LEADER) trial, fewer people developed the composite outcome of cardiovascular mortality, nonfatal myocardial infarction, and nonfatal stroke in the liraglutide arm compared with placebo (HR 0.87, 95% CI 0.78–0.97).[33] This trial was conducted in patients with type 2 diabetes and high cardiovascular risk to maximize the outcome measure. A similar result was reported in the Trial to Evaluate Cardiovascular and Other Long-term Outcomes with Semaglutide in Subjects with Type 2 Diabetes (SUSTAIN-6).[34] In this study, the HR for the composite outcome of cardiovascular death, nonfatal myocardial infarction, or nonfatal stroke was 0.74 (95% CI 0.58–0.95).

Once-weekly exenatide and once-daily lixisenatide were noninferior compared with placebo in terms of cardiovascular outcome.[35,36] In the large Exenatide Study of Cardiovascular Event Lowering (EXSCEL) trial ($n = 14,752$), once-weekly exenatide was compared with placebo in patients with type 2 diabetes, with or without previous cardiovascular disease, and the incidence of major adverse cardiovascular events (cardiovascular death, nonfatal myocardial infarction, or nonfatal stroke) did not differ significantly in the two groups.[35] Compared with placebo, there was no excess incidence of serious adverse events with once-weekly exenatide in the EXSCEL trial, and the rate of severe hypoglycemia was comparable (1.0 and 0.9 events per 100 subject-years in the trial and placebo groups, respectively).

GLP-1 agonists also cause a modest reduction in systolic blood pressure of approximately 2 to 3 mm Hg.[37,38] The mechanism by which GLP-1 agonists reduce blood pressure is not well-understood but, unlike the SGLT-2 inhibitors, blood pressure reduction with GLP-1 agonists is accompanied by an increase in heart rate,[39] suggesting that sympathetic inhibition is probably not the mechanism. Furthermore, the correlation between blood pressure reduction and weight loss is weak, and mechanisms other than weight loss are being investigated.[40]

Effect on Glycemic Outcomes

Outside of insulin, GLP-1 agonist is probably among the most effective classes of glucose-lowering medications. In the semaglutide (SUSTAIN-6) trial, the HbA1c achieved in semaglutide group was 7.3%, which was 1.0% points lower than that achieved with placebo.[34] A meta-analysis reported a reduction of HbA1c of approximately 1% with all GLP-1 agonists compared with placebo.[41] Similar to SGLT-2 inhibitors, however, GLP-1 agonists have metabolic benefits beyond reduction in HbA1c.

GLP-1 agonists are associated with weight reduction of approximately 1.5 to 2.5 kg.[41,42] GLP-1 agonists are frequently used in weight management clinics to treat obese individuals who do not have diabetes. Higher dose liraglutide is currently approved in Australia to be used for this purpose. In a randomized trial involving 3700 subjects without diabetes, liraglutide at a dosage of 3.0 mg daily resulted in 5.6 kg more weight loss compared with placebo over 56 weeks.[43] Liraglutide must continue to be used to maintain its weight-lowering effects, and the main adverse events were nausea and diarrhea.

Effect on Renal Outcomes

There have been no trials designed specifically to look at renal outcome with GLP-1 agonists. In trials assessing cardiovascular outcome, which looked at renal outcome as their secondary endpoint, GLP-1 agonists have beneficial effect on renal outcome compared with placebo. In the LEADER trial, fewer patients taking liraglutide reached the secondary endpoint, which was a composite of new-onset persistent macroalbuminuria, persistent doubling of the serum creatinine, endstage renal disease, or death due to renal disease.[44] Similar findings were found in SUSTAIN-6 trial, which reported lower rates of new or worsening nephropathy with semaglutide.[34] More recently, once-weekly dulaglutide was demonstrated to be safe for use in patients with type 2 diabetes and stage 3 to 4 chronic kidney disease.[45] Dulaglutide was noninferior to insulin glargine in achieving glycemic control in these patients, and may widen the treatment options for people with more advanced kidney disease. The cardiovascular outcome trial for dulaglutide is currently still underway.[46]

Safety Considerations

One of the most prominent, and often dose-limiting, side effects of GLP-1 agonists is the gastrointestinal side effects; 10% to 50% of patients experience nausea, vomiting, or diarrhea.[41] These adverse events are usually worst in the beginning and tend to improve after several weeks of treatment. Because of this, the short-acting forms of GLP-1 agonist, such as exenatide immediate-release and liraglutide, require uptitration. Postmarketing reports have also suggested an association between GLP-1 agonist and risk of pancreatitis, although there are currently insufficient data to say whether or not there is a causal relationship. Regardless, GLP-1 agonist should be avoided in patients who have a history of pancreatitis.

A potential association with use of semaglutide was worsening of diabetic retinopathy. The SUSTAIN-6 trial reported higher rates of retinopathy complications (vitreous hemorrhage, blindness, the need for treatment with intravitreal agent or photocoagulation) with semaglutide compared with placebo.[34] A subsequent analysis of the SUSTAIN-1 to SUSTAIN-5 trials did not reveal excess diabetic retinopathy complications[47] and it is thought that the excess retinopathy in SUSTAIN-6 was probably due to an ultrarapid reduction in HbA1c, which has been associated with retinopathy.[48] Although the mechanism is not well-elucidated, some proposed hypotheses for worsening retinopathy include increased insulin-like growth factor (IGF)-1 level due to increased availability of insulin (either endogenous or exogenous).[48] IGF-1, in turn, could potentially promote angiogenesis and proliferative retinopathy. Another hypothesis is that the expression of vascular endothelial growth factor may increase following normalization of blood glucose level, which then drives angiogenesis.

DIPEPTIDYL PEPTIDASE-4 INHIBITORS
Mechanism of Action

DPP-4 is an enzyme that deactivates GLP-1 and, therefore, allows endogenous GLP-1 and other incretins to exert their effects on glucose control (see **Fig. 2**). As previously discussed, GLP-1 stimulates glucose-dependent insulin release from the pancreas. Similar to GLP-1 agonists, DPP-4 inhibitors by themselves do not cause hypoglycemia unless they are used in combination with other agents such as sulfonylureas or insulin. The DPP-4 inhibitors that are available on the market include sitagliptin, linagliptin, saxagliptin, alogliptin, and vildagliptin.

Effect on Cardiovascular Outcomes

The DPP-4 inhibitors have a largely neutral effect on cardiovascular outcomes. In the Trial Evaluating Cardiovascular Outcomes with Sitagliptin,[49] sitagliptin was noninferior to placebo for the composite outcome of cardiovascular death, nonfatal myocardial infarction, nonfatal stroke, or hospitalization for unstable angina. There was also no difference in the rate of hospitalization for heart failure. However, in the trial assessing the efficacy of saxagliptin, there was an excess risk of hospitalization for heart failure in the trial arm compared with placebo.[50] Similar concern was raised with alogliptin. Although the mechanism of heart failure with these drugs is not clear, the FDA suggests avoidance of medications containing saxagliptin or alogliptin in patients who have heart failure.[51]

Effect on Glycemic Outcomes

DPP-4 inhibitors have a modest effect in reducing HbA1c by approximately 0.50% to 0.70%.[52,53] All of the DPP-4 inhibitors seem to have similar efficacy, although there are few head-to-head trials comparing the different agents. In a trial comparing the addition of either saxagliptin or sitagliptin with metformin, the reduction in HbA1c was −0.52% and −0.62%, respectively (between group difference was 0.09%, demonstrating noninferiority).[53] An advantage of DPP-4 inhibitors is that they do not cause hypoglycemia unless used in conjunction with other agents that can induce hypoglycemia. However, unlike the GLP-1 agonists and SGLT-2 inhibitors, the DPP-4 inhibitors do not have a weight-reduction effect and are considered weight neutral.[52]

Effect on Renal Outcomes

There is some evidence of renoprotective effect with the use of DPP-4 inhibitors. In a trial comparing the addition of linagliptin or placebo to renin-angiotensin-aldosterone blockade, the addition of linagliptin led to a significant reduction in albuminuria in patients with type 2 diabetes with preexisting albuminuria.[54] Retrospective studies also suggested a reduction in the rate of decline of estimated glomerular filtration with the use of DPP-4 inhibitors.[55,56] Most DPP-4 inhibitors are renally cleared and, therefore, require dose adjustment in chronic kidney disease. The exception to this is linagliptin, which is mostly eliminated via the enterohepatic pathway and can, therefore, be used in patients with chronic kidney disease without dose reduction.

Safety Considerations

The DPP-4 inhibitors are generally well-tolerated. They can cause some gastrointestinal side effects, although not to the extent caused by GLP-1 agonists. There have been reports of pancreatitis in patients taking DPP-4 inhibitors, although the causal relationship has not been definitively established.[57] In postmarketing reports, the DPP-4 inhibitors have also been associated with hypersensitivity reactions, including anaphylaxis and angioedema.[58] The proposed mechanism is reduced clearance of bradykinin because DPP-4 is an enzyme that is involved in bradykinin metabolism. DPP-4 inhibitor use is, therefore, contraindicated in patients with history of hypersensitivity reactions.

SUMMARY

Treatment options for type 2 diabetes have undergone a Renaissance in the last decade. The 3 newer classes of agents are the SGLT-2 inhibitors, GLP-1 agonists, and DPP-4 inhibitors. Following the new FDA guidelines, these agents need to demonstrate cardiovascular safety in addition to glycemic efficacy. In cardiovascular outcome trials, some of the SGLT-2 inhibitors and GLP-1 agonists have not only demonstrated noninferiority but also superiority, which has been widely welcomed in the diabetes community. Although metformin still remains the first-line agent of choice in treating type 2 diabetes, the choice of a second-line agent depends on various factors such as the patient's cardiovascular risk profile, weight, and renal function. When making a selection for diabetes treatment, clinicians currently need to consider not only the glycemic efficacy of the agent but also all the other potential benefits, balanced by the potential adverse effects. This article has summarized the key points with regard to the benefit and safety considerations of new agents for the treatment of type 2 diabetes.

REFERENCES

1. World Health Organisation. Global Report on Diabetes 2016. Available at: http://apps.who.int/iris/bitstream/handle/10665/204871/9789241565257_eng.pdf; jsessionid=6A969076FC8BC0008CF09A23291FE5C6?sequence=1. Accessed June, 2018.
2. Sola D, Rossi L, Schianca GP, et al. Sulfonylureas and their use in clinical practice. Arch Med Sci 2015;11(4):840–8.
3. Bailey CJ. Metformin: historical overview. Diabetologia 2017;60(9):1566–76.
4. Nesto RW, Bell D, Bonow RO, et al. Thiazolidinedione use, fluid retention, and congestive heart failure: a consensus statement from the American Heart Association and American Diabetes Association. Diabetes Care 2004;27(1):256–63.
5. Nissen SE, Wolski K. Effect of rosiglitazone on the risk of myocardial infarction and death from cardiovascular causes. N Engl J Med 2007;356(24):2457–71.
6. Food and Drug Administration. Diabetes mellitus - evaluating cardiovascular risk in new antidiabetic therapies to treat type 2 diabetes 2008. Available at: https://www.fda.gov/downloads/Drugs/GuidanceComplianceRegulatoryInformation/Guidances/UCM071627.pdf. Accessed, 2018.
7. Zheng SL, Roddick AJ, Aghar-Jaffar R, et al. Association between use of sodium-glucose cotransporter 2 inhibitors, glucagon-like peptide 1 agonists, and dipeptidyl peptidase 4 inhibitors with all-cause mortality in patients with type 2 diabetes: a systematic review and meta-analysis. JAMA 2018;319(15):1580–91.

8. Gallo LA, Wright EM, Vallon V. Probing SGLT2 as a therapeutic target for diabetes: basic physiology and consequences. Diab Vasc Dis Res 2015;12(2): 78–89.
9. Tabatabai NM, Sharma M, Blumenthal SS, et al. Enhanced expressions of sodium-glucose cotransporters in the kidneys of diabetic Zucker rats. Diabetes Res Clin Pract 2009;83(1):e27–30.
10. Vallon V, Rose M, Gerasimova M, et al. Knockout of Na-glucose transporter SGLT2 attenuates hyperglycemia and glomerular hyperfiltration but not kidney growth or injury in diabetes mellitus. Am J Physiol Renal Physiol 2013;304(2): F156–67.
11. Zinman B, Wanner C, Lachin JM, et al, EMPA-REG OUTCOME Investigators. Empagliflozin, cardiovascular outcomes, and mortality in type 2 diabetes. N Engl J Med 2015;373(22):2117–28.
12. Abdul-Ghani M, Del Prato S, Chilton R, et al. SGLT2 Inhibitors and cardiovascular risk: lessons learned from the EMPA-REG OUTCOME Study. Diabetes Care 2016; 39(5):717–25.
13. Ferrannini E, Mark M, Mayoux E. CV protection in the EMPA-REG outcome trial: a "thrifty substrate" hypothesis. Diabetes Care 2016;39(7):1108–14.
14. Neal B, Perkovic V, Mahaffey KW, et al, CANVAS Program Collaborative Group. Canagliflozin and cardiovascular and renal events in type 2 diabetes. N Engl J Med 2017;377(7):644–57.
15. Kosiborod M, Cavender MA, Fu AZ, et al. Lower risk of heart failure and death in patients initiated on sodium-glucose cotransporter-2 inhibitors versus other glucose-lowering drugs: the CVD-REAL study (comparative effectiveness of cardiovascular outcomes in new users of sodium-glucose cotransporter-2 inhibitors). Circulation 2017;136(3):249–59.
16. Liu XY, Zhang N, Chen R, et al. Efficacy and safety of sodium-glucose cotransporter 2 inhibitors in type 2 diabetes: a meta-analysis of randomized controlled trials for 1 to 2years. J Diabetes Complications 2015;29(8):1295–303.
17. Sun YN, Zhou Y, Chen X, et al. The efficacy of dapagliflozin combined with hypoglycaemic drugs in treating type 2 diabetes mellitus: meta-analysis of randomised controlled trials. BMJ Open 2014;4(4):e004619.
18. Schernthaner G, Gross JL, Rosenstock J, et al. Canagliflozin compared with sitagliptin for patients with type 2 diabetes who do not have adequate glycemic control with metformin plus sulfonylurea: a 52-week randomized trial. Diabetes Care 2013;36(9):2508–15.
19. Nauck MA, Del Prato S, Meier JJ, et al. Dapagliflozin versus glipizide as add-on therapy in patients with type 2 diabetes who have inadequate glycemic control with metformin: a randomized, 52-week, double-blind, active-controlled noninferiority trial. Diabetes Care 2011;34(9):2015–22.
20. Wanner C, Inzucchi SE, Lachin JM, et al. Empagliflozin and progression of kidney disease in type 2 diabetes. N Engl J Med 2016;375(4):323–34.
21. Food and Drug Administration 2016. Available at: https://www.accessdata.fda.gov/drugsatfda_docs/label/2016/204042s015s019lbl.pdf. Accessed, 2018.
22. Fralick M, Schneeweiss S, Patorno E. Risk of diabetic ketoacidosis after initiation of an SGLT2 inhibitor. N Engl J Med 2017;376(23):2300–2.
23. Erondu N, Desai M, Ways K, et al. Diabetic ketoacidosis and related events in the canagliflozin type 2 diabetes clinical program. Diabetes Care 2015;38(9):1680–6.
24. Taylor SI, Blau JE, Rother KI. SGLT2 inhibitors may predispose to ketoacidosis. J Clin Endocrinol Metab 2015;100(8):2849–52.

25. Rosenstock J, Ferrannini E. Euglycemic diabetic ketoacidosis: a predictable, detectable, and preventable safety concern with sglt2 inhibitors. Diabetes Care 2015;38(9):1638–42.

26. Tang H, Li D, Wang T, et al. Effect of sodium-glucose cotransporter 2 inhibitors on diabetic ketoacidosis among patients with type 2 diabetes: a meta-analysis of randomized controlled trials. Diabetes Care 2016;39(8):e123–4.

27. Milder DA, Milder TY, Kam PCA. Sodium-glucose co-transporter type-2 inhibitors: pharmacology and peri-operative considerations. Anaesthesia 2018;73(8): 1008–18.

28. Australian Diabetes Society. Alert: Severe euglycaemic ketoacidosis with SGLT2 inhibitor use in the perioperative period [press release]. 2018.

29. Sung J, Padmanabhan S, Gurung S, et al. SGLT2 inhibitors and amputation risk: real-world data from a diabetes foot wound clinic. J Clin Transl Endocrinol 2018; 13:46–7.

30. Lee YS, Jun HS. Anti-diabetic actions of glucagon-like peptide-1 on pancreatic beta-cells. Metabolism 2014;63(1):9–19.

31. Vilsboll T, Krarup T, Deacon CF, et al. Reduced postprandial concentrations of intact biologically active glucagon-like peptide 1 in type 2 diabetic patients. Diabetes 2001;50(3):609–13.

32. Kim W, Egan JM. The role of incretins in glucose homeostasis and diabetes treatment. Pharmacol Rev 2008;60(4):470–512.

33. Marso SP, Daniels GH, Brown-Frandsen K, et al. Liraglutide and cardiovascular outcomes in type 2 diabetes. N Engl J Med 2016;375(4):311–22.

34. Marso SP, Bain SC, Consoli A, et al. Semaglutide and cardiovascular outcomes in patients with type 2 diabetes. N Engl J Med 2016;375(19):1834–44.

35. Holman RR, Bethel MA, Mentz RJ, et al. Effects of once-weekly exenatide on cardiovascular outcomes in type 2 diabetes. N Engl J Med 2017;377(13):1228–39.

36. Pfeffer MA, Claggett B, Diaz R, et al. Lixisenatide in patients with type 2 diabetes and acute coronary syndrome. N Engl J Med 2015;373(23):2247–57.

37. Sun F, Wu S, Guo S, et al. Impact of GLP-1 receptor agonists on blood pressure, heart rate and hypertension among patients with type 2 diabetes: a systematic review and network meta-analysis. Diabetes Res Clin Pract 2015;110(1):26–37.

38. Ferdinand KC, White WB, Calhoun DA, et al. Effects of the once-weekly glucagon-like peptide-1 receptor agonist dulaglutide on ambulatory blood pressure and heart rate in patients with type 2 diabetes mellitus. Hypertension 2014; 64(4):731–7.

39. Robinson LE, Holt TA, Rees K, et al. Effects of exenatide and liraglutide on heart rate, blood pressure and body weight: systematic review and meta-analysis. BMJ Open 2013;3(1) [pii:e001986].

40. Okerson T, Chilton RJ. The cardiovascular effects of GLP-1 receptor agonists. Cardiovasc Ther 2012;30(3):e146–55.

41. Shyangdan DS, Royle P, Clar C, et al. Glucagon-like peptide analogues for type 2 diabetes mellitus. Cochrane Database Syst Rev 2011;(10):CD006423.

42. Potts JE, Gray LJ, Brady EM, et al. The effect of glucagon-like peptide 1 receptor agonists on weight loss in type 2 diabetes: a systematic review and mixed treatment comparison meta-analysis. PLoS One 2015;10(6):e0126769.

43. Pi-Sunyer X, Astrup A, Fujioka K, et al. A randomized, controlled trial of 3.0 mg of liraglutide in weight management. N Engl J Med 2015;373(1):11–22.

44. Mann JFE, Orsted DD, Brown-Frandsen K, et al. Liraglutide and renal outcomes in type 2 diabetes. N Engl J Med 2017;377(9):839–48.

45. Tuttle KR, Lakshmanan MC, Rayner B, et al. Dulaglutide versus insulin glargine in patients with type 2 diabetes and moderate-to-severe chronic kidney disease (AWARD-7): a multicentre, open-label, randomised trial. Lancet Diabetes Endocrinol 2018;6(8):605–17.

46. Gerstein HC, Colhoun HM, Dagenais GR, et al. Design and baseline characteristics of participants in the Researching cardiovascular Events with a Weekly INcretin in Diabetes (REWIND) trial on the cardiovascular effects of dulaglutide. Diabetes Obes Metab 2018;20(1):42–9.

47. Vilsboll T, Bain SC, Leiter LA, et al. Semaglutide, reduction in glycated haemoglobin and the risk of diabetic retinopathy. Diabetes Obes Metab 2018;20(4):889–97.

48. Feldman-Billard S, Larger E, Massin P. Early worsening of diabetic retinopathy after rapid improvement of blood glucose control in patients with diabetes. Diabetes Metab 2018;44(1):4–14.

49. Green JB, Bethel MA, Armstrong PW, et al. Effect of sitagliptin on cardiovascular outcomes in type 2 diabetes. N Engl J Med 2015;373(3):232–42.

50. Scirica BM, Bhatt DL, Braunwald E, et al. Saxagliptin and cardiovascular outcomes in patients with type 2 diabetes mellitus. N Engl J Med 2013;369(14):1317–26.

51. Food and Drug Administration. Safety Communication: FDA adds warnings about heart failure risk to labels of type 2 diabetes medicines containing saxagliptin and alogliptin 2014. Available at: https://www.fda.gov/Drugs/DrugSafety/ucm486096.htm.

52. Amori RE, Lau J, Pittas AG. Efficacy and safety of incretin therapy in type 2 diabetes: systematic review and meta-analysis. JAMA 2007;298(2):194–206.

53. Scheen AJ, Charpentier G, Ostgren CJ, et al. Efficacy and safety of saxagliptin in combination with metformin compared with sitagliptin in combination with metformin in adult patients with type 2 diabetes mellitus. Diabetes Metab Res Rev 2010;26(7):540–9.

54. Groop PH, Cooper ME, Perkovic V, et al. Linagliptin lowers albuminuria on top of recommended standard treatment in patients with type 2 diabetes and renal dysfunction. Diabetes Care 2013;36(11):3460–8.

55. Esaki H, Tachi T, Goto C, et al. Renoprotective effect of dipeptidyl peptidase-4 inhibitors in patients with type 2 diabetes mellitus. Front Pharmacol 2017;8:835.

56. Kim YG, Byun J, Yoon D, et al. Renal protective effect of DPP-4 inhibitors in type 2 diabetes mellitus patients: a cohort study. J Diabetes Res 2016;2016:1423191.

57. Pinto LC, Rados DV, Barkan SS, et al. Dipeptidyl peptidase-4 inhibitors, pancreatic cancer and acute pancreatitis: a meta-analysis with trial sequential analysis. Sci Rep 2018;8(1):782.

58. Karagiannis T, Boura P, Tsapas A. Safety of dipeptidyl peptidase 4 inhibitors: a perspective review. Ther Adv Drug Saf 2014;5(3):138–46.

Melatonin in Critical Care

Annachiara Marra, MD, PhD[a], Tracy J. McGrane, MD, MPH[b],
Christopher Patrick Henson, DO[b], Pratik P. Pandharipande, MD, MSCI, FCCM[b],*

KEYWORDS

- Critical care • Delirium • Melatonin • Neuroprotection • Sepsis • Sleep

KEY POINTS

- Melatonin regulates a variety of physiologic functions, such as circadian rhythm, immune regulation, prooxidant and antioxidant activity, and neuroprotection.
- Melatonin secretion in critically ill patients has been investigated in several studies but with conflicting results. Some studies reported abolished melatonin secretion pattern in sedated critically ill patients, whereas other studies reported a preserved circadian periodicity.
- An increase in duration and quality of sleep has been associated with the administration of exogenous melatonin; however, larger randomized controlled trials are necessary before its routine use can be recommended.
- Perioperative melatonin supplementation resulted in shorter delirium duration. This could be the result of the chronobiotic properties of melatonin, which resets the sleep–wake cycle through its influence on the biological clock. Alternatively, it may play a direct role in the pathophysiology of delirium.
- Melatonin may have a role in preventing septic shock. In addition to action at the local sites of inflammation, melatonin also acts as immunomodulator, antioxidant, and antiapoptotic agent.

INTRODUCTION

Melatonin (N-acetyl-5-hydroxytryptamine) is a hormone that is secreted primarily by the pineal gland, with the most secretion occurring in times of darkness and paralleling the light–dark cycle (**Figs. 1** and **2**). Endogenous melatonin is released at night beginning around 21:00 with peak release between 2:00 and 4:00, and it is inhibited typically between 7:00 and 9:00, coinciding with the peak secretion of endogenous cortisol.

Disclosures and Funding Sources: Dr P.P. Pandharipande has received a research grant from Hospira Inc, in collaboration with the NIH. Other authors have nothing to disclose relevant to this article.
[a] Department of Neurosciences, Reproductive and Odontostomatological Sciences, University of Naples, Federico II, Via S. Pansini 5, Naples 80138, Italy; [b] Department of Anesthesiology, Division of Anesthesiology Critical Care Medicine, Vanderbilt University Medical Center, 1211 21st Avenue South, Medical Arts Building, Suite 422, Nashville, TN 37212, USA
* Corresponding author.
E-mail address: pratik.pandharipande@vanderbilt.edu

Crit Care Clin 35 (2019) 329–340
https://doi.org/10.1016/j.ccc.2018.11.008
0749-0704/19/© 2018 Elsevier Inc. All rights reserved.

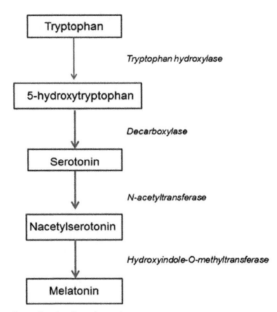

Fig. 1. Pineal gland synthesis of melatonin.

Norepinephrine stimulates the rhythmic secretion of endogenous melatonin via both β1 and α1 receptors.[1] The pineal gland does not have the ability to store melatonin, so plasma melatonin levels closely reflect the synthetic activity of the gland.[2] The melatonin receptors (MTs) 1 and 2 are G-protein–coupled receptors. MT1 receptor activation is implicated in sleep induction; MT2 receptor activation is involved in the regulation of circadian rhythms.[3] Endogenous and exogenous melatonin is metabolized by the liver to 6-hydroxymelatonin, which is then conjugated with either sulfuric acid to 6-sulfatoxymelatonin (SMT) or glucuronic acid. Orally administered melatonin is subject to extensive first-pass metabolism, and absolute bioavailability is reported to be approximately 15%, although highly variable[4] owing to interindividual differences of expression and activity of hepatic cytochrome P450 1A2 (CYP1A2).[5] The conjugated metabolites are renally excreted and, in healthy subjects, 6-SMT urinary excretion parallels melatonin secretion.[6] Melatonin has an elimination half-life of 30 to 45 minutes, which is extended to approximately 100 minutes in cirrhotic patients.[7] Critically ill patients have an impeded elimination probably due to altered liver and kidney function.[8]

Melatonin secretion in critical care patients has been investigated in several studies reporting conflicting results. Some studies have reported disruption of the natural melatonin secretion pattern in sedated critically ill patients,[9–13] and a disturbed melatonin excretion pattern and absence of nocturnal rise in all critically ill patients,[14] whereas other studies reported a preserved circadian periodicity.[10,15] Boyko and colleagues[16] observed phase-delayed diurnal variation of melatonin secretion in critically ill patients, probably explained by evening light exposure in the intensive care unit (ICU) setting during procedures.

The role of the level or the type of sedation on melatonin secretion is not completely understood.[16] The choice of sedative seemed to have little influence on melatonin and 6-SMT levels.[11,15,17] In some studies, benzodiazepines administration (mostly midazolam) was associated with a slightly higher 6-SMT excretion.[17] Conversely, Riutta

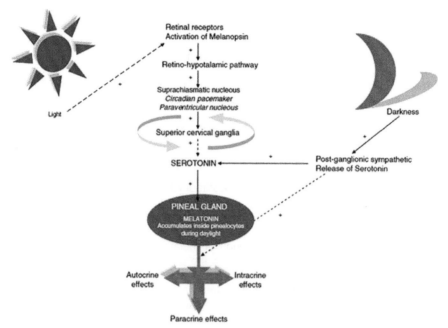

Fig. 2. Physiologic pathways for the synthesis of melatonin. Direct light activates melanopsin (a photopigment within the retina), leading to pupillary constriction, suppression of circadian rhythms, photoentrainment, regulation of alertness, and cognitive functions, with suppression of the release of melatonin. Light inhibits the release of melatonin from the pineal gland and promotes its storage during dark cycles. Darkness stimulates postganglionic serotonin. (*From* Bellapart J, Boots R. Potential use of melatonin in sleep and delirium in the critically ill. Br J Anaesth 2012;108(4):574; with permission.)

and colleagues[18] found maintained diurnal pattern of melatonin secretion in nonseptic critically ill patients, and benzodiazepines did not affect the diurnal variation of 6-SMT excretion.

Exogenous melatonin has been administered for possible regulation of sleep and delirium in critically ill patients.[1] Its use has also demonstrated anxiolytic, analgesic, and antioxidative properties.[19–21]

This article reviews the principal properties of melatonin and how these could find clinical applications in critical care.

SLEEP DISORDERS AND DELIRIUM IN CRITICALLY ILL PATIENTS

Sleep deprivation and delirium are major problems in the ICU.[22] Although the relationship between sleep disturbance and delirium has not been well-established, the literature suggests that these phenomena share similarity of mechanisms, such as neurohormonal changes, imbalances in neurotransmitters, and similar sites of action in the central nervous system.[22,23] Clinical characteristics associated with delirium, such as inattention, fluctuating mental status, and cognitive dysfunction may also be present in patients with disrupted sleep.[23] Moreover, the risk factors for the development of sleep deprivation in critically ill overlap with those of delirium.[23]

Sleep disturbances in critically ill patients are characterized by severe fragmentation, and by frequent arousals and awakenings.[24] Sleep architecture is disrupted with a dominance of stage-1 and stage-2 nonrapid eye movement sleep, with reduced deeper phases of sleep slow-wave sleep (SWS) and rapid eye movement (REM) sleep.[24] Sleep deprivation has several documented adverse effects somatically and psychologically, such as deranging immune function, prolonging mechanical ventilation, and provoking ICU delirium.[23]

The administration and the sudden discontinuation of many medications can influence the wake–sleep-regulatory system by a direct effect on neurotransmitter and hormone activity. Benzodiazepines and opioids can reduce both SWS and REM sleep via γ-aminobutyric (GABA) type A and opioid μ-receptor stimulation, respectively. Additionally, opioids can cause delirium by decreasing acetylcholine and increasing dopamine and glutamate activity. Propofol suppresses the REM sleep stage and further worsens the poor sleep quality of these patients, and might be associated with short-term (delirium) and long-term (posttraumatic stress disorder) effects in critically ill patients.[25]

Environmental factors, mechanical ventilation, critical illness itself, and medication play an important role in sleep disruption in critically ill patients.[26–28] Multiple studies indicated that impaired secretion of melatonin was observed in critically ill patients, which may be associated with the development of sleep deprivation and delirium.

Pharmacologic treatment of sleep disturbances of patients in critical care units is problematic, in terms of both drug efficacy and adverse effects, especially on the architecture of normal sleep.[29] The efficacy of exogenous melatonin to improve sleep in critically ill patients has been studied in a variety of doses and preparations.[1] Shilo and colleagues[30] found increased sleep duration (6.3 h $\pm$ 1.1 standard deviation) and sleep quality, assessed by actigraph, with 3 mg melatonin in critically ill patients with chronic obstructive pulmonary disease. At the same dose, Ibrahim and colleagues[31] found no differences in subjectively assessed sleep in 2 groups of tracheostomized, critically ill patients. Bourne and colleagues[8] reported improved sleep efficiency, monitored by Bispectral Index (BIS), with 10 mg melatonin in mechanically ventilated, critically ill patients in the weaning period.

Selective melatonin receptor agonists have been used for the treatment of insomnia and circadian rhythm. Currently, 2 agents, ramelteon and tasimelteon, are available in the United States and a third agent, agomelatine, has been used in Europe for the treatment of major depressive episodes owing to its additional serotonin antagonist properties.[32] Ramelteon is the only agent that has been studied in the ICU setting, and it seems to enhance sleep by shortening sleep latency and extending the total duration of sleep through diminishing arousal signals generated by the suprachiasmatic nucleus.[33] Ramelteon has been shown to have no abuse potential, less sedating effects, and minimal cognitive impairment effects.[34]

Significant questions remain regarding the application of melatonin treatment of sleep disorders in critically ill patients and larger randomized controlled trials are necessary to confirm the benefits, dosage, timing, and necessary duration of administration of melatonin therapy in improving sleep in patients recovering from critical illness before its routine use can be recommended.[7]

Delirium is a common and challenging complication in ICU patients[35] and is a strong predictor of increased length of mechanical ventilation, longer ICU stays, increased cost, long-term cognitive impairment, and mortality.[36–40] Although proof of a causal relation is still lacking, evidence has shown an association between melatonin abnormalities and delirium,[11,14,41–43] and recent randomized controlled clinical trials have indicated that melatonin can prevent delirium.[42,44,45] de Jonghe and colleagues[43] evaluated the effect of prophylactic melatonin, at dose of 3 mg, on the incidence of delirium in subjects requiring hip surgery and found no significant difference (29.6%, 55/186) in the melatonin group versus (25.5%, 49/192) the placebo group (absolute difference 4.1%, 95% CI −0.05–13.1). There were no between-group differences in mortality or cognitive or functional outcomes at 3-months follow-up. However, there was some indication that perioperative melatonin supplementation resulted in fewer subjects having a long duration (>2 days) of delirium.[43] This could be the result of the chronobiotic properties of melatonin that resets the sleep–wake cycle through its influence on the biological clock. Alternatively, it may play a direct role in the pathophysiology of delirium.[43] (**Fig. 3**).

The use of ramelteon was associated with a lower risk of delirium and a decrease of delirium duration and ICU length of stay.[42,46] From the current findings, it is unclear whether the preventive effects of ramelteon on delirium are associated with its sleep-promoting activity.[42]

Further studies are needed and the 2018 clinical practice guidelines for the management of pain, agitation, and delirium in adult patients in the intensive care unit include no specific recommendations for delirium prophylaxis using any particular medication.[47]

SEPSIS

Oxidative stress is important in the pathophysiology of cellular injury in sepsis, and there is some evidence that pharmacologic doses of melatonin may be beneficial in the treatment of sepsis.[7]

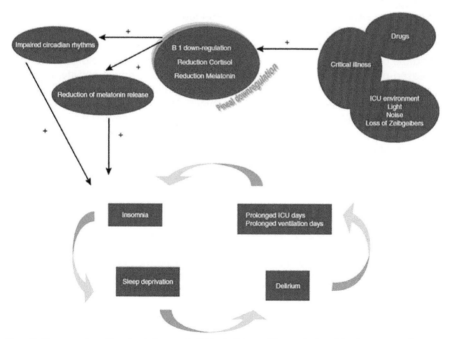

Fig. 3. Proposed pathophysiology of ICU delirium. The relationship between the ICU environment and the development of delirium shows an altered release of melatonin and a fragmentation of biological and circadian rhythms. (*From* Bellapart J, Boots R. Potential use of melatonin in sleep and delirium in the critically ill. Br J Anaesth 2012;108(4):576; with permission.)

It is unknown whether physiologic levels of melatonin have sufficient direct antioxidant activity to attenuate the development or severity of sepsis; however, in vitro models show that melatonin and its major hydroxylated metabolite, 6-hydroxymelatonin, are both effective at reducing the levels of key inflammatory cytokines, oxidative stress, and mitochondrial dysfunction in sepsis.[48]

In animal models, melatonin has been identified as protective against bacterial, viral, and parasitic infections, presumably through a variety of immunomodulatory and antioxidant mechanisms.[49] Melatonin is a powerful antioxidant that scavenges superoxide radicals, as well as other radical oxygen species (ROS) and radical nitrogen species, which gives rise to a cascade of metabolites that share its antioxidant properties. Melatonin also acts indirectly to promote gene expression of antioxidant enzymes and to inhibit gene expression of prooxidant enzymes.[50] Melatonin exhibits significant antiinflammatory properties presumably by decreasing the synthesis of proinflammatory cytokines such as tumor necrosis factor (TNF)-α and by suppressing inducible nitric oxide synthase (iNOS) gene expression. Melatonin also exerts a strong antiapoptotic effect.[50]

In animal experiments, melatonin administered to rats before and after administration of lipopolysaccharide (LPS)-reduced lipid peroxidation, increased glutathione levels, and reduced polymorphonuclear neutrophil infiltration of the liver compared with a placebo-treated group.[51] Another study exposed rats to LPS endotoxin 4 hours after melatonin (10 mg/kg) or placebo was administered,[52] demonstrating a reversal of the reduction in erythrocyte deformability and significantly increasing levels of glutathione peroxidase in the treatment group compared with the placebo group. This study suggests that melatonin may also attenuate the decrease in capillary perfusion that occurs in sepsis. Melatonin prevents LPS-induced endotoxemia, presumably by reducing circulating TNF-α levels, superoxide production in the aorta, and iNOS in the liver.[53] Melatonin (10 mg/kg, intraperitoneal [IP]) given 30 minutes before LPS prevented the decrease in Pao_2 and the lung injury caused by the endotoxin. Melatonin decreased pulmonary edema, the elevated lung myeloperoxidase activity, and lipid peroxidation after LPS.[49] The increase of the proinflammatory cytokine TNF-α levels in pulmonary tissue given by LPS was also prevented by melatonin, whereas the levels of the antiinflammatory cytokine interleukin (IL)-10 were augmented.[49] In another study, rats receiving melatonin (10 mg/kg IP) before and 6 hours after induction of sepsis by cecal ligation and perforation showed reduced lipid peroxidation and neutrophil infiltration of their intestinal and bladder tissues, relative to placebo group, and avoided the reduction of glutathione seen in the placebo group.[54]

In an experimental model for septic shock, the massive release of proinflammatory mediators TNF-α, IL-6, prostaglandins, nitric oxide (NO), and ROS observed with the zymosan A, was ameliorated with simultaneous administration of melatonin (0.8 mg/kg), and resulted in only 27% mortality rate compared with 100% with zymosan A alone.[55] Melatonin has also demonstrated protection against myocardial ischemia when administered to rats before isoproterenol-induced injury.[56] These results are difficult to extrapolate; however, it does not preclude further investigation of melatonin as a preemptive therapy in situations in which ischemic reperfusion injury is predictable (eg, hepatic resection).

Several clinical studies performed have shown that melatonin reduces oxidative stress in newborns with sepsis or other conditions in which there is excessive ROS production. In a study of 20 septic newborns, the melatonin-treatment group had statistically significant reduced white cell counts, neutrophil counts, and C-reactive protein levels, as well as raised platelet levels, compared with the placebo group.[20] Additionally, the melatonin group had statistically lower levels of lipid peroxidation products 1 hour and 4 hours after treatment. Although there had been a clinical improvement in the daily sepsis score in the melatonin group, the study was too small to demonstrate a statistically significant difference in patient mortality. Although melatonin has antioxidant effects, it also shows prooxidative properties. These oxidative effects are considered responsible for the antimicrobial properties of melatonin.[57] It has been shown that melatonin reduces viremia, delays the natural history of viral disease and reduces mortality in animal models.[57] Melatonin also exhibits antimicrobial effects by reducing bacterial lipid content and by having iron-binding properties, leading to bacterial substrates depletion.[58]

Larger randomized controlled trials are necessary to confirm the suggested benefits of melatonin in different populations of septic patients, with the necessary longer term morbidity and mortality data, before this treatment can be recommended. Also, the potential immunostimulatory and suppressive actions of melatonin need to be considered in terms of current knowledge of the pathophysiology of sepsis.[20]

Melatonin is a substance with therapeutic potential for the treatment of systemic inflammation, including sepsis, because it may act at the earliest step of activation of the oxidative and proinflammatory cascade.[49]

The potential effect of melatonin in preventing septic shock is complex. Apart from acting on the local sites of inflammation, melatonin also exerts its beneficial actions through a multifactorial pathway, including its effects as immunomodulator, antioxidant, and antiapoptotic agent.[49]

The dose needed for antioxidant action is thought to be considerably higher than that given for modulation of the sleep–wake cycle; however, the actual dose required in humans is unclear, primarily because the major bioactive effects of oral melatonin in the context of inflammation are likely to be mediated by metabolite levels.[48,49]

SEDATION AND ANALGESIA

Melatonin is a neuroprotective agent with sedative, hypnotic, and analgesic properties without any respiratory depressant effect, which makes it an attractive adjuvant for sedation in the ICU.[59,60] The antinociceptive effects of melatonin have been shown in several animal models.[61,62]

In clinical studies, melatonin has been shown to have analgesic benefits in patients with chronic pain, such as fibromyalgia, irritable bowel syndrome, and migraine,[60] and those with extensive tissue injuries.[63]

The physiologic mechanisms underlying the analgesic actions of melatonin have not been clarified and may be linked to G(i)-coupled melatonin receptors, to G(i)-coupled opioid μ-receptor or GABA receptors, with unknown downstream changes, leading to a consequential reduction in anxiety and pain. Also, the repeated administration of melatonin improves sleep and, thereby, may reduce anxiety, which leads to lower levels of pain.[60,64] The melatonin dose with analgesic potential is undefined.[65]

Deep sedation in patients who are critically ill is associated with poor clinical outcomes, including prolonged mechanical ventilation and death.[66] The clinical practice guidelines for the prevention and management of pain, agitation/sedation, delirium, immobility, and sleep disruption in adult patients in the ICU recommend clinicians should target a light rather than deep level of sedation in their intubated, critically ill adult patients unless deeper sedation is clinically indicated. In critically ill, intubated adults, daily sedative interruption protocols and nursing-protocolized targeted sedation are safe, and no differences exist between them in achieving and maintaining a light level of sedation.[47] Patients in whom ongoing agitation complicates the sedation minimization processes may benefit from nonsedative adjuvant agents. Mistraletti and colleagues[67] evaluated whether nocturnal melatonin supplementation (3 + 3 mg at 20:00 and midnight) from the third ICU day until ICU discharge would reduce the need for sedation in patients with critical illness. The administration of melatonin as a supplement in critically ill patients was associated with a decrease in the consumption of enteral hydroxyzine, shorter duration of mechanical ventilation, improved neurologic indicators, and cost-reduction. The difference in mechanical ventilation weaning between groups became evident after a week of melatonin administration, suggesting that the clinical role of melatonin is mediated by a cumulative effect in the reduction of sedatives and by its immune-modulating effect, both requiring time to become clinically relevant. In another study, Gitto and colleagues[64] evaluated the analgesic activity of melatonin during endotracheal intubation of the newborn by using the Neonatal Infant Pain Scale (NIPS) and Premature Infant Pain Profile (PIPP) score. Sixty preterm infants were enrolled in the study and were randomly divided into 2 groups: 30 infants treated with melatonin plus common sedation and analgesia (group 1) and 30 infants treated with only common sedation and analgesia.[64] The reduction in pain score (NIPS) was similar in both groups at an early phase, whereas the PIPP score was lower in the melatonin-treated group infants than in the other newborns at a late phase, during intubation, and mechanical ventilation. The differences were statistically significant at 12, 24, 48, and 72 hours ($P<.001$).[64] This study suggests positive benefits with the use of melatonin as an adjunct analgesic therapy during procedural pain, especially when an inflammatory component is involved.[64]

The low-risk profile of melatonin, along with its positive effect on clinical outcomes for critically ill patients, makes it a potentially attractive strategy to reduce the sedation requirements of critically ill patients with agitation. Further multicenter evaluations are required to confirm these results with different sedation protocols.

NEUROPROTECTION

Models of traumatic brain injury suggest that melatonin may have neuroprotective effects mediated through the inhibition of excitotoxic damage and prevention of ischemia–reperfusion injury.[68] Melatonin has also been shown to reduce body temperature in humans,[69] which has been associated with improved neurologic outcome after cardiac arrest, in addition to improved regional cerebral blood flow in animal models.[70] By its antioxidant properties, melatonin protects against oxidative stress, prevents neuronal damage associated with epilepsy, has putative neuroprotective effects, and can be used as an anticonvulsant.[71]

TREATMENT AND PREVENTION OF STRESS-INDUCED GASTRIC ULCERS

Melatonin is generated in the gastrointestinal tract and serves as a local antioxidant and protective factor.[72] Melatonin has ulcer healing and gastroprotective effects. This involves hyperemia at the ulcer margin and numerous mechanisms, including activation of brain gut axis, sensory afferent nerves, and certain gut hormones, especially gastrin.[73]

SUMMARY

The naturally produced hormone melatonin contributes to numerous therapeutic benefits associated with normalization of the sleep–wake cycle, reduction of inflammation, and protection of the gastrointestinal tract. Therapeutic doses of exogenous melatonin may have more profound effects as therapy for prevention of septic shock, organ protection following injury, and analgesia for acute and chronic pain syndromes.

The potential clinical effects and general safety profile suggest that it may be an excellent supplement to other analgesics, hypnotics, sedatives, and antiinflammatory drugs used in the treatment of critically ill patients; however, larger randomized controlled trials are necessary to confirm the benefits, dosage, timing, and necessary duration of administration of melatonin therapy before its routine use can be recommended.

REFERENCES

1. Bellapart J, Boots R. Potential use of melatonin in sleep and delirium in the critically ill. Br J Anaesth 2012;108(4):572–80.
2. Claustrat B, Brun J, Chazot G. The basic physiology and pathophysiology of melatonin. Sleep Med Rev 2005;9(1):11–24.
3. Johnsa JD, Neville MW. Tasimelteon: a melatonin receptor agonist for non-24-hour sleep-wake disorder. Ann Pharmacother 2014;48(12):1636–41.
4. Di WL, Kadva A, Johnston A, et al. Variable bioavailability of oral melatonin. N Engl J Med 1997;336(14):1028–9.
5. Hartter S, Ursing C, Morita S, et al. Orally given melatonin may serve as a probe drug for cytochrome P450 1A2 activity in vivo: a pilot study. Clin Pharmacol Ther 2001;70(1):10–6.
6. Bojkowski CJ, Arendt J, Shih MC, et al. Melatonin secretion in humans assessed by measuring its metabolite, 6-sulfatoxymelatonin. Clin Chem 1987;33(8):1343–8.
7. Bourne RS, Mills GH. Melatonin: possible implications for the postoperative and critically ill patient. Intensive Care Med 2006;32(3):371–9.
8. Bourne RS, Mills GH, Minelli C. Melatonin therapy to improve nocturnal sleep in critically ill patients: encouraging results from a small randomised controlled trial. Crit Care 2008;12(2):R52.
9. Paul T, Lemmer B. Disturbance of circadian rhythms in analgosedated intensive care unit patients with and without craniocerebral injury. Chronobiol Int 2007; 24(1):45–61.
10. Mundigler G, Delle-Karth G, Koreny M, et al. Impaired circadian rhythm of melatonin secretion in sedated critically ill patients with severe sepsis. Crit Care Med 2002;30(3):536–40.
11. Olofsson K, Alling C, Lundberg D, et al. Abolished circadian rhythm of melatonin secretion in sedated and artificially ventilated intensive care patients. Acta Anaesthesiol Scand 2004;48(6):679–84.
12. Perras B, Meier M, Dodt C. Light and darkness fail to regulate melatonin release in critically ill humans. Intensive Care Med 2007;33(11):1954–8.
13. Verceles AC, Silhan L, Terrin M, et al. Circadian rhythm disruption in severe sepsis: the effect of ambient light on urinary 6-sulfatoxymelatonin secretion. Intensive Care Med 2012;38(5):804–10.
14. Shilo L, Dagan Y, Smorjik Y, et al. Patients in the intensive care unit suffer from severe lack of sleep associated with loss of normal melatonin secretion pattern. Am J Med Sci 1999;317(5):278–81.
15. Gehlbach BK, Chapotot F, Leproult R, et al. Temporal disorganization of circadian rhythmicity and sleep-wake regulation in mechanically ventilated patients receiving continuous intravenous sedation. Sleep 2012;35(8):1105–14.
16. Boyko Y, Holst R, Jennum P, et al. Melatonin secretion pattern in critically ill patients: a pilot descriptive study. Crit Care Res Pract 2017;2017:7010854.
17. Frisk U, Olsson J, Nylen P, et al. Low melatonin excretion during mechanical ventilation in the intensive care unit. Clin Sci (Lond) 2004;107(1):47–53.

18. Riutta A, Ylitalo P, Kaukinen S. Diurnal variation of melatonin and cortisol is maintained in non-septic intensive care patients. Intensive Care Med 2009;35(10): 1720-7.

19. Andersen LP, Werner MU, Rosenberg J, et al. A systematic review of perioperative melatonin. Anaesthesia 2014;69(10):1163-71.

20. Gitto E, Karbownik M, Reiter RJ, et al. Effects of melatonin treatment in septic newborns. Pediatr Res 2001;50(6):756-60.

21. Gitto E, Romeo C, Reiter RJ, et al. Melatonin reduces oxidative stress in surgical neonates. J Pediatr Surg 2004;39(2):184-9 [discussion: 184-9].

22. Figueroa-Ramos MI, Arroyo-Novoa CM, Lee KA, et al. Sleep and delirium in ICU patients: a review of mechanisms and manifestations. Intensive Care Med 2009; 35(5):781-95.

23. Weinhouse GL, Schwab RJ, Watson PL, et al. Bench-to-bedside review: delirium in ICU patients - importance of sleep deprivation. Crit Care 2009;13(6):234.

24. Watson PL, Pandharipande P, Gehlbach BK, et al. Atypical sleep in ventilated patients: empirical electroencephalography findings and the path toward revised ICU sleep scoring criteria. Crit Care Med 2013;41(8):1958-67.

25. Kondili E, Alexopoulou C, Xirouchaki N, et al. Effects of propofol on sleep quality in mechanically ventilated critically ill patients: a physiological study. Intensive Care Med 2012;38(10):1640-6.

26. Gabor JY, Cooper AB, Crombach SA, et al. Contribution of the intensive care unit environment to sleep disruption in mechanically ventilated patients and healthy subjects. Am J Respir Crit Care Med 2003;167(5):708-15.

27. Fanfulla F, Ceriana P, D'Artavilla Lupo N, et al. Sleep disturbances in patients admitted to a step-down unit after ICU discharge: the role of mechanical ventilation. Sleep 2011;34(3):355-62.

28. Cooper AB, Thornley KS, Young GB, et al. Sleep in critically ill patients requiring mechanical ventilation. Chest 2000;117(3):809-18.

29. Bourne RS, Mills GH. Sleep disruption in critically ill patients - pharmacological considerations. Anaesthesia 2004;59(4):374-84.

30. Shilo L, Dagan Y, Smorjik Y, et al. Effect of melatonin on sleep quality of COPD intensive care patients: a pilot study. Chronobiol Int 2000;17(1):71-6.

31. Ibrahim MG, Bellomo R, Hart GK, et al. A double-blind placebo-controlled randomised pilot study of nocturnal melatonin in tracheostomised patients. Crit Care Resusc 2006;8(3):187-91.

32. Laudon M, Frydman-Marom A. Therapeutic effects of melatonin receptor agonists on sleep and comorbid disorders. Int J Mol Sci 2014;15(9):15924-50.

33. Neubauer DN. A review of ramelteon in the treatment of sleep disorders. Neuropsychiatr Dis Treat 2008;4(1):69-79.

34. Mo Y, Scheer CE, Abdallah GT. Emerging role of melatonin and melatonin receptor agonists in sleep and delirium in intensive care unit patients. J Intensive Care Med 2016;31(7):451-5.

35. Pandharipande P, Costabile S, Cotton B, et al. Prevalence of delirium in surgical ICU patients. Crit Care Med 2005;33(12 Suppl):A45.

36. Ely EW, Shintani A, Truman B, et al. Delirium as a predictor of mortality in mechanically ventilated patients in the intensive care unit. JAMA 2004;291(14):1753-62.

37. Jackson JC, Hart RP, Gordon SM, et al. Six-month neuropsychological outcome of medical intensive care unit patients. Crit Care Med 2003;31(4):1226-34.

38. Lin SM, Liu CY, Wang CH, et al. The impact of delirium on the survival of mechanically ventilated patients. Crit Care Med 2004;32(11):2254-9.

39. Ely EW, Baker AM, Dunagan DP, et al. Effect on the duration of mechanical venti-lation of identifying patients capable of breathing spontaneously. N Engl J Med 1996;335(25):1864–9.

40. Salluh JI, Wang H, Schneider EB, et al. Outcome of delirium in critically ill pa-tients: systematic review and meta-analysis. BMJ 2015;350:h2538.

41. Miyazaki T, Kuwano H, Kato H, et al. Correlation between serum melatonin circa-dian rhythm and intensive care unit psychosis after thoracic esophagectomy. Sur-gery 2003;133(6):662–8.

42. Hatta K, Kishi Y, Wada K, et al. Preventive effects of ramelteon on delirium: a ran-domized placebo-controlled trial. JAMA Psychiatry 2014;71(4):397–403.

43. de Jonghe A, van Munster BC, Goslings JC, et al. Effect of melatonin on inci-dence of delirium among patients with hip fracture: a multicentre, double-blind randomized controlled trial. CMAJ 2014;186(14):E547–56.

44. Sultan SS. Assessment of role of perioperative melatonin in prevention and treat-ment of postoperative delirium after hip arthroplasty under spinal anesthesia in the elderly. Saudi J Anaesth 2010;4(3):169–73.

45. Al-Aama T, Brymer C, Gutmanis I, et al. Melatonin decreases delirium in elderly patients: a randomized, placebo-controlled trial. Int J Geriatr Psychiatry 2011; 26(7):687–94.

46. Nishikimi M, Numaguchi A, Takahashi K, et al. Effect of administration of ramel-teon, a melatonin receptor agonist, on the duration of stay in the ICU: a single-center randomized placebo-controlled trial. Crit Care Med 2018;46(7):1099–105.

47. Devlin JW, Skrobik Y, Gelinas C, et al. Clinical practice guidelines for the preven-tion and management of pain, agitation/sedation, delirium, immobility, and sleep disruption in adult patients in the ICU. Crit Care Med 2018;46(9):e825–73.

48. Galley HF, Lowes DA, Allen L, et al. Melatonin as a potential therapy for sepsis: a phase I dose escalation study and an ex vivo whole blood model under condi-tions of sepsis. J Pineal Res 2014;56(4):427–38.

49. Srinivasan V, Pandi-Perumal SR, Spence DW, et al. Melatonin in septic shock: some recent concepts. J Crit Care 2010;25(4):656.e1-6.

50. Reiter RJ, Paredes SD, Manchester LC, et al. Reducing oxidative/nitrosative stress: a newly-discovered genre for melatonin. Crit Rev Biochem Mol Biol 2009;44(4):175–200.

51. Sewerynek E, Melchiorri D, Reiter RJ, et al. Lipopolysaccharide-induced hepato-toxicity is inhibited by the antioxidant melatonin. Eur J Pharmacol 1995;293(4): 327–34.

52. Yerer MB, Aydogan S, Yapislar H, et al. Melatonin increases glutathione peroxi-dase activity and deformability of erythrocytes in septic rats. J Pineal Res 2003;35(2):138–9.

53. Wu CC, Chiao CW, Hsiao G, et al. Melatonin prevents endotoxin-induced circula-tory failure in rats. J Pineal Res 2001;30(3):147–56.

54. Paskaloglu K, Sener G, Kapucu C, et al. Melatonin treatment protects against sepsis-induced functional and biochemical changes in rat ileum and urinary bladder. Life Sci 2004;74(9):1093–104.

55. Reynolds FD, Dauchy R, Blask D, et al. The pineal gland hormone melatonin im-proves survival in a rat model of sepsis/shock induced by zymosan A. Surgery 2003;134(3):474–9.

56. Acikel M, Buyukokuroglu ME, Aksoy H, et al. Protective effects of melatonin against myocardial injury induced by isoproterenol in rats. J Pineal Res 2003; 35(2):75–9.

57. Ben-Nathan D, Maestroni GJ, Lustig S, et al. Protective effects of melatonin in mice infected with encephalitis viruses. Arch Virol 1995;140(2):223–30.
58. Tekbas OF, Ogur R, Korkmaz A, et al. Melatonin as an antibiotic: new insights into the actions of this ubiquitous molecule. J Pineal Res 2008;44(2):222–6.
59. Kurdi MS, Patel T. The role of melatonin in anaesthesia and critical care. Indian J Anaesth 2013;57(2):137–44.
60. Wilhelmsen M, Amirian I, Reiter RJ, et al. Analgesic effects of melatonin: a review of current evidence from experimental and clinical studies. J Pineal Res 2011; 51(3):270–7.
61. Onal SA, Inalkac S, Kutlu S, et al. Intrathecal melatonin increases the mechanical nociceptive threshold in the rat. Agri 2004;16(4):35–40.
62. Yu CX, Zhu CB, Xu SF, et al. Selective MT(2) melatonin receptor antagonist blocks melatonin-induced antinociception in rats. Neurosci Lett 2000;282(3):161–4.
63. Caumo W, Torres F, Moreira NL Jr, et al. The clinical impact of preoperative melatonin on postoperative outcomes in patients undergoing abdominal hysterectomy. Anesth Analg 2007;105(5):1263–71 [table of contents].
64. Gitto E, Aversa S, Salpietro CD, et al. Pain in neonatal intensive care: role of melatonin as an analgesic antioxidant. J Pineal Res 2012;52(3):291–5.
65. Ismail SA, Mowafi HA. Melatonin provides anxiolysis, enhances analgesia, decreases intraocular pressure, and promotes better operating conditions during cataract surgery under topical anesthesia. Anesth Analg 2009;108(4):1146–51.
66. Shehabi Y, Bellomo R, Reade MC, et al. Early intensive care sedation predicts long-term mortality in ventilated critically ill patients. Am J Respir Crit Care Med 2012;186(8):724–31.
67. Mistraletti G, Umbrello M, Sabbatini G, et al. Melatonin reduces the need for sedation in ICU patients: a randomized controlled trial. Minerva Anestesiol 2015;81(12):1298–310.
68. Reiter RJ, Tan DX, Gitto E, et al. Pharmacological utility of melatonin in reducing oxidative cellular and molecular damage. Pol J Pharmacol 2004;56(2):159–70.
69. Cagnacci A, Elliott JA, Yen SS. Melatonin: a major regulator of the circadian rhythm of core temperature in humans. J Clin Endocrinol Metab 1992;75(2): 447–52.
70. Capsoni S, Stankov BM, Fraschini F. Reduction of regional cerebral blood flow by melatonin in young rats. Neuroreport 1995;6(9):1346–8.
71. Sanchez-Barcelo EJ, Mediavilla MD, Reiter RJ. Clinical uses of melatonin in pediatrics. Int J Pediatr 2011;2011:892624.
72. Sutherland ER, Martin RJ, Ellison MC, et al. Immunomodulatory effects of melatonin in asthma. Am J Respir Crit Care Med 2002;166(8):1055–61.
73. Konturek SJ, Konturek PC, Brzozowski T. Melatonin in gastroprotection against stress-induced acute gastric lesions and in healing of chronic gastric ulcers. J Physiol Pharmacol 2006;57(Suppl 5):51–66.

Incretin Physiology and Pharmacology in the Intensive Care Unit

Mark P. Plummer, MBBS, PhD[a,b,*], Jeroen Hermanides, MD, PhD[c], Adam M. Deane, MBBS, PhD[a,b]

KEYWORDS

- Diabetes mellitus • Glucose-dependent insulinotropic polypeptide • GIP
- Glucagon-like peptide-1 • GLP-1 • Hyperglycemia • ICU

KEY POINTS

- The incretin effect refers to the increased insulin secretory response to an oral glucose load when compared with an isoglycemic intravenous glucose infusion, and is mediated by the enterohormones glucagon-like peptide-1 (GLP-1) and glucose-dependent insulinotropic polypeptide (GIP).
- Drugs that stimulate the GLP-1 receptor (termed GLP-1 receptor agonists) and inhibit dipeptidyl peptidase-4 (which is responsible for the metabolism of endogenously secreted GLP-1 and GIP; termed DPP-IV inhibitors) are the incretin-based therapies and have recently been incorporated into standard treatment algorithms for the management of type 2 diabetes.
- Patients with diabetes are frequently admitted to intensive care units (ICUs) and an increasing number of patients take incretin-based medications. Accordingly, the intensive care clinician should have a basic understanding of incretin physiology and pharmacology.
- Incretin-based therapies have a unique glucose-dependent mechanism of action such that the risk of hypoglycemia is negligible. This has driven interest in the potential for incretin-based agents to be used in the management of acute hyperglycemia in the critically ill.
- Although the evidence to date in the critically ill is limited to small single-center randomized controlled trials, preliminary efficacy and safety data are promising.

Disclosure Statement: The authors have no conflict of interest to declare.
[a] Intensive Care Unit, Royal Melbourne Hospital, 300 Grattan Street, Parkville, Victoria 3050, Australia; [b] Intensive Care, University of Melbourne, 300 Grattan Street, Parkville, Victoria 3050, Australia; [c] Department of Anaesthesiology, Amsterdam UMC, University of Amsterdam, Meibergdreef 9, Postbus 22660, Amsterdam 1105 AZ, The Netherlands
* Corresponding author.
E-mail address: mark.philip.plummer@gmail.com

INCRETIN PHYSIOLOGY
Incretin Effect

The insulin secretory response to an oral glucose load is approximately three-fold greater than the response to an isoglycemic (ie, resulting in the same blood glucose concentrations) intravenous glucose infusion (**Fig. 1**).[1] This phenomenon is called the incretin effect and is attributed to nutrient-stimulated release of the incretin hormones, glucose-dependent insulinotropic polypeptide (GIP), and glucagon-like peptide-1 (GLP-1) from specialized enteroendocrine cells in the gut.[2,3] Plasma concentrations of these hormones rise within minutes of ingesting nutrient and act on the islets of Langerhans in the pancreas to increase insulin and decrease glucagon secretion when the plasma glucose concentration is greater than approximately 6 mmol/L.[4]

The Incretin Hormones

First identified in 1971, GIP was originally named gastric inhibitory polypeptide because it inhibited gastric acid secretion in dogs, only later gaining the more relevant autonym of GIP.[5] GIP is a single 42-amino acid peptide and a member of a family of structurally related hormones including secretin, glucagon, and vasoactive intestinal polypeptide. It is synthesized and stored in specialized enteroendocrine cells, known as K cells, primarily located in the proximal small intestine, and released in response to enteral fat and carbohydrate.[2]

GLP-1 is synthesized and stored in vesicles within enteroendocrine L cells located in the distal ileum and colon, and is released in response to luminal fat, carbohydrate, bile acids, and protein.[6–9] Plasma concentrations of GIP and GLP-1 are low in the fasting state but these rapidly rise following nutrient intake in the setting of normal gastric emptying.[10] Following nutrient ingestion, GIP levels reach a peak after approximately

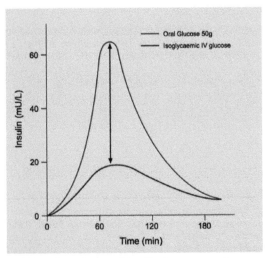

Fig. 1. The incretin effect. The release of insulin in response to an oral glucose load is approximately three-fold greater than following an isoglycemic intravenous infusion of glucose. The difference between the plasma insulin (*arrow*) is the incretin effect and is mediated by the enterohormones glucagon-like peptide 1 and glucose-dependent insulinotropic polypeptide. (*Adapted from* Nauck M, Stockmann F, Ebert R, et al. Reduced incretin effect in type 2 (non-insulin-dependent) diabetes. Diabetologia 1986;29(1):49; with permission.)

1 hour and fall back to basal concentrations over several hours, whereas GLP-1 has a biphasic response with an early peak after 15 minutes and a prolonged second phase over an hour.[10,11] Given the more distal location of the GLP-1 secreting L cells, the near parallel rise in GIP and GLP-1 within minutes of eating suggests autonomic neuron-mediated stimulation of GLP-1 release in this early phase with the prolonged phase attributed to nutrient reaching the L cells in the distal gut.[3]

Once secreted GLP-1 and GIP are degraded by di-peptidyl peptidase 4 (DPP-IV), an enzyme that is bound to lymphocytes and endothelial cells of the gut and liver vascu-lature, and is present in a soluble form within the circulation. This ubiquity in expres-sion of DPP-IV limits the plasma half-life of endogenously secreted GLP-1 and GIP to minutes.[12] Both GLP-1 and GIP are cleaved to inactive metabolites, which are then subsequently cleared by the kidney.

Role of Incretin Hormones in Glucose Homeostasis

The overall effect of the incretin hormones is glucose-dependent glucose lowering via stimulation of insulin and suppression of glucagon secretion and slowing of gastric emptying.[10] Islet ß cells express GIP and GLP-1 G-protein coupled receptors.[13] The binding of each ligand to its respective receptor cannot initiate insulin secretion *de novo* but rather augments clinically significant insulin release in a dose-dependent fashion higher than a glucose threshold of approximately 6 mmol/L.[14] In addition to glucose-dependent insulinotropy, GIP and GLP-1 promote insulin biosynthesis and potentiate ß-cell proliferation thereby augmenting insulin reserve.[12] In health, the rela-tive contributions of GIP and GLP-1 to overall insulinotropy depends on the rate of gastric emptying with GIP the dominant effector at lower rates of nutrient delivery to the small intestine ($\leq$2 kcal/min) and GLP-1 of greater importance at higher rates.[15] The pancreatic alpha-cell express GIP but not GLP-1 receptors. GIP stimulates glucagon secretion in the setting of low plasma glucose, whereas GLP-1 indirectly suppresses glucagon secretion during hyperglycemia leading to reduced hepatic gluconeogenesis.[10,12] Finally, GLP-1 causes marked slowing of the gastric emptying rate, which potently attenuates postprandial glycemic excursions by limiting the deliv-ery of nutrients for absorption in the small intestine.[2,16] Unlike its effects on the islet cell, GLP-1-induced slowing of gastric emptying occurs independently of plasma glucose concentration.[17,18]

INCRETINS IN TYPE 2 DIABETES
Incretin Hormone Pathophysiology in Type 2 Diabetes

The secretion of GIP and GLP-1 is maintained in patients with long-standing type 2 diabetes, whereas the incretin effect is markedly diminished to absent.[19] This is pri-marily attributed to the failure of the endocrine pancreas to respond to GIP, a phenom-enon that persists even when GIP is administered exogenously at supraphysiologic concentrations.[20,21] Slower rates of gastric emptying with decreased delivery of nutri-ents to the small intestine in type 2 diabetes are also thought to be contributory.[15] Conversely, the insulinotropic and glucagonostatic effects of GLP-1 are well pre-served; however because GIP is an important component of the incretin effect, the resulting response is persistent hyperglycemia, perpetuating beta-cell failure.[10,20]

Therapeutic Manipulation of Glucagon-Like Peptide-1 for the Management of Type 2 Diabetes

The preservation of the glucose-lowering ability of GLP-1 during chronic hyperglyce-mia stimulated interest in the development of GLP-1-based pharmacologic therapy for the management of type 2 diabetes.[22] Initial proof-of-principle studies used supraphysiologic doses of exogenous GLP-1 administered subcutaneously or by continuous intravenous infusion, demonstrating a pronounced glucose-dependent glucose lowering effect via enhanced insulin secretion, inhibition of glucagon secretion, and delayed gastric emptying.[14,23,24] Furthermore, via stimulation of hypothalamic GLP-1 receptors, exogenous GLP-1 regulates satiety resulting in reduced caloric intake and sustained weight loss in obesity, which is frequently a desirable outcome for patients with type 2 diabetes who are overweight.[25]

An intervention that increased insulin and decreased glucagon secretion without causing hypoglycemia, and that stimulated weight loss, in this cohort was appealing. However, the clinical utility of exogenous GLP-1 was limited by its short half-life because of rapid degradation by DPP-IV, necessitating continuous intravenous infusions. The fragility of GLP-1 *in vivo* has been overcome by the development of stable DPP-IV-resistant GLP-1 receptor agonists (GLP-1 RAs), and DPP-IV inhibitors, which protect native GLP-1 (and GIP) from enzymatic degradation, thereby increasing systemic and intestinal concentrations to supraphysiologic levels.[26] These two classes of GLP-1-based therapy have been incorporated into standard treatment algorithms for the management of type 2 diabetes and are now frequently prescribed.[27] Approximately 25% of adult patients admitted to the intensive care unit (ICU) have type 2 diabetes.[28] Accordingly, the intensivist should have a basic working knowledge of the action of glucose-lowering medication, including incretin-based therapies.

Commercially Available Incretin Therapies

Glucagon-like peptide-1 receptor agonists

In the United States and Europe there are currently seven GLP-1 RAs approved for the treatment of type 2 diabetes (**Table 1**). In their vanguard herpetologic work, Eng and colleagues[29] identified the first GLP-1 receptor agonist, exendin-4, in the salivary venom of the North American Gila Monster (*Heloderma suspectum*). This lizard peptide has 53% amino acid sequence homology to human GLP-1 and acts as a full agonist at the GLP-1 receptor with the variations in amino acid structure imparting resistance against DPP-IV, extending the plasma half-life to 2.4 hours.[30] Exenatide was developed as the synthetic replica of exendin-4 and in 2005 was the first incretin-based therapy approved for the treatment of type 2 diabetes. Since then, a further four GLP-1 RAs (liraglutide, exenatide XR, lixisenatide, and dulaglutide) have reached the market in Australia and these are broadly categorized as short- or long-acting.

Because of limited oral bioavailability, all are given subcutaneously and safely decrease HbA$_{1c}$ with a low risk of hypoglycaemia.[31] Nausea, vomiting, and diarrhea occur frequently but decrease with time and the magnitude of these gastrointestinal side effects is reduced by gradual titration of dose.[32,33] All GLP-1 RAs lower blood glucose by stimulating insulin and decreasing glucagon in a glucose-dependent fashion; however, there are important differences in fasting and post-prandial glucose control between the short- and long-acting compounds. Exenatide, liraglutide, and lixisenatide are short-acting GLP-1 RAs that require daily or twice-daily dosing with resultant large fluctuations in circulating plasma concentrations.[34] The primary mechanism of glucose lowering with short-acting GLP-1 RAs is mediated via slowing of gastric emptying, decreasing nutrient delivery into the small intestine, thereby attenuating post-prandial glycemic excursions.[35] Accordingly, short-acting GLP-1 RAs should be administered before meals for improved efficacy.[31] These agents are recommended as monotherapy for patients with type 2 diabetes who are intolerant of metformin and as adjunctive therapy in patients with inadequately controlled type 2

Table 1
Marketed GLP-1 receptor agonists

	Exenatide	Liraglutide	Lixisenatide	Exenetaide XR	Albiglutide	Dulaglutide	Semaglutide
Trade name	Byetta	Victoza	Lyumia	Bydureon	Eperzan	Trulicity	Ozempic
Dose	5–10 µg SC BD	0.6–1.8 mg SC OD	10–20 µg SC BD	2 mg SC weekly	30–50 mg SC weekly	0.75–1.5 mg SC weekly	0.25–1 mg weekly
Half-life (t1/2)	2.4 h	13 h	3 h	2.4 h (once released)	5 d	4.5–4.7 d	7 d
Fixed-dose insulin combination	No	Yes	Yes	No	No	No	No
Precautions	ESRD	ESRD, MEN 2, MTC	ESRD	ESRD, MEN 2, MTC	ESRD, Men 2, MTC	ESRD, MEN 2, MTC	MEN 2, MTC

Abbreviations: BD, twice daily; ESRD, end-stage renal disease; MEN 2, multiple endocrine neoplasia syndrome type 2; MTC, medullary thyroid carcinoma; OD, once daily; SC, subcutaneous.

diabetes on oral hypoglycemic agents, basal insulin, or both.[27] By lowering post-prandial glycaemia they confer complementary glycemic control when combined with basal insulin, which primarily targets fasting glucose. Compared with basal-bolus insulin regimens, combination therapy with a short-acting GLP-1 RAs is associated with equivalent reductions in HbA_{1c}, fewer episodes of hypoglycemia, and weight loss as opposed to weight gain.[36] Capitalizing on this ideal trifecta in diabetic treatment there are currently two Food and Drug Administration approved once-daily combination products containing basal insulin plus a short-acting GLP-1 receptor agonist: insulin glargine/lixisenatide and insulin degludec/liraglutide.[27]

Long-acting formulations of GLP-1 RAs have been achieved by encapsulating exenatide into slow-degradable polymeric microspheres (Exenatide-XR), or fusing GLP-1 with human albumin (albiglutide and semaglutide) or heavy chain human immunoglobulin (dulaglutide) allowing for once-weekly subcutaneous dosing. Compared with short-acting GLP-1 RAs they achieve greater reductions in fasting glucose and have little effect on gastric emptying, which has been attributed to gastromotor tachyphylaxis to continuous GLP-1 stimulation.[34] Accordingly, their clinical utility lies in patients with fasting hyperglycemia, and compared with basal insulin they have greater reductions in HbA_{1c}.[37]

Finally, although the approved GLP-1 RA all require subcutaneous administration, semaglutide has recently been combined with an absorption enhancer that allows oral administration, which is currently in phase 3 trials for the treatment of type 2 diabetes.[38]

Di-peptidyl peptidase 4 inhibitors, incretin effect amplifiers

The DPP-IV inhibitors, etymologically identified by the suffix "–gliptin-," are administered orally and glycemic control is primarily mediated locally within the gut via inhibition of intestinal DPP-IV activity, activation of gastric autonomic neural pathways, and amplified stimulation of pancreatic GLP-1 receptors rather than a systemic increase in incretin plasma concentrations.[26] They are approved for use as first-line monotherapy in patients intolerant of metformin and in combination with oral hypoglycemic and/or insulin in patients with recalcitrant hyperglycemia (**Table 2**).[27] In keeping with the inherent safety of incretin-based therapies, the risk of hypoglycemia is negligible when used as monotherapy and low when combined with sulphonylureas and insulin.[39] Compared with GLP-1 RAs they are marginally less efficacious in lowering HbA_{1c} and are weight neutral; however, they are generally better tolerated with fewer adverse events (particularly gastrointestinal) and lower rates of discontinuation because of patient intolerance.[39] Initial concerns were raised because of the presence of DPP-IV on T lymphocytes and macrophages, with enzyme inhibition posing a theoretic risk of immune dysfunction.[40] Adding merit to these concerns was a nested case-control of the Vigibase World Health Organization database reporting an increase in postmarketing reports of upper-respiratory tract infection with DPP-IV therapy.[41] However, this association has subsequently been refuted in a large systematic review.[39]

Safety of Incretin Therapies in Type 2 Diabetes

Early rodent studies suggested an increased risk of thyroid hyperplasia and medullary thyroid carcinoma with GLP-1 receptor stimulation.[42] However, this has not eventuated in human clinical trial data, likely reflective of the low to absent expression of the GLP-1 receptor in normal human thyroid unlike in rodents.[31] Nevertheless, GLP-1 receptor agonists are not recommended for patients at risk of medullary thyroid carcinoma.[43]

Table 2
Marketed DPP-IV inhibitors

	Sitagliption	Vildagliptin	Alogliptin	Saxagliptin	Linagliptin
Trade name	Januvia	Galvus	Nesina	Onglyza	Trajenta
Dose, mg	25–100 PO OD	50 PO BD	25 PO OD	2.5–5 PO OD	5 PO OD
Half-life (t1/2), h	10–12	2	21	27	12
Available fixed-dose combination with metformin	Yes	No	Yes	No	No
Precautions	ESRD	ESRD, hepatic impairment	ESRD	ESRD	—

Abbreviations: BD, twice daily; ESRD, end-stage renal disease; OD, once daily; PO, per oral.

There have also been postmarketing reports raising the possibility of an association between GLP-1 receptor agonists and pancreatitis and pancreatic cancer.[44] An independent review of observational and toxicologic data by European and North American governing bodies did not demonstrate any causal relationship between incretin-based therapies and either pancreatitis or pancreatic cancer and recent large, prospective longer-term outcome studies have also reported no increase in risk.[45–48]

Cardiovascular Effects of Incretin Therapies in Type 2 Diabetes

The US Federal Drug Administration–mandated cardiovascular safety trials for all new diabetic medications has recently provided insights into the cardiovascular safety of incretin therapies.[46–52] GLP-1 RAs (lixisenatide, liraglutide, semaglutide, and extended-release exenatide) were reported to be safe and decrease the risk of major cardiovascular outcomes including cardiovascular death, myocardial infarction, and stroke.[52,53] DPP-IV inhibitors (saxagliptin, alogliptin, and sitagliptin) neither increase nor decrease the risk of major cardiovascular outcomes.[54] Putative mechanisms contributing to the protective cardiovascular effect of the GLP-1 agonists include direct and indirect cardiac mechanisms. In addition to improved glycemic control and weight loss, GLP-1 receptor agonists have been demonstrated to decrease systolic blood pressure, vascular inflammation, and platelet aggregation and improve endothelial function, plaque stability, blood lipid profile, and myocardial contractility independently of myocardial oxygen demand.[54] These manifold cardiovascular qualities have fostered interest in the therapeutic potential of GLP-1-based therapies for the management of hyperglycemia in the setting of cardiovascular surgery.

RECOMMENDATIONS FOR INCRETIN-BASED THERAPIES IN THE CRITICALLY ILL

Although widely adopted in the treatment of type-2 diabetes in the community, incretin-based therapies have been infrequently studied in the critically ill and formal recommendations on their use during critical illness are lacking. Intuitively, critical illness may attenuate absorption of these oral and subcutaneously administered drugs and metabolism and excretion will be altered in the setting of hepatic and renal dysfunction, with resultant unpredictable half-lives and clearance (see **Tables 1** and **2**).[55] For these reasons, outside of a clinical trial, we recommended that incretin-based drugs are discontinued when critically ill patients with diabetes are admitted to the ICU.[56]

In patients who remain hyperglycemic and are transitioning from ICU to ward-level care, current recommended practice is to commence scheduled subcutaneous basal-bolus insulin regimens.[57] The role for commencing incretin-based therapies in previously naive patients is an area of active research. Two recent open-label randomized controlled trials in ward-based elective surgical patients have demonstrated that a DPP-IV inhibitor (sitagliptin and saxagliptin) combined with basal insulin, is noninferior to basal-bolus insulin and is associated with decreased insulin requirements and reduced glycemic variability.[58,59] Although GLP-1 receptor agonists in the noncritically ill hospitalized patient show promise, proof of safety and efficacy should be informed by well-conducted randomized controlled trials.[57]

INCRETINS IN INTENSIVE CARE UNIT
Incretin Physiology in Critical Illness

The illness or injury that results in ICU admission is frequently associated with disordered glucose metabolism. Up to one-half of critically ill patients with normal glucose tolerance preceding their ICU admission develop stress-induced hyperglycemia and 25% of patients have pre-existing diabetes.[28] By infusing glucose directly into the small intestine, thereby by-passing the confounding variable of gastric emptying, our group has demonstrated that the secretion of GLP-1 and GIP is preserved in critically ill patients with stress-induced hyperglycaemia.[60] Nielsen and colleagues[61] quantified the impaired incretin response in critical illness by comparing oral glucose tolerance tests and matched isoglycemic intravenous glucose infusions between healthy volunteers and critically ill patients. Despite comparable GLP-1 and GIP levels, the incretin effect was markedly diminished in the critically ill cohort.[61] These data suggest that impaired beta-cell secretory response to circulating incretin hormones may be a contributing mechanism underlying stress hyperglycemia.

Rationale for the Use of Incretin Therapies in Critical Illness

Management of hyperglycemia in critically ill patients with and without diabetes primarily involves intravenous infusions of short-acting insulin with the dose titrated according to intermittent measurement of blood glucose.[62] Although effective, this strategy is complicated, labor intensive, and increases the risk of hypoglycemia and glycemic variability, which are associated with increased morbidity and mortality.[63–68] The performance and safety of incretin therapies in ambulant type 2 diabetes has fostered enthusiasm for these agents as adjuncts or alternatives to insulin for glycemic control in the critically ill.[56] Potential advantages of incretin therapies include the following;

- Glucose-dependent mechanism of action and the inherently low risk of hypoglycemia
- Decreased glycemic variability
- Reduced administration of exogenous insulin (which may be advantageous given that insulin suppresses autophagy in this cohort[69])
- Amenable to continuous infusions without the need for frequent dose titration
- Minimal impact on plasma electrolytes
- Cardioprotective qualities
- Organ-independent metabolism for exogenous infusions of human GLP-1 and GIP

At present, exogenous infusions of the human peptides are prohibitively expensive; however, intravenous infusions of synthetic short-acting GLP-1 agonists should provide a more cost-effective option.[70,71] The oral route of the DPP-IV inhibitors and subsequent unpredictable absorption is likely to limit the clinical utility of these agents in the critically ill, at least in the acute phase, although they have been investigated as a glycemic control strategy post coronary artery bypass graft and major surgery.[58,72,73]

Incretin-Based Therapy Trials in Critical Illness

Surgical and mixed intensive care unit populations

In their vanguard study in 2004, Meier and colleagues[74] compared glycemic control over 8 hours between continuous intravenous GLP-1 (1.2 pmol/kg/min) and placebo in eight patients with type 2 diabetes who had undergone major surgery. GLP-1 normalized blood glucose (<7 mmol/L) and significantly increased plasma insulin and glucagon levels compared with placebo without causing hypoglycaemia.[74]

Our group subsequently assessed continuous intravenous infusions of GLP-1 over 3 to 6 hours in a series of blinded randomized controlled crossover trials in mixed medical-surgical cohorts of mechanically ventilated patients.[75–78] Using the same infusion rate as Meier and colleagues,[74] GLP-1 attenuated post-prandial hyperglyce-mia in patients with stress-induced hyperglycemia and in patients with type 2 dia-betes, albeit to a lesser extent in the latter.[75–78] Furthermore, GLP-1 slowed gastric emptying when baseline emptying rate was normal but had no additive slowing effect when emptying was already delayed.[76]

GLP-1 has also been assessed as an adjunct to insulin. Galiatsatos and col-leagues[79] compared extended infusions of GLP-1 (over 72 hours) with placebo in 20 critically ill patients receiving intensive insulin therapy in a parallel group double-blind randomized controlled trial, reporting no difference in mean blood glucose, hypoglycemia, or insulin requirements between groups, but significantly reduced gly-cemic variability in the intervention arm.

Unlike the profound incretin effect of GIP in health, but paralleling diabetic physi-ology, our group has also demonstrated that intravenous infusions of GIP had no detectable effect on glycaemia in mechanically ventilated patients with stress-induced hyperglycemia and no additive glucose lowering effect when combined with GLP-1.[80,81]

Incretin-based therapy in the cardiac intensive care unit population

Beneficial cardiac effects from incretin axis stimulation reported in preclinical murine and small mammal studies include positive inotropy, improved coronary and myocar-dial blood flow, rate control, lowered systolic blood pressure, and attenuated platelet aggregation.[54,82] Furthermore, exogenous GLP-1 has been demonstrated to improve left ventricular ejection fraction, myocardial oxygen uptake, and 6-minute-walk dis-tance in ambulant patients with cardiac failure.[83] Together, these data provide a persuasive rationale to test GLP-1-based therapies in the setting of cardiac surgery. Several studies have assessed the effect of GLP-1 receptor stimulation as an adjunct to insulin during and following coronary artery bypass graft surgery. In prospective double-blind placebo-controlled randomized controlled trials, exogenous GLP-1 infused at 1.5 pmol/kg/min has been shown to reduce intraoperative mean blood glucose and exogenous insulin requirements without increasing the risk of hypoglyce-mia.[84,85] Infusion rates up to 3.6 pmol/kg/min have been well tolerated with no epi-sodes of nausea, vomiting, or hypoglycemia.[86] Similar results have been replicated in trials of the short-acting GLP-1 receptor agonists (exenatide and liraglutide) in the setting of coronary artery bypass graft.[71,87]

Future Directions

Because of the limitations of continuous intravenous insulin there is a compelling ratio-nale to seek alternative strategies for glycemic control in the critically ill. Data from the aforementioned single-center randomized controlled trials provide preliminary evidence that GLP-1-based therapies may be a feasible option with mechanistic plausibility and safety. Further studies, ideally methodologically rigorous adequately powered randomized controlled trials, are required to define (1) the population most likely to benefit (medical, surgical, diabetic, nondiabetic), (2) the optimal drug (exogenous GLP-1 vs GLP-1 RA), (3) the optimal dose, and (4) the side effect profile in patients with deranged physiology.

SUMMARY

With incretin-bases therapies now incorporated into standard treatment algorithms for patients with type 2 diabetes living in the community and the number of patients with type 2 diabetes requiring admission to the ICU continuing to rise, it is increasingly likely that the intensive care physician will manage patients who were using these medications before their acute illness. At present, there are insufficient safety data to advocate routinely continuing these medications on admission to the ICU. Nevertheless, the negligible risk of hypoglycemia, reduced glycemic variability, and potential for cardioprotective benefits has fostered enthusiasm for the potential role of incretin therapies, particularly GLP-1, in the management of acute hyperglycemia during critical illness. There is an increasing body of evidence from small single-center studies reporting promising efficacy and safety data but further research in this area is urgently needed to characterize the patient groups most likely to benefit, and the optimal agent, dose and regimen.

REFERENCES

1. Perley MJ, Kipnis DM. Plasma insulin responses to oral and intravenous glucose: studies in normal and diabetic subjects. J Clin Invest 1967;46(12):1954–62.
2. Deane A, Chapman MJ, Fraser RJ, et al. Bench-to-bedside review: the gut as an endocrine organ in the critically ill. Crit Care 2010;14(5):228.
3. Brubaker PL. Regulation of intestinal proglucagon-derived peptide secretion by intestinal regulatory peptides. Endocrinology 1991;128(6):3175–82.
4. Meier JJ, Nauck MA. Glucagon-like peptide 1(GLP-1) in biology and pathology. Diabetes Metab Res Rev 2005;21(2):91–117.
5. Brown JC, Dryburgh JR. A gastric inhibitory polypeptide. II. The complete amino acid sequence. Can J Biochem 1971;49(8):867–72.
6. Schirra J, Katschinski M, Weidmann C, et al. Gastric emptying and release of incretin hormones after glucose ingestion in humans. J Clin Invest 1996;97(1): 92–103.
7. Parker HE, Wallis K, le Roux CW, et al. Molecular mechanisms underlying bile acid-stimulated glucagon-like peptide-1 secretion. Br J Pharmacol 2012;165(2): 414–23.
8. Fujita Y, Chui JW, King DS, et al. Pax6 and Pdx1 are required for production of glucose-dependent insulinotropic polypeptide in proglucagon-expressing L cells. Am J Physiol Endocrinol Metab 2008;295(3):E648–57.
9. Hutchison AT, Feinle-Bisset C, Fitzgerald PC, et al. Comparative effects of intraduodenal whey protein hydrolysate on antropyloroduodenal motility, gut hormones, glycemia, appetite, and energy intake in lean and obese men. Am J Clin Nutr 2015;102(6):1323–31.
10. Nauck MA, Meier JJ. Incretin hormones: their role in health and disease. Diabetes Obes Metab 2018;20(Suppl 1):5–21.

11. Herrmann C, Goke R, Richter G, et al. Glucagon-like peptide-1 and glucose-dependent insulin-releasing polypeptide plasma levels in response to nutrients. Digestion 1995;56(2):117–26.

12. Kim W, Egan JM. The role of incretins in glucose homeostasis and diabetes treatment. Pharmacol Rev 2008;60(4):470–512.

13. Holst JJ, Gromada J. Role of incretin hormones in the regulation of insulin secretion in diabetic and nondiabetic humans. Am J Physiol Endocrinol Metab 2004; 287(2):E199–206.

14. Nauck MA, Heimesaat MM, Behle K, et al. Effects of glucagon-like peptide 1 on counterregulatory hormone responses, cognitive functions, and insulin secretion during hyperinsulinemic, stepped hypoglycemic clamp experiments in healthy volunteers. J Clin Endocrinol Metab 2002;87(3):1239–46.

15. Marathe CS, Rayner CK, Bound M, et al. Small intestinal glucose exposure determines the magnitude of the incretin effect in health and type 2 diabetes. Diabetes 2014;63(8):2668–75.

16. Deane AM, Nguyen NQ, Stevens JE, et al. Endogenous glucagon-like peptide-1 slows gastric emptying in healthy subjects, attenuating postprandial glycemia. J Clin Endocrinol Metab 2010;95(1):215–21.

17. Plummer MP, Jones KL, Annink CE, et al. Glucagon-like peptide 1 attenuates the acceleration of gastric emptying induced by hypoglycemia in healthy subjects. Diabetes Care 2014;37(6):1509–15.

18. Plummer MP, Jones KL, Cousins CE, et al. Hyperglycemia potentiates the slowing of gastric emptying induced by exogenous GLP-1. Diabetes Care 2015;38(6): 1123–9.

19. Nauck M, Stockmann F, Ebert R, et al. Reduced incretin effect in type 2 (non-insulin-dependent) diabetes. Diabetologia 1986;29(1):46–52.

20. Nauck MA, Heimesaat MM, Orskov C, et al. Preserved incretin activity of glucagon-like peptide 1 [7-36 amide] but not of synthetic human gastric inhibitory polypeptide in patients with type-2 diabetes mellitus. J Clin Invest 1993;91(1): 301–7.

21. Vilsboll T, Krarup T, Madsbad S, et al. Defective amplification of the late phase insulin response to glucose by GIP in obese type II diabetic patients. Diabetologia 2002;45(8):1111–9.

22. Hermansen K, Vaaler S, Madsbad S, et al. Postprandial glycemic control with biphasic insulin aspart in patients with type 1 diabetes. Metabolism 2002;51(7): 896–900.

23. Kreymann B, Williams G, Ghatei MA, et al. Glucagon-like peptide-1 7-36: a physiological incretin in man. Lancet 1987;2(8571):1300–4.

24. Nauck MA, Niedereichholz U, Ettler R, et al. Glucagon-like peptide 1 inhibition of gastric emptying outweighs its insulinotropic effects in healthy humans. Am J Physiol 1997;273(5 Pt 1):E981–8.

25. Verdich C, Flint A, Gutzwiller JP, et al. A meta-analysis of the effect of glucagon-like peptide-1 (7-36) amide on ad libitum energy intake in humans. J Clin Endocrinol Metab 2001;86(9):4382–9.

26. Waget A, Cabou C, Masseboeuf M, et al. Physiological and pharmacological mechanisms through which the DPP-4 inhibitor sitagliptin regulates glycemia in mice. Endocrinology 2011;152(8):3018–29.

27. Marathe PH, Gao HX, Close KL. American Diabetes Association standards of medical care in diabetes 2017. J Diabetes 2017;9(4):320–4.

28. Plummer MP, Bellomo R, Cousins CE, et al. Dysglycaemia in the critically ill and the interaction of chronic and acute glycaemia with mortality. Intensive Care Med 2014;40(7):973–80.

29. Eng J, Kleinman WA, Singh L, et al. Isolation and characterization of exendin-4, an exendin-3 analogue, from Heloderma suspectum venom. Further evidence for an exendin receptor on dispersed acini from Guinea pig pancreas. J Biol Chem 1992;267(11):7402–5.

30. Bhavsar S, Mudaliar S, Cherrington A. Evolution of exenatide as a diabetes therapeutic. Curr Diabetes Rev 2013;9(2):161–93.

31. Aroda VR. A review of GLP-1 receptor agonists: evolution and advancement, through the lens of randomised controlled trials. Diabetes Obes Metab 2018; 20(Suppl 1):22–33.

32. Holst JJ, Vilsboll T, Deacon CF. The incretin system and its role in type 2 diabetes mellitus. Mol Cell Endocrinol 2009;297(1–2):127–36.

33. Neumiller JJ. Clinical pharmacology of incretin therapies for type 2 diabetes mellitus: implications for treatment. Clin Ther 2011;33(5):528–76.

34. Meier JJ. GLP-1 receptor agonists for individualized treatment of type 2 diabetes mellitus. Nat Rev Endocrinol 2012;8(12):728–42.

35. Linnebjerg H, Park S, Kothare PA, et al. Effect of exenatide on gastric emptying and relationship to postprandial glycemia in type 2 diabetes. Regul Pept 2008; 151(1–3):123–9.

36. Eng C, Kramer CK, Zinman B, et al. Glucagon-like peptide-1 receptor agonist and basal insulin combination treatment for the management of type 2 diabetes: a systematic review and meta-analysis. Lancet 2014;384(9961):2228–34.

37. Singh S, Wright EE Jr, Kwan AY, et al. Glucagon-like peptide-1 receptor agonists compared with basal insulins for the treatment of type 2 diabetes mellitus: a systematic review and meta-analysis. Diabetes Obes Metab 2017;19(2):228–38.

38. Davies M, Pieber TR, Hartoft-Nielsen ML, et al. Effect of oral semaglutide compared with placebo and subcutaneous semaglutide on glycemic control in patients with type 2 diabetes: a randomized clinical trial. JAMA 2017;318(15): 1460–70.

39. Goossen K, Graber S. Longer term safety of dipeptidyl peptidase-4 inhibitors in patients with type 2 diabetes mellitus: systematic review and meta-analysis. Diabetes Obes Metab 2012;14(12):1061–72.

40. Mentlein R. Dipeptidyl-peptidase IV (CD26): role in the inactivation of regulatory peptides. Regul peptides 1999;85(1):9–24.

41. Willemen MJ, Mantel-Teeuwisse AK, Straus SM, et al. Use of dipeptidyl peptidase-4 inhibitors and the reporting of infections: a disproportionality analysis in the World Health Organization VigiBase. Diabetes Care 2011;34(2): 369–74.

42. Bjerre Knudsen L, Madsen LW, Andersen S, et al. Glucagon-like peptide-1 receptor agonists activate rodent thyroid C-cells causing calcitonin release and C-cell proliferation. Endocrinology 2010;151(4):1473–86.

43. Aroda VR, Ratner R. The safety and tolerability of GLP-1 receptor agonists in the treatment of type 2 diabetes: a review. Diabetes Metab Res Rev 2011;27(6): 528–42.

44. Bain SC, Stephens JW. Exenatide and pancreatitis: an update. Expert Opin Drug Saf 2008;7(6):643–4.

45. Egan AG, Blind E, Dunder K, et al. Pancreatic safety of incretin-based drugs: FDA and EMA assessment. N Engl J Med 2014;370(9):794–7.

46. Pfeffer MA, Claggett B, Diaz R, et al. Lixisenatide in patients with type 2 diabetes and acute coronary syndrome. N Engl J Med 2015;373(23):2247–57.
47. Marso SP, Daniels GH, Brown-Frandsen K, et al. Liraglutide and cardiovascular outcomes in type 2 diabetes. N Engl J Med 2016;375(4):311–22.
48. Holman RR, Bethel MA, Mentz RJ, et al. Effects of once-weekly exenatide on cardiovascular outcomes in type 2 diabetes. N Engl J Med 2017;377(13):1228–39.
49. Green JB, Bethel MA, Armstrong PW, et al. Effect of sitagliptin on cardiovascular outcomes in type 2 diabetes. N Engl J Med 2015;373(3):232–42.
50. White WB, Cannon CP, Heller SR, et al. Alogliptin after acute coronary syndrome in patients with type 2 diabetes. N Engl J Med 2013;369(14):1327–35.
51. Scirica BM, Bhatt DL, Braunwald E, et al. Saxagliptin and cardiovascular outcomes in patients with type 2 diabetes mellitus. N Engl J Med 2013;369(14):1317–26.
52. Marso SP, Bain SC, Consoli A, et al. Semaglutide and cardiovascular outcomes in patients with type 2 diabetes. N Engl J Med 2016;375(19):1834–44.
53. Bethel MA, Patel RA, Merrill P, et al. Cardiovascular outcomes with glucagon-like peptide-1 receptor agonists in patients with type 2 diabetes: a meta-analysis. Lancet Diabetes Endocrinol 2018;6(2):105–13.
54. Nauck MA, Meier JJ, Cavender MA, et al. Cardiovascular actions and clinical outcomes with glucagon-like peptide-1 receptor agonists and dipeptidyl peptidase-4 inhibitors. Circulation 2017;136(9):849–70.
55. Smith BS, Yogaratnam D, Levasseur-Franklin KE, et al. Introduction to drug pharmacokinetics in the critically ill patient. Chest 2012;141(5):1327–36.
56. Plummer MP, Chapman MJ, Horowitz M, et al. Incretins and the intensivist: what are they and what does an intensivist need to know about them? Crit Care 2014;18(2):205.
57. American Diabetes Association. 14. Diabetes care in the hospital. Diabetes Care 2017;40(Suppl 1):S120–7.
58. Pasquel FJ, Gianchandani R, Rubin DJ, et al. Efficacy of sitagliptin for the hospital management of general medicine and surgery patients with type 2 diabetes (Sita-Hospital): a multicentre, prospective, open-label, non-inferiority randomised trial. Lancet Diabetes Endocrinol 2017;5(2):125–33.
59. Garg R, Schuman B, Hurwitz S, et al. Safety and efficacy of saxagliptin for glycemic control in non-critically ill hospitalized patients. BMJ Open Diabetes Res Care 2017;5(1):e000394.
60. Deane AM, Rayner CK, Keeshan A, et al. The effects of critical illness on intestinal glucose sensing, transporters, and absorption. Crit Care Med 2014;42(1):57–65.
61. Nielsen ST, Janum S, Krogh-Madsen R, et al. The incretin effect in critically ill patients: a case-control study. Crit Care 2015;19:402.
62. American Diabetes Association. 13. Diabetes care in the hospital. Diabetes Care 2016;39(Suppl 1):S99–104.
63. Krinsley JS, Egi M, Kiss A, et al. Diabetic status and the relation of the three domains of glycemic control to mortality in critically ill patients: an international multicenter cohort study. Crit Care 2013;17(2):R37.
64. Egi M, Bellomo R, Stachowski E, et al. Hypoglycemia and outcome in critically ill patients. Mayo Clinic Proc 2010;85(3):217–24.
65. Krinsley JS, Schultz MJ, Spronk PE, et al. Mild hypoglycemia is independently associated with increased mortality in the critically ill. Crit Care 2011;15(4):R173.
66. Ali NA, O'Brien JM Jr, Dungan K, et al. Glucose variability and mortality in patients with sepsis. Crit Care Med 2008;36(8):2316–21.

67. Plummer MP, Finnis ME, Horsfall M, et al. Prior exposure to hyperglycaemia attenuates the relationship between glycaemic variability during critical illness and mortality. Crit Care Resusc 2016;18(3):189–97.

68. Hermanides J, Vriesendorp TM, Bosman RJ, et al. Glucose variability is associated with intensive care unit mortality. Crit Care Med 2010;38(3):838–42.

69. Vanhorebeek I, Gunst J, Derde S, et al. Insufficient activation of autophagy allows cellular damage to accumulate in critically ill patients. J Clin Endocrinol Metab 2011;96(4):E633–45.

70. Lips M, Mraz M, Klouckova J, et al. Effect of continuous exenatide infusion on cardiac function and peri-operative glucose control in patients undergoing cardiac surgery: a single-blind, randomized controlled trial. Diabetes Obes Metab 2017;19(12):1818–22.

71. Besch G, Perrotti A, Mauny F, et al. Clinical effectiveness of intravenous exenatide infusion in perioperative glycemic control after coronary artery bypass graft surgery: a phase II/III randomized trial. Anesthesiology 2017;127(5):775–87.

72. Brackbill ML, Rahman A, Sandy JS, et al. Adjunctive sitagliptin therapy in postoperative cardiac surgery patients: a pilot study. Int J Endocrinol 2012;2012: 810926.

73. Umpierrez GE, Gianchandani R, Smiley D, et al. Safety and efficacy of sitagliptin therapy for the inpatient management of general medicine and surgery patients with type 2 diabetes: a pilot, randomized, controlled study. Diabetes Care 2013; 36(11):3430–5.

74. Meier JJ, Weyhe D, Michaely M, et al. Intravenous glucagon-like peptide 1 normalizes blood glucose after major surgery in patients with type 2 diabetes. Crit Care Med 2004;32(3):848–51.

75. Deane AM, Chapman MJ, Fraser RJ, et al. The effect of exogenous glucagon-like peptide-1 on the glycaemic response to small intestinal nutrient in the critically ill: a randomised double-blind placebo-controlled cross over study. Crit Care 2009; 13(3):R67.

76. Deane AM, Chapman MJ, Fraser RJ, et al. Effects of exogenous glucagon-like peptide-1 on gastric emptying and glucose absorption in the critically ill: relationship to glycemia. Crit Care Med 2010;38(5):1261–9.

77. Deane AM, Summers MJ, Zaknic AV, et al. Exogenous glucagon-like peptide-1 attenuates the glycaemic response to postpyloric nutrient infusion in critically ill patients with type-2 diabetes. Crit Care 2011;15(1):R35.

78. Miller A, Deane AM, Plummer MP, et al. Exogenous glucagon-like peptide-1 attenuates glucose absorption and reduces blood glucose concentration after small intestinal glucose delivery in critical illness. Crit Care Resusc 2017;19(1): 37–42.

79. Galiatsatos P, Gibson BR, Rabiee A, et al. The glucoregulatory benefits of glucagon-like peptide-1 (7-36) amide infusion during intensive insulin therapy in critically ill surgical patients: a pilot study. Crit Care Med 2014;42(3):638–45.

80. Lee MY, Fraser JD, Chapman MJ, et al. The effect of exogenous glucose-dependent insulinotropic polypeptide in combination with glucagon-like peptide-1 on glycemia in the critically ill. Diabetes Care 2013;36(10):3333–6.

81. Kar P, Cousins CE, Annink CE, et al. Effects of glucose-dependent insulinotropic polypeptide on gastric emptying, glycaemia and insulinaemia during critical illness: a prospective, double blind, randomised, crossover study. Crit Care 2015;19:20.

82. Ussher JR, Drucker DJ. Cardiovascular actions of incretin-based therapies. Circ Res 2014;114(11):1788–803.

83. Sokos GG, Nikolaidis LA, Mankad S, et al. Glucagon-like peptide-1 infusion improves left ventricular ejection fraction and functional status in patients with chronic heart failure. J Card Fail 2006;12(9):694–9.

84. Sokos GG, Bolukoglu H, German J, et al. Effect of glucagon-like peptide-1 (GLP-1) on glycemic control and left ventricular function in patients undergoing coronary artery bypass grafting. Am J Cardiol 2007;100(5):824–9.

85. Kohl BA, Hammond MS, Cucchiara AJ, et al. Intravenous GLP-1 (7-36) amide for prevention of hyperglycemia during cardiac surgery: a randomized, double-blind, placebo-controlled study. J Cardiothorac Vasc Anesth 2014;28(3):618–25.

86. Mussig K, Oncu A, Lindauer P, et al. Effects of intravenous glucagon-like peptide-1 on glucose control and hemodynamics after coronary artery bypass surgery in patients with type 2 diabetes. Am J Cardiol 2008;102(5):646–7.

87. Polderman JAW, van Steen SCJ, Thiel B, et al. Peri-operative management of patients with type-2 diabetes mellitus undergoing non-cardiac surgery using liraglutide, glucose-insulin-potassium infusion or intravenous insulin bolus regimens: a randomised controlled trial. Anaesthesia 2018;73(3):332–9.

Therapeutic Opportunities for Hepcidin in Acute Care Medicine

Lakhmir S. Chawla, MD[a,b,*], Blaire Beers-Mulroy, MS[b], George F. Tidmarsh, MD, PhD[b,c]

KEYWORDS

- Hepcidin • Catalytic free iron • Macrophage polarization • Siderotherapy
- Iron homeostasis • Infections • Ferroportin • Transferrin saturation

KEY POINTS

- Acute injury mechanisms increase catalytic free iron.
- The natural inflammatory response stimulates hepcidin production to induce serum hypo-ferremia to reduce the pathologic effects of increased catalytic free iron.
- Exogenous hepcidin may provide a more rapid and pronounced therapeutic benefit in the prevention and treatment of iron-induced injury during acute disease.

INTRODUCTION

Iron is a critical nutrient that is required for basic metabolic processes in cells. However, iron is a reactive transition metal and its availability in the body is carefully regulated because excess iron can increase the production of oxygen free radicals, which can cause cellular damage.[1] As such, a tight control of iron availability, concentration, and tissue distribution is essential. Hepcidin is the principal regulator of iron in the body.[2–4] The mature bioactive form of hepcidin is a 25 amino acid peptide that derives from the 84 amino acid precursor preprohepcidin, which undergoes two enzymatic cleavages. Ferroportin is a transmembrane protein that exports iron from inside to the outside of a cell. This channel is the primary mechanism by which iron is exported out of cells, and the regulation of ferroportin allows control of iron in cells, the plasma, extracellular space, and absorption of iron from the gut. Hepcidin exerts

Disclosure Statement: L.S. Chawla, B. Beers-Mulroy, and G.F. Tidmarsh are employees of La Jolla Pharmaceutical.
[a] Department of Medicine, Veterans Affairs Medical Center, La Jolla, CA 92161, USA; [b] La Jolla Pharmaceutical Company, 4550 Towne Centre Court, San Diego, CA 92121, USA; [c] Department of Pediatrics, Stanford University School of Medicine, Palo Alto, CA 94305, USA
* Corresponding author. San Diego Veterans Hospital, 3350 La Jolla Village Drive, San Diego, CA 92161.
E-mail address: minkchawla@gmail.com

Crit Care Clin 35 (2019) 357–374
https://doi.org/10.1016/j.ccc.2018.11.014   criticalcare.theclinics.com
0749-0704/19/© 2018 The Authors. Published by Elsevier Inc. This is an open access article under the CC BY-NC-ND license (http://creativecommons.org/licenses/by-nc-nd/4.0/).

its control over iron by its interaction with ferroportin. Hepcidin attaches to ferroportin, which causes the internalization and degradation of ferroportin, thereby blocking the export of iron from reticuloendothelial macrophages, hepatocytes, immune cells, and duodenal enterocytes.[4] Therefore, administration of hepcidin has the therapeutic potential to be used for the treatment of illnesses associated with acute or chronic iron excess.

HISTORY OF DISCOVERY

In 2000, two independent research groups identified a novel defensin-like disulfide-bonded 25 amino acid peptide with antimicrobial activity using a mass spectrometric assay in human ultrafiltrate and urine.[5,6] Krause and colleagues[5] named the novel peptide liver-expressed antimicrobial peptide (LEAP-1) after determining the expression pattern is highest in the liver and identifying its dose-dependent antimicrobial effect against bacteria and yeast. While purifying cysteine-rich antimicrobial peptides from human urine, Park and colleagues[6] identified the same peptide and isolated two other amino-terminal shortened forms. The peptide was named hepcidin and determined to contain eight disulfide bonded cysteines forming a structure of β-turns, loops, and distorted β-sheets.[6]

The first connection between hepcidin and iron was made with the identification of dose-dependent hepcidin mRNA transcript induction by suppressive subtractive hybridization between iron-overloaded and control mice.[2] This link was strengthened when Nicolas and colleagues[3] demonstrated that in the absence of hepcidin, iron accumulated primarily in the liver and pancreas; moderately to the heart; that serum iron increased; and splenic iron stores depleted. These studies suggested that hepcidin could be the regulatory signal maintaining iron balance. Taken together with the identification of two mutations (93delG and 166C → T) in hepcidin on 19q13 in patients with juvenile hemochromatosis, Roetto and colleagues,[7] linked hepcidin inactivation and iron dysregulation in humans.

The mechanism by which hepcidin mediates iron homeostasis was identified in 2004 when Nemeth and colleagues[4] added hepcidin to fluorescently labeled ferroportin and observed the altered distribution of ferroportin from the cell membrane to intracellular lysosomes. This internalization and degradation of ferroportin blocked the iron exportation from duodenal enterocytes, macrophages, and hepatocytes, providing the basis for regulating the concentration and tissue distribution of iron.

HEPCIDIN MECHANISM OF ACTION

The mechanism by which hepcidin regulates iron homeostasis is well understood.[8–10] Hepcidin binds to ferroportin, induces covalent modification, and causes its internalization and degradation in lysosomes, which blocks the export of iron from reticuloendothelial macrophages, hepatocytes, and duodenal enterocytes.[4] Hepcidin reduces the concentration of ferroportin molecules on the cell surface thereby inhibiting the entry of iron into plasma. Limiting iron efflux from cells coupled with the ongoing iron uptake of erythropoiesis by the bone marrow results in decreased serum iron and a decreased transferrin (TF) saturation (**Fig. 1**). Prolonged high levels of hepcidin can result in insufficient serum iron for erythropoiesis and lead to iron-restricted anemias.[11,12]

Synthesis of hepcidin from hepatocytes is stimulated by elevated serum iron and by increased inflammation, and downregulated by anemia and hypoxia.[10,13] Regulation of hepcidin by iron occurs through TF-bound signaling extracellularly and by hepatic iron stores. In high extracellular TF-bound iron states, human hemochromatosis protein preferentially binds TF receptor-2, which activates the BMP/SMAD pathway,

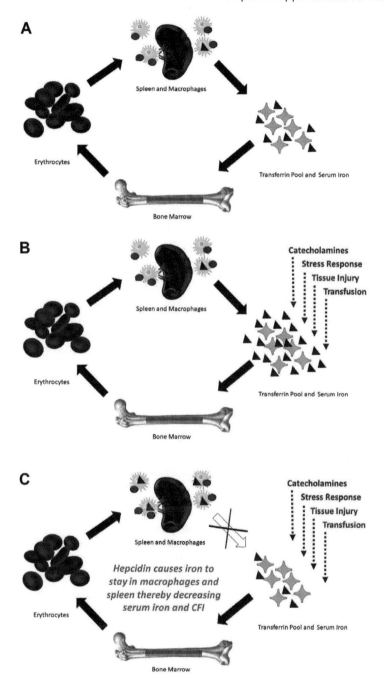

Fig. 1. Iron dynamic equilibrium in the normal and acute injury state. (*A*) In the normal state, serum iron is bound and held under tight control by transferrin. Most serum iron is transported to the bone marrow where it is used for heme synthesis. Splenic macrophages recycle senescent erythrocytes and store iron or release it back into circulation via ferroportin. (*B*) During stress response, catecholamines, tissue injury, and transfusion all contribute to the acute stress iron state marked by a dramatic increase in catalytic free iron. (*C*) Hepcidin degrades ferroportin and effectively blocks the efflux of iron from splenic macrophages, reducing the transferrin saturation. CFI, catalytic free iron.

ultimately inducing hepcidin expression.[14,15] High hepatocellular iron states increase BMP6 expression, which acts as an autocrine factor, binding the hemojuvelin and bone morphogenic protein receptor complex on hepatocytes thereby activating the SMAD pathway and inducing hepcidin expression.[15–18] In iron-depleted states, transmembrane protease serine 6 degrades hemojuvelin, inhibiting hepcidin transcription.[19,20]

Hepcidin is also regulated by inflammation with the increase in hepcidin expression predominantly stimulated by interleukin (IL)-6. Under noninflammatory conditions, serum iron levels largely determine the serum hepcidin concentration; however, the stimulation of IL-6 to increase hepcidin supersedes the signaling from the serum iron levels. Thus, inflamed patients can often have elevated serum hepcidin levels and a low serum iron concentration. IL-6 acts as an autocrine or paracrine factor binding the IL-6 receptor on hepatocytes or reticuloendothelial macrophages, which activates the janus kinase and STAT3 signaling pathway, inducing hepcidin expression, and reducing serum iron.[21] Activation of the BMP/SMAD pathway also influences hepcidin production during the inflammatory response.[18] Studies have shown that an infusion of IL-6 in humans caused an increase in hepcidin associated with an average 34% decrease in serum iron and 33% decrease in TF saturation within a few hours following infusion.[22] When levels of inflammatory cytokines remain elevated in cases of chronic inflammation, hepcidin expression remains elevated, depleting serum iron required for erythropoiesis and resulting in anemia of chronic disease. Conversely, low serum iron, anemia, and hypoxia all decrease hepcidin production, resulting in a greater export of iron through ferroportin into plasma (**Box 1**).[10,13]

CATALYTIC FREE IRON IN ACUTE ILLNESS

Iron is a critical nutrient and under normal physiologic conditions catalytic free iron (CFI) is undetectable and plasma iron is tightly bound to TF. CFI, which can be thought of as unbound iron, is a promiscuous molecule that functions as a "bad-actor." When CFI is in its ferrous state (Fe^{2+}), CFI can initiate the Fenton reactions or when iron is unbound in its ferric state (Fe^{3+}) CFI can initiate Haber-Weiss reactions (**Fig. 2**). These reactions generate oxygen free radicals, such as hydroxyl radical (OH^-), peroxynitrite ($ONOO^-$), superoxide free radical anion (O_2^-), and hydrogen peroxide (H_2O_2).[23,24] These oxygen free radicals are often referred to as reactive oxygen species (ROS) and can damage important macromolecules. ROS have been shown to cause lipid peroxidation, endothelial injury, protein oxidation, mitochondrial injury, erythrocyte damage, and DNA damage (**Fig. 3**).[23] As such, human physiologic systems

---

Box 1
Mechanisms of hepcidin therapy in acute illness

1. Decrease catalytic free iron
   a. Decreases reactive oxygen species
   b. Decreases iron availability to pathogens

2. Increase serum ferritin

3. Increase intracellular H-type ferritin

4. Induce protective acute phase reactant proteins

5. Alter immune cells favorably
   a. Decreases inflammatory response
   b. Adjusts polarization of macrophages to M2 phenotype

$$Fe^{3+} + O_2^{-} \longleftrightarrow Fe^{2+} + O_2$$

$$Fe^{2+} + H_2O_2 \longrightarrow Fe^{3+} + HO^{\cdot} + OH^{-} \quad \text{(Fenton reaction)}$$

$$O_2^{-} + H_2O_2 \longleftrightarrow O_2 + HO^{\cdot} + OH^{-} \quad \text{(Haber-Weiss reaction)}$$

Fig. 2. Fenton and Haber-Weiss reactions are a source of oxidative stress. The generation of oxygen free radicals occurs first with the reduction of ferric to ferrous iron and then by the Fenton reaction with ferrous iron catalyzing the breakdown of hydrogen peroxide to hydroxyl radical and hydroxyl. The net reaction is termed the Haber-Weiss reaction.

orchestrate a careful balance of iron acquisition and binding to avoid injury while still effectively delivering iron to tissues as a critical nutrient.

Iron is acquired from the gut and absorbed through enterocytes. Through the portal system, iron is transported to the liver and then enters the circulation. TF is the plasma protein responsible for transporting iron in the plasma and then into the tissues. In addition to iron transport, TF has high affinity for free iron and functions as the body's natural iron chelator, effectively binding iron and preventing the formation of CFI. Iron is received by the tissues via the TF receptor. The largest consumer of iron in the body is the bone marrow where TF delivers iron via TF receptor for the production of erythrocytes. TF also delivers iron to tissues for the production of myoglobin, cytochromes, and other iron-containing enzymes.

In acute illness, iron homeostasis is often significantly disrupted such that CFI is produced and begins to contribute to tissue injury and pathologic effects.[25] Many mechanisms contribute to an increase in CFI during acute illness, such as catecholamine surges, metabolic acidosis, tissue injury, hemolysis, and bleeding.[26–30] Because CFI rapidly induces an increase in ROS, which causes more tissue injury leading to the release of cell-free heme and other iron-containing products, the liberation of CFI is self-sustaining and further exacerbates acute injury.[25,31] Thus, CFI has been implicated as a critical injury pathway in many acute illnesses, such as myocardial infarction, sepsis, stroke, acute kidney injury (AKI), traumatic injuries, lung injury, stem cell

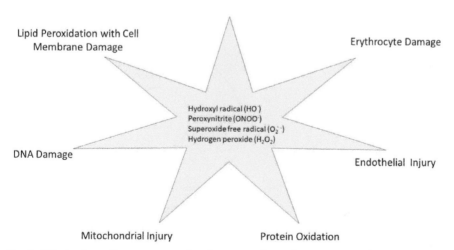

Fig. 3. Effects of reactive oxygen species. An excess of reactive oxygen species causes tissue-specific oxidative damage. Reactive oxygen species can damage DNA, proteins, and lipids, altering their structure and affecting function, ultimately contributing to various pathologies.

transplantation, and reperfusion injury.[27,30,32–38] The increase in CFI in acute illness is further exacerbated by the fact that iron is also a key nutrient for microorganisms that proliferate and induce virulence factors in the presence of iron.[39,40] Thus, noninfectious acute injuries increase the risk of infection because of increased CFI, and infection-mediated injuries (ie, sepsis) are worsened by the increase in CFI.

The typical sequence of events is as follows. First, an injurious event causes a stress response. The classic fight or flight response is induced by increased sympathetic tone and a catecholamine surge. Catecholamines effectively cause the release of free-iron from hepatocytes and myocytes such that serum iron levels are increased rapidly.[41] Although this response is likely adaptive (ie, increasing nutrient availability during stress), the increase in background iron is then exacerbated by the iron release that is caused by tissue injury from noninfectious or infectious insult. This rapid double-hit creates iron levels that exceed the binding capacity of TF leading to increased CFI levels thereby increasing ROS. During significant levels of injury, the induction of ROS can initiate a vicious cycle (see **Fig. 3**; **Fig. 4**).

The inflammatory response leads to hepcidin production and other acute-phase reactants to be produced that help ameliorate the iron-associated injury. Because hepcidin is induced by IL-6, many studies show that hepcidin is associated with worse outcomes and some have suggested that hepcidin has negative impacts.[42,43] In the view of the authors, that is akin to judging firemen to be negative actors because more firemen are seen at larger fires. In the estimation of the authors, it is noteworthy that many of the acute-phase reactants are proteins that protect against iron-associated injury. For instance, the acute-phase proteins include hemopexin, haptoglobin, ferritin, lactoferrin, ceruloplasmin, NGAL, and hepcidin, all of which are involved in iron or iron-complexed macromolecule protective functions.[22,44–50]

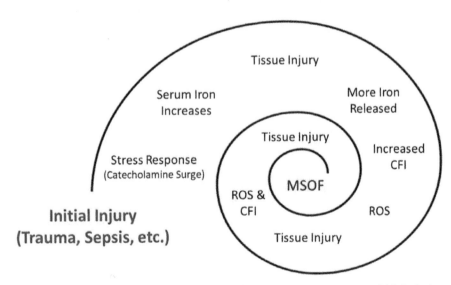

Fig. 4. Cycle of oxidative damage. An initial insult causes a stress response, which includes a surge of catecholamines that facilitates the release of iron from storage organs and increases serum iron. The dramatic increase of catalytic free iron participates in Fenton chemistry, generates reactive oxygen species, and causes tissue-specific oxidative damage. The tissue injury causes more iron to be released and the vicious cycle continues with the potential to result in multisystem organ failure. MSOF, multisystem organ failure.

Initial placebo-controlled studies in healthy volunteers demonstrate that exogenous hepcidin induces a rapid increase in the acute-phase protein serum ferritin in addition to hypoferremia.[51] The authors hypothesize that other iron-related acute-phase reactants are also increased by the administration of exogenous hepcidin. If this hypothesis is verified, exogenous hepcidin might be used to augment the natural iron injury defense system of the host to more rapidly and forcefully treat iron and cell-free hemoglobin-induced injury during acute illness. In essence, exogenous hepcidin may be a method to initiate a broad iron protective response that we denote as "siderotherapy."

HEPCIDIN AS AN AGENT FOR SIDEROTHERAPY

Hepcidin is the body's master regulator of iron and when induced, rapidly and effectively reduces plasma iron and initiates intracellular signaling for intracellular iron protective processes. Hepcidin induces hypoferremia by decreasing the TF saturation thereby activating the body's natural chelator. Hepcidin in the plasma causes the rapid degradation of ferroportin in macrophages in the liver, spleen, and plasma space. Under normal conditions, more than 90% of the daily iron supply is derived from macrophages.[15,52] In addition, the degradation of ferroportin in enterocytes prevents further iron absorption in the gut. Thus, the supply of iron into the plasma is shut off. Because the bone marrow is in a constant state of iron uptake to generate erythrocytes to replace the senescent erythrocytes, the combination of bone marrow demand and reduced supply from hepcidin degradation of ferroportin results in a rapid drop in the serum iron and the TF saturation (see **Fig. 1**).

The pharmacodynamics of hepcidin show that parenteral hepcidin results in a rapid decrease in serum iron and TF saturation with a nadir at 8 to 12 hours.[53] As such, hepcidin could have a role as a preventive agent and as a therapeutic agent after the acute injury has occurred.

In addition to inducing plasma hypoferremia and hyperferritinemia, hepcidin has been demonstrated in preclinical studies to induce intracellular ferritin, often referred to as H-ferritin.[38] Ferritin is a highly conserved protein across mammalian species and has two key functions. First, ferritin is effective at sequestering and storing iron in its nonreactive form. Second, ferritin is a ferroxidase and rapidly converts ferrous (Fe^{2+}, very toxic) to ferric (Fe^{3+}, somewhat less toxic) iron.[45,46] Ferric iron is rapidly loaded onto TF in the plasma and ferric iron is also sequestered into ferritin.[46] In general, ferritin is made up of light (L) and heavy (H) subunits. In the plasma, the ferritin has a higher proportion of L-subunits, whereas intracellular ferritin is largely made of H subunits. Both L-rich and H-rich ferritins have ferroxidase activity. L-rich ferritins are slower to incorporate iron but can hold more, whereas H-rich ferritins can rapidly incorporate iron but can store less.[45,46]

The degradation of ferroportin by hepcidin prevents iron egress from the cell, thus increasing the intracellular iron concentration. Increased intracellular iron levels sets off a series of events that signals the cell to detoxify and rapidly store iron. The presence of H-rich ferritin is cytoprotective and allows cells to withstand injury, making them more resistant to apoptosis and necroptosis.[38,54] Preclinical studies demonstrate that induction or administration of hepcidin improves survival and decreases injury scores in preclinical models of AKI.[38,55]

An easy way to understand the effects of hepcidin is seen in the syndrome known as anemia of chronic disease, which is caused by high serum levels of hepcidin.[56] This syndrome is most commonly encountered in patients with chronic inflammation (ie, uremia, rheumatoid arthritis, osteomyelitis). Although classically seen in inflammation, this syndrome almost certainly evolved as an adaptive response to chronic infection. The host's response to a chronic infection is to inflame and to make iron as scarce as possible because microbes require iron to survive. The syndrome is characterized by hypoferremia, low TF saturation, high ferritin, decreased iron absorption, and high levels of macrophage iron.[56] This syndrome manifests as a microcytic anemia but is more accurately described as an iron scarcity syndrome. Thus, increasing levels of hepcidin may accelerate the body's conversion to an iron-scarce environment during acute injury to protect the host from CFI-induced damage with various acute diseases. If the level of injury during the acute insult is limited, the consequent inflammation may be reduced, and outcomes improved (see **Fig. 4**).

USE OF HEPCIDIN IN ACUTE ILLNESS
Infectious Diseases

All eukaryotic and prokaryotic cells require iron to live, reproduce, and flourish. Bacteria, fungi, and parasites have all evolved strategies to acquire iron from the environment and/or the host to thrive. Certain infectious microbes are more vulnerable to the iron scarcity effects of hepcidin. The notion that hypoferremic interventions can improve outcomes in infected patients is not new.[39] However, the treatments currently available to lower iron are all iron chelators. The main limitation of all the available iron-chelators is that the chelator-iron complex may deliver iron to microbes and exacerbate the infection.[39,57] In addition, available iron chelators have significant toxicity, which includes but is not limited to neutropenia, kidney injury, and liver injury. Because hepcidin uses the body's natural hypoferremic pathways, we postulate that this approach would be safer and more effective than iron chelation therapy. This section reviews the various potential opportunities to use hepcidin as an adjuvant agent in the treatment of acute infections. Hepcidin itself has antimicrobial properties, but the most logical way to use hepcidin may be as adjuvant treatment alongside standard antimicrobials for the treatment of infectious disease.

Enteric gram-negative bacilli

Patients with iron overload, such as hemochromatosis, transfusional iron overload, and cirrhosis, are more susceptible to certain gram-negative bacilli, particularly siderophilic bacilli (**Box 2**).[58,59] Deadly infections with siderophilic gram-negative bacilli, such as Yersinia enterocolitica, Vibrio vulnificus, and Klebsiella pneumoniae, have been reported in patients with iron overload.[60,61] Nonclinical models of these infectious agents demonstrate that increased CFI increases the lethality of these

| Box 2 |
Siderophilic pathogens
Vibrio vulnificus
Listeria monocytogenes
Yersenia enterocolitica
Salmonella enterica
Klebsiella pneumoniae
Escherichia coli
Rhizopus arrhizus
Mucor

infections.[62–64] In these models, hepcidin agonists rapidly decreased iron levels and improved survival.[62–64] Hepcidin added to standard therapy has the potential to improve outcomes in these infections particularly among those patients with iron overload.

It should be noted that hepcidin therapy added to standard antimicrobial therapy for bacterial infections may be useful. The early phase of injury and stress causes increased levels of endogenous catecholamines, which facilitates the release of iron. Because exogenous catecholamines (ie, norepinephrine, dopamine) are part of the standard care of patients with septic shock it is likely that clinicians may unwittingly worsen the infection by providing more iron via catecholamine therapy.[65] Thus, adding hepcidin therapy when patients first present to medical care, before or soon after the initiation of antimicrobial and/or catecholamine therapy, may prove beneficial.

Another potential use for hepcidin therapy is in patients who are infected with highly resistant gram-negative bacilli, such as *Acinetobacter baumannii*, *K. pneumoniae*, and other similar siderophilic bacilli. There are two key concepts that inform this hypothesis. First, the acquisition of resistance for a micro-organism is not free. Resistance involves altering the normal intracellular machinery of a bacterium and hence the bacterium must pay a fitness cost for this resistance attribute.[66] This concept of fitness was discovered because of the observation that when resistant microorganisms (bacteria, fungi, or parasites) are moved into an environment without antibiotic pressure, they are outcompeted by nonresistant microbes that can acquire nutrients and divide faster unencumbered by resistance machinery.[66] Second, in animal models of resistant bacteria, the addition of antimicrobial agents improves survival even if the microbe is resistant to that agent.[67,68] Some investigators have postulated that even if the microbe is resistant, the presence of the antimicrobial in the environment forces the pathogen to behave in a way that either lessens virulence or allows for a more efficient immune response.[39] We postulate that because resistant organisms are less fit, they may be more susceptible to an approach that rapidly removes a critical nutrient from their environment. Moreover, because none of the available antibiotics or other antimicrobial therapeutics target iron acquisition, induction of hypoferremia may be a thoughtful vulnerability to exploit. Because hepcidin induces extracellular and intracellular iron scarcity, the addition of robust hypoferremia may be particularly effective for patients infected with resistant organisms who have few alternative therapies available.

Fungal infections

Although all fungi require iron to thrive, certain pathogenic fungi are more siderophilic and thus may be more sensitive to hypoferremic interventions. Preclinical and clinical studies demonstrate that iron overload favors the development of fungal infections and may increase pathogen virulence.[69–71]

Patients who undergo myeloablative or bone marrow conditioning therapies are at risk for iron overload because these therapies decrease the demand from the bone marrow. As such, the continued egress of iron from macrophages and splenocytes from erythrophagocytosis exceeds that bone marrow uptake, which results in high TF saturation and increased CFI (see **Fig. 1**).[37,72] These patients are susceptible to infection in part because of increased iron availability and immune dysfunction, notably the presence of neutropenia. Consequently, these patients tend to become infected with siderophilic bacteria and fungi. The fungi that are most common and pathogenic are *Candida* spp, *Aspergillus*, and *Mucor*. Although iron-chelation therapy has not shown any benefit in clinical studies of fungal infection, this type of hypoferremic therapy is confounded by the potential enhanced delivery of iron to the microbes.[73] For patients with iron overload manifested by an increased TF saturation, hepcidin-induced hypoferremia may have an important role as a prophylactic agent and may also have a role as a therapeutic in patients who are infected.

Malaria

A complete discussion about hepcidin and malaria is beyond the scope of this article. In brief, hepcidin has potentially three key roles in the treatment of malaria. First is as a prophylaxis of liver stage malaria. Plasmodium species have a complex life cycle and after being bitten by a mosquito, plasmodium schizonts must first invade the liver and go through a liver stage before being able to infect the blood and continue the infection.[74] A nonclinical study suggests that prior ongoing malaria infection may cause enough hepcidin production to prevent coinfections with other strains of malaria.[75] This is likely because hepcidin generates a brisk hypoferremic effect within hepatocytes thereby making them less conducive to infection and propagation. We postulate that because of this effect, exogenous hepcidin may have a role as a prophylactic medication for infections with plasmodium species especially for people traveling to areas with endemic malaria. Hepcidin could also be used to facilitate live-schizont vaccination regimens.[76] Specifically, live-schizont vaccine therapies are predicated on creating a moat around the liver preventing systemic infection and allowing the immune system to become activated and develop immunity. However, this approach would not work for forms of malaria that develop chronic liver stage infection. Exogenous hepcidin given before *Plasmodium vivax* or *Plasmodium falciparum* schizont inoculation may prevent liver stage infection and allow the immune system to develop durable immunity.

A second opportunity for hepcidin involves the treatment of the liver stage of malaria. Certain plasmodium species have hypnozoites, which are forms of malaria that can lay dormant in the liver for years and then reactivate. The authors propose that hepcidin may have capacity as a drug to help eradicate liver stage plasmodium species similar to the use of the drug tafenoquine.[77] Tafenoquine has been shown to be effective in radical cure of *P vivax*, but tafenoquine is associated with toxicity. We suggest that hepcidin may be used in conjunction with tafenoquine allowing for a decreased dose that may improve synergy and decrease toxicity.

The third potential role for hepcidin in malaria is related to resistance. Plasmodia species that infect humans are efficient at developing resistance. New strains of plasmodia have emerged that are resistant to artemisinin and quinine antimicrobials. Because plasmodia species also pay a fitness cost for the acquisition of resistance, we believe that the addition of hepcidin to current antimalarial regimens may restore artemisinin and/or quinine sensitivity.[78,79]

Sepsis

Preclinical studies assessing a multitude of sepsis models indicate that hepcidin is protective.[36,80,81] Although most studies identify the reduction of CFI as the key mechanism for improving outcomes, particularly in models that assess siderophilic or enteric organisms, it seems that the protective mechanism is not exclusively related to iron. Other nonclinical studies show that hepcidin also has effects on immune cells.[82,83] One example is that hepcidin favors the M2 over M1 polarization of macrophages, which may be a more optimal distribution of macrophage phenotype in end-organ outcomes.[84,85] The non-iron immune cell effects of hepcidin are reviewed extensively elsewhere and are beyond the scope of this review.[82,83] Nonetheless, the key message is that hepcidin evolved as the key regulator of iron to help protect against infection. Therefore, it is logical that hepcidin would have other pleiotropic effects that augment the host's ability to respond to infection.[86]

Noninfectious Diseases

Acute kidney injury

Iron-mediated oxidative stress is implicated in the pathogenesis of renal ischemia reperfusion injury ([IRI] a major cause of AKI), and multiple animal models have demonstrated that catalytic iron is a key mediator of AKI.[33,38,87] In disease states, such as acute kidney diseases, after IRI, sepsis, and myocardial infarction, CFI is increased.[35] This is caused by a decrease in pH or free radical–induced reduction of iron that causes dissociation of bound intracellular iron, yielding free iron that can serve as a catalyst for vulnerable situations of oxidative stress.[88] During operations that require cardiopulmonary bypass (CPB; which is inherently a high CFI environment caused by surgical stress) extracorporeally circulated blood exposed to nonphysiologic surfaces and shear forces may injure red blood cells, releasing free hemoglobin and free iron; association with adverse postoperative outcomes is observed with CFI.[33] Moreover, in patients who are undergoing surgery requiring CPB, TF saturation routinely exceeds 50% during surgery and consequently plasma CFI increases, which is strongly linked to AKI.[29,33,38,87,89] In addition, significant elevations in CFI, but not other iron parameters, have been observed in patients after cardiac surgery and were directly associated with CPB time and number of packed red blood cell transfusions.[33]

Interventional studies to reduce CFI levels are hypothesized to prevent AKI.[33,38] Endogenous hepcidin regulates iron absorption and recycling, provides protection from reactive iron species, and is a biomarker for iron-related pathophysiology.

It has been observed in murine models that hepcidin is freely filtered by the glomerulus and reabsorbed in the proximal tubule cells by megalin-dependent endocytosis.[55,90] In animal models of AKI, CFI has been implicated in nephrotoxicity resulting from a wide range of insults including ischemia/reperfusion, aminoglycosides, rhabdomyolysis, and hemoglobinuria. Iron chelators, such as deferiprone and deferoxamine, have been demonstrated to protect against experimental cardiac IRI in diverse animal models, establishing a cause and effect relationship.[35] Animal models have also shown that hepcidin-deficient mice demonstrated increased susceptibility to IRI compared with wild-type mice and that reconstitution with exogenous hepcidin induced hepatic iron sequestration; attenuated reduction of renal tissue ferritin; and reduced oxidative stress, apoptosis, inflammation, and tubular injury. Similar models have shown that hepcidin treatment restores iron homeostasis and reduces inflammation to mediate protection in renal IRI.[38]

Overall, the authors suggest that pretreatment with hepcidin before surgeries requiring CPB may have five key effects[38]:

1. Prevents initial surge of iron from the spleen and liver via degradation of ferroportin in macrophages, hepatocytes, and splenocytes.
2. Reduction of TF saturation in preparation for CPB, thereby forming an iron buffer (TF is the body's natural chelator) that can accommodate the free iron liberated by CPB and transfusion.
3. Induction of intracellular H-ferritin in the proximal convoluted tubule cells from filtered hepcidin uptake before cardiopulmonary surgeries requiring CPB, thereby inducing a cytoprotective response in the kidney.
4. Increase in serum ferritin providing more rapid loading of free iron onto TF and providing a sink for free iron.
5. Induction of a more favorable immune response.

Taken together, the central biologic role of hepcidin in iron metabolism and the possible importance of iron in the pathogenesis of CPB-associated AKI identify hepcidin as a potential treatment in preventing AKI in patients undergoing surgery requiring CPB.

Trauma and transfusion

Patients with severe trauma often require massive blood transfusion.[91] Because banked blood becomes more fragile over time when stored, a significant proportion of the transfused blood is removed from the circulation rapidly and undergoes extravascular hemolysis.[92] When this process occurs, the iron from the phagocytosed red cells is released into the bloodstream thereby increasing CFI.[93] This release of free iron after transfusion is consistent and even occurs in healthy volunteers receiving autologous blood.[94] The increased CFI environment seen in patients with trauma receiving massive blood transfusion is exacerbated because many trauma patients require catecholamine infusions (which increase serum iron) and suffer severe anemia from hemorrhage, which leads to the release of erythropoietin, which suppresses hepcidin generation thereby increasing CFI.[13,26,41,95] As a consequence, severe trauma is often exacerbated by high levels of CFI. Thus, patients with trauma requiring massive blood transfusion leading to high-levels of CFI may benefit from hepcidin-induced hypoferremia. Ideally, hepcidin therapy would be initiated immediately on presentation to hospital to maximize the potential benefits of counteracting the increased CFI seen in trauma patients requiring massive blood transfusion.

Cardioprotection

Iron plays a key role in the injury associated with reperfusion.[96] Thus, there have been multiple investigations assessing hypoferremic modalities in myocardial infarction and cardioprotection. Preclinical studies indicate that myocardial reperfusion injury is ameliorated by hypoferremia induced by iron chelation therapy.[97–99] Clinical trials in humans after bypass surgery supported these findings by demonstrating that treatment with the iron chelator deferoxamine ameliorated lipid peroxidation and protected the myocardium from reperfusion injury.[100,101] The addition of deferoxamine to vasoplegia solution has been shown to offer better cardioprotection in large mammal studies of CPB.[102] In a large cohort trial, higher levels of CFI were associated with increased risk of death in patients with acute coronary syndrome.[27]

In aggregate, these data suggest that the safe and rapid induction of hypoferremia by hepcidin may protect against reperfusion injury and offer myocardial protection in acute coronary syndrome and CPB.

Liver disease

The source of plasma hepcidin is largely liver-derived and patients with advanced liver disease lose synthetic function of liver proteins.[103,104] The loss of synthetic function results in low plasma levels of TF and low levels of hepcidin, which leads to increased CFI.[103,104] Iron overloaded states in nonalcoholic fatty liver disease, indicated by elevated serum ferritin, are associated with increased hepatic iron deposition, advancement of hepatic fibrosis, and a diagnosis of nonalcoholic steatohepatitis.[105] As such, patients with severe liver disease often suffer from complications that are found in patients with chronic iron overload. As an example, patients with cirrhosis are susceptible to siderophilic gram-negative bacilli, such as V vulnificus and enteric bacilli.[106,107] As evidence of excess iron and risk, cohort studies have shown that dysregulated iron homeostasis is associated with multiorgan failure and early mortality in acute-on-chronic liver failure.[104,108] The main risk factors identified were low serum TF levels, elevated TF saturation, and decreased hepcidin levels. An environment of increased CFI makes the host more vulnerable to infection and makes the risk of severe ROS associated with infection more likely.

Exogenous hepcidin hypoferremic effects could be used for prevention in patients with advanced liver disease and might also have an adjunctive role in treating infections in patients with cirrhosis, particularly those caused by siderophilic bacilli.

SUMMARY

Acute diseases tend to worsen when CFI is increased. Iron chelators can induce rapid hypoferremia but have significant toxicity. Hepcidin, the body's master regulator of iron, has the capacity to induce hypoferremia, initiate cytoprotective pathways, and favorably affect the immune response. Thus, exogenous hepcidin may have a role in the treatment of acute diseases associated with elevated CFI.

REFERENCES

1. Kell DB. Iron behaving badly: inappropriate iron chelation as a major contributor to the aetiology of vascular and other progressive inflammatory and degenerative diseases. BMC Med Genomics 2009;2:2.
2. Pigeon C, Ilyin G, Courselaud B, et al. A new mouse liver-specific gene, encoding a protein homologous to human antimicrobial peptide hepcidin, is overexpressed during iron overload. J Biol Chem 2001;276(11):7811–9.
3. Nicolas G, Bennoun M, Devaux I, et al. Lack of hepcidin gene expression and severe tissue iron overload in upstream stimulatory factor 2 (USF2) knockout mice. PNAS 2001;98(15):6.
4. Nemeth E, Tuttle MS, Powelson J, et al. Hepcidin regulates cellular iron efflux by binding to ferroportin and inducing its internalization. Science 2004;306:4.
5. Krause A, Neitz S, Magert H, et al. LEAP-1, a novel highly disulfide-bonded human peptide, exhibits antimicrobial activity. FEBS Lett 2000;480:4.
6. Park CH, Valore EV, Waring AJ, et al. Hepcidin, a urinary antimicrobial peptide synthesized in the liver. J Biol Chem 2001;276(11):7806–10.
7. Roetto A, Papanikolaou G, Politou M, et al. Mutant antimicrobial peptide hepcidin is associated with severe juvenile hemochromatosis. Nat Genet 2003;33(1):21–2.
8. Ganz T. Hepcidin and iron regulation, 10 years later. Blood 2011;117(17):4425–33.
9. Ganz T, Nemeth E. Iron metabolism: interactions with normal and disordered erythropoiesis. Cold Spring Harb Perspect Med 2012;2(5):a011668.
10. Nemeth E, Ganz T. Regulation of iron metabolism by hepcidin. Annu Rev Nutr 2006;26:323–42.
11. Nicolas G, Bennoun M, Porteu A, et al. Severe iron deficiency anemia in transgenic mice expressing liver hepcidin. Proc Natl Acad Sci U S A 2002;99(7):4596–601.
12. Weinstein DA, Roy CN, Fleming MD, et al. Inappropriate expression of hepcidin is associated with iron refractory anemia: implications for the anemia of chronic disease. Blood 2002;100(10):3776–81.
13. Nicolas G, Chauvet C, Viatte L, et al. The gene encoding the iron regulatory peptide hepcidin is regulated by anemia, hypoxia, and inflammation. J Clin Invest 2002;110(7):1037–44.
14. D'Alessio F, Hentze MW, Muckenthaler MU. The hemochromatosis proteins HFE, TfR2, and HJV form a membrane-associated protein complex for hepcidin regulation. J Hepatol 2012;57(5):1052–60.
15. Hentze MW, Muckenthaler MU, Galy B, et al. Two to tango: regulation of mammalian iron metabolism. Cell 2010;142(1):24–38.

16. Andriopoulos B Jr, Corradini E, Xia Y, et al. BMP6 is a key endogenous regulator of hepcidin expression and iron metabolism. Nat Genet 2009;41(4):482–7.

17. Babitt JL, Huang FW, Wrighting DM, et al. Bone morphogenetic protein signaling by hemojuvelin regulates hepcidin expression. Nat Genet 2006; 38(5):531–9.

18. Casanovas G, Mleczko-Sanecka K, Altamura S, et al. Bone morphogenetic protein (BMP)-responsive elements located in the proximal and distal hepcidin promoter are critical for its response to HJV/BMP/SMAD. J Mol Med (Berl) 2009; 87(5):471–80.

19. Du X, She E, Gelbart T, et al. The serine protease TMPRSS6 is required to sense iron deficiency. Science 2008;320(5879):5.

20. Silvestri L, Pagani A, Nai A, et al. The serine protease matriptase-2 (TMPRSS6) inhibits hepcidin activation by cleaving membrane hemojuvelin. Cell Metab 2008;8(6):502–11.

21. Wrighting DM, Andrews NC. Interleukin-6 induces hepcidin expression through STAT3. Blood 2006;108(9):3204–9.

22. Nemeth E, Rivera S, Gabayan V, et al. IL-6 mediates hypoferremia of inflammation by inducing the synthesis of the iron regulatory hormone hepcidin. J Clin Invest 2004;113(9):6.

23. Kehrer JP. The Haber-Weiss reaction and mechanisms of toxicity. Toxicology 2000;149(1):43–50.

24. Wardman P, Candeias LP. Fenton chemistry: an introduction. Radiat Res 1996; 145(5):523–31.

25. Halliwell B, Gutteridge JM. Role of free radicals and catalytic metal ions in human disease: an overview. Methods Enzymol 1990;186:1–85.

26. Sandrini SM, Shergill R, Woodward J, et al. Elucidation of the mechanism by which catecholamine stress hormones liberate iron from the innate immune defense proteins transferrin and lactoferrin. J Bacteriol 2010;192(2):587–94.

27. Lele SS, Mukhopadhyay BN, Mardikar MM, et al. Impact of catalytic iron on mortality in patients with acute coronary syndrome exposed to iodinated radiocontrast: the Iscom Study. Am Heart J 2013;165(5):744–51.

28. Baliga R, Zhang Z, Baliga M, et al. Evidence for cytochrome P-450 as a source of catalytic iron in myoglobinuric acute renal failure. Kidney Int 1996;49(2): 362–9.

29. Pepper JR, Mumby S, Gutteridge JM. Sequential oxidative damage, and changes in iron-binding and iron-oxidising plasma antioxidants during cardiopulmonary bypass surgery. Free Radic Res 1994;21(6):377–85.

30. Fuernau G, Traeder F, Lele SS, et al. Catalytic iron in acute myocardial infarction complicated by cardiogenic shock: a biomarker substudy of the IABP-SHOCK II-trial. Int J Cardiol 2017;227:83–8.

31. Balla G, Vercellotti GM, Muller-Eberhard U, et al. Exposure of endothelial cells to free heme potentiates damage mediated by granulocytes and toxic oxygen species. Lab Invest 1991;64(5):648–55.

32. Lagan AL, Melley DD, Evans TW, et al. Pathogenesis of the systemic inflammatory syndrome and acute lung injury: role of iron mobilization and decompartmentalization. Am J Physiol Lung Cell Mol Physiol 2008;294(2):L161–74.

33. Leaf DE, Rajapurkar M, Lele SS, et al. Increased plasma catalytic iron in patients may mediate acute kidney injury and death following cardiac surgery. Kidney Int 2015;87(5):1046–54.

34. Haase M, Bellomo R, Haase-Fielitz A. Novel biomarkers, oxidative stress, and the role of labile iron toxicity in cardiopulmonary bypass-associated acute kidney injury. J Am Coll Cardiol 2010;55(19):2024–33.

35. Shah SV, Rajapurkar MM, Baliga R. The role of catalytic iron in acute kidney injury. Clin J Am Soc Nephrol 2011;6(10):2329–31.

36. Chen QX, Song SW, Chen QH, et al. Silencing airway epithelial cell-derived hepcidin exacerbates sepsis induced acute lung injury. Crit Care 2014;18(4):470.

37. Pullarkat V. Iron overload in patients undergoing hematopoietic stem cell transplantation. Adv Hematol 2010;2010 [pii:345756].

38. Scindia Y, Dey P, Thirunagari A, et al. Hepcidin mitigates renal ischemia-reperfusion injury by modulating systemic iron homeostasis. J Am Soc Nephrol 2015;26(11):2800–14.

39. Cassat JE, Skaar EP. Iron in infection and immunity. Cell Host Microbe 2013; 13(5):509–19.

40. Hood MI, Skaar EP. Nutritional immunity: transition metals at the pathogen-host interface. Nat Rev Microbiol 2012;10(8):525–37.

41. Tapryal N, Vivek GV, Mukhopadhyay CK. Catecholamine stress hormones regulate cellular iron homeostasis by a posttranscriptional mechanism mediated by iron regulatory protein: implication in energy homeostasis. J Biol Chem 2015; 290(12):7634–46.

42. Xiong XY, Liu L, Wang FX, et al. Toll-like receptor 4/MyD88-mediated signaling of hepcidin expression causing brain iron accumulation, oxidative injury, and cognitive impairment after intracerebral hemorrhage. Circulation 2016;134(14): 1025–38.

43. Wagner M, Ashby DR, Kurtz C, et al. Hepcidin-25 in diabetic chronic kidney disease is predictive for mortality and progression to end stage renal disease. PLoS One 2015;10(4):e0123072.

44. Smith A, McCulloh RJ. Hemopexin and haptoglobin: allies against heme toxicity from hemoglobin not contenders. Front Physiol 2015;6:187.

45. Mehlenbacher M, Poli M, Arosio P, et al. Iron oxidation and core formation in recombinant heteropolymeric human ferritins. Biochemistry 2017;56(30):3900–12.

46. Harrison PM, Arosio P. The ferritins: molecular properties, iron storage function and cellular regulation. Biochim Biophys Acta 1996;1275(3):161–203.

47. Baker HM, Baker EN. A structural perspective on lactoferrin function. Biochem Cell Biol 2012;90(3):320–8.

48. Attieh ZK, Mukhopadhyay CK, Seshadri V, et al. Ceruloplasmin ferroxidase activity stimulates cellular iron uptake by a trivalent cation-specific transport mechanism. J Biol Chem 1999;274(2):1116–23.

49. Bao G, Clifton M, Hoette TM, et al. Iron traffics in circulation bound to a siderocalin (NGAL)-catechol complex. Nat Chem Biol 2010;6(8):602–9.

50. Goetz DH, Holmes MA, Borregaard N, et al. The neutrophil lipocalin NGAL is a bacteriostatic agent that interferes with siderophore-mediated iron acquisition. Mol Cell 2002;10(5):1033–43.

51. A phase 1, randomized, double-blind, two-arm, placebo-controlled, single and multiple dose escalation study to assess the safety and tolerability of LJPC-401 in healthy adults. 2018. LJ401-NHV02. Available at: https://learningcenter. ehaweb.org/eha/2018/stockholm/214475/vip.viprakasit.a.phase.1.open-label. study.to.determine.the.safety.tolerability.html?f=topic=1574*media=3.

52. Pantopoulos K, Porwal SK, Tartakoff A, et al. Mechanisms of mammalian iron homeostasis. Biochemistry 2012;51(29):5705–24.

53. Yeager D, Piga A, Lai A, et al. A phase 1, placebo-controlled study to determine the safety, tolerability, and pharmacokinetics of escalating subcutaneous doses of LJPC-401 (synthetic human hepcidin) in healthy adults. 23rd European Hematology Association Congress. Stockholm, June 15, 2018.

54. Zarjou A, Bolisetty S, Joseph R, et al. Proximal tubule H-ferritin mediates iron trafficking in acute kidney injury. J Clin Invest 2013;123(10):4423–34.

55. van Swelm RP, Wetzels JF, Verweij VG, et al. Renal handling of circulating and renal-synthesized hepcidin and its protective effects against hemoglobin-mediated kidney injury. J Am Soc Nephrol 2016;27(9):2720–32.

56. Weiss G, Goodnough LT. Anemia of chronic disease. N Engl J Med 2005; 352(10):1011–23.

57. Kim CM, Park YJ, Shin SH. A widespread deferoxamine-mediated iron-uptake system in *Vibrio vulnificus*. J Infect Dis 2007;196(10):1537–45.

58. Casu C, Nemeth E, Rivella S. Hepcidin agonists as therapeutic tools. Blood 2018;131(16):1790–4.

59. Khan FA, Fisher MA, Khakoo RA. Association of hemochromatosis with infectious diseases: expanding spectrum. Int J Infect Dis 2007;11(6):482–7.

60. Gerhard GS, Levin KA, Price Goldstein J, et al. *Vibrio vulnificus* septicemia in a patient with the hemochromatosis HFE C282Y mutation. Arch Pathol Lab Med 2001;125(8):1107–9.

61. Chung BH, Ha SY, Chan GC, et al. Klebsiella infection in patients with thalassemia. Clin Infect Dis 2003;36(5):575–9.

62. Stefanova D, Raychev A, Arezes J, et al. Endogenous hepcidin and its agonist mediate resistance to selected infections by clearing non-transferrin-bound iron. Blood 2017;130(3):245–57.

63. Arezes J, Jung G, Gabayan V, et al. Hepcidin-induced hypoferremia is a critical host defense mechanism against the siderophilic bacterium *Vibrio vulnificus*. Cell Host Microbe 2015;17(1):47–57.

64. Michels KR, Zhang Z, Bettina AM, et al. Hepcidin-mediated iron sequestration protects against bacterial dissemination during pneumonia. JCI Insight 2017; 2(6):e92002.

65. Lyte M, Freestone PP, Neal CP, et al. Stimulation of *Staphylococcus epidermidis* growth and biofilm formation by catecholamine inotropes. Lancet 2003; 361(9352):130–5.

66. Andersson DI, Hughes D. Antibiotic resistance and its cost: is it possible to reverse resistance? Nat Rev Microbiol 2010;8(4):260–71.

67. McPherson CJ, Aschenbrenner LM, Lacey BM, et al. Clinically relevant gram-negative resistance mechanisms have no effect on the efficacy of MC-1, a novel siderophore-conjugated monocarbam. Antimicrob Agents Chemother 2012; 56(12):6334–42.

68. Pramanik A, Stroeher UH, Krejci J, et al. Albomycin is an effective antibiotic, as exemplified with *Yersinia enterocolitica* and *Streptococcus pneumoniae*. Int J Med Microbiol 2007;297(6):459–69.

69. Saikia S, Oliveira D, Hu G, et al. Role of ferric reductases in iron acquisition and virulence in the fungal pathogen *Cryptococcus neoformans*. Infect Immun 2014; 82(2):839–50.

70. Iglesias-Osma C, Gonzalez-Villaron L, San Miguel J, et al. Iron metabolism and fungal infections in patients with haematological malignancies. J Clin Pathol 1995;48(3):3.

71. Alexander J, Limaye AP, Ko CW, et al. Association of hepatic iron overload with invasive fungal infection in liver transplant recipients. Liver Transpl 2006;12(12): 1799–804.
72. Sahlstedt L, von Bonsdorff L, Ebeling F, et al. Non-transferrin-bound iron in haematological patients during chemotherapy and conditioning for autologous stem cell transplantation. Eur J Haematol 2009;83(5):455–9.
73. Spellberg B, Ibrahim AS, Chin-Hong PV, et al. The Deferasirox-AmBisome Therapy for Mucormycosis (DEFEAT Mucor) study: a randomized, double-blinded, placebo-controlled trial. J Antimicrob Chemother 2012;67(3):715–22.
74. Prudencio M, Rodriguez A, Mota MM. The silent path to thousands of merozoites: the *Plasmodium* liver stage. Nat Rev Microbiol 2006;4(11):849–56.
75. Portugal S, Carret C, Recker M, et al. Host-mediated regulation of superinfection in malaria. Nat Med 2011;17(6):732–7.
76. Mordmuller B, Surat G, Lagler H, et al. Sterile protection against human malaria by chemoattenuated PfSPZ vaccine. Nature 2017;542(7642):445–9.
77. Rajapakse S, Rodrigo C, Fernando SD. Tafenoquine for preventing relapse in people with *Plasmodium vivax* malaria. Cochrane Database Syst Rev 2015;(4):CD010458.
78. Rosenthal PJ. The interplay between drug resistance and fitness in malaria parasites. Mol Microbiol 2013;89(6):1025–38.
79. Spottiswoode N, Duffy PE, Drakesmith H. Iron, anemia and hepcidin in malaria. Front Pharmacol 2014;5:125.
80. Stefanova D, Raychev A, Deville J, et al. Hepcidin protects against lethal *Escherichia coli* sepsis in mice inoculated with isolates from septic patients. Infect Immun 2018;86(7):12.
81. Zeng C, Chen Q, Zhang K, et al. Hepatic hepcidin protects against polymicrobial sepsis in mice by regulating host iron status. Anesthesiology 2015;122(2): 374–86.
82. Pagani A, Nai A, Corna G, et al. Low hepcidin accounts for the proinflammatory status associated with iron deficiency. Blood 2011;118(3):736–46.
83. Riba M, Rausa M, Sorosina M, et al. A strong anti-inflammatory signature revealed by liver transcription profiling of Tmprss6-/- mice. PLoS One 2013;8(7): e69694.
84. Agoro R, Taleb M, Quesniaux VFJ, et al. Cell iron status influences macrophage polarization. PLoS One 2018;13(5):e0196921.
85. Martinez FO, Gordon S. The M1 and M2 paradigm of macrophage activation: time for reassessment. F1000prime Rep 2014;6:13.
86. Michels K, Nemeth E, Ganz T, et al. Hepcidin and host defense against infectious diseases. PLoS Pathog 2015;11(8):e1004998.
87. Walker VJ, Agarwal A. Targeting iron homeostasis in acute kidney injury. Semin Nephrol 2016;36(1):62–70.
88. Martines AM, Masereeuw R, Tjalsma H, et al. Iron metabolism in the pathogenesis of iron-induced kidney injury. Nat Rev Nephrol 2013;9(7):385–98.
89. Pepper JR, Mumby S, Gutteridge JM. Blood cardioplegia increases plasma iron overload and thiol levels during cardiopulmonary bypass. Ann Thorac Surg 1995;60(6):1735–40.
90. Peters HP, Laarakkers CM, Pickkers P, et al. Tubular reabsorption and local production of urine hepcidin-25. BMC Nephrol 2013;14:70.
91. Como JJ, Dutton RP, Scalea TM, et al. Blood transfusion rates in the care of acute trauma. Transfusion 2004;44(6):809–13.

92. Rapido F, Brittenham GM, Bandyopadhyay S, et al. Prolonged red cell storage before transfusion increases extravascular hemolysis. J Clin Invest 2017;127(1): 375–82.

93. Brittenham GM. Iron-chelating therapy for transfusional iron overload. N Engl J Med 2011;364(2):146–56.

94. Hod EA, Brittenham GM, Billote GB, et al. Transfusion of human volunteers with older, stored red blood cells produces extravascular hemolysis and circulating non-transferrin-bound iron. Blood 2011;118(25):6675–82.

95. Pak M, Lopez MA, Gabayan V, et al. Suppression of hepcidin during anemia requires erythropoietic activity. Blood 2006;108(12):3730–5.

96. Halliwell B. Superoxide, iron, vascular endothelium and reperfusion injury. Free Radic Res Commun 1989;5(6):315–8.

97. Ambrosio G, Zweier JL, Jacobus WE, et al. Improvement of postischemic myocardial function and metabolism induced by administration of deferoxamine at the time of reflow: the role of iron in the pathogenesis of reperfusion injury. Circulation 1987;76(4):906–15.

98. van der Kraaij AM, Mostert LJ, van Eijk HG, et al. Iron-load increases the susceptibility of rat hearts to oxygen reperfusion damage. Protection by the antioxidant (+)-cyanidanol-3 and deferoxamine. Circulation 1988;78(2):442–9.

99. Williams RE, Zweier JL, Flaherty JT. Treatment with deferoxamine during ischemia improves functional and metabolic recovery and reduces reperfusion-induced oxygen radical generation in rabbit hearts. Circulation 1991;83(3):1006–14.

100. Paraskevaidis IA, Iliodromitis EK, Vlahakos D, et al. Deferoxamine infusion during coronary artery bypass grafting ameliorates lipid peroxidation and protects the myocardium against reperfusion injury: immediate and long-term significance. Eur Heart J 2005;26(3):263–70.

101. Ferreira R, Burgos M, Milei J, et al. Effect of supplementing cardioplegic solution with deferoxamine on reperfused human myocardium. J Thorac Cardiovasc Surg 1990;100(5):708–14.

102. Veres G, Radovits T, Merkely B, et al. Custodiol-N, the novel cardioplegic solution reduces ischemia/reperfusion injury after cardiopulmonary bypass. J Cardiothorac Surg 2015;10:27.

103. Tan TC, Crawford DH, Franklin ME, et al. The serum hepcidin:ferritin ratio is a potential biomarker for cirrhosis. Liver Int 2012;32(9):1391–9.

104. Bruns T, Nuraldeen R, Mai M, et al. Low serum transferrin correlates with acute-on-chronic organ failure and indicates short-term mortality in decompensated cirrhosis. Liver Int 2017;37(2):232–41.

105. Kowdley KV, Belt P, Wilson LA, et al. Serum ferritin is an independent predictor of histologic severity and advanced fibrosis in patients with nonalcoholic fatty liver disease. Hepatology 2012;55(1):77–85.

106. Ascione T, Di Flumeri G, Boccia G, et al. Infections in patients affected by liver cirrhosis: an update. Infez Med 2017;25(2):91–7.

107. Haq SM, Dayal HH. Chronic liver disease and consumption of raw oysters: a potentially lethal combination. A review of Vibrio vulnificus septicemia. Am J Gastroenterol 2005;100(5):1195–9.

108. Maras JS, Maiwall R, Harsha HC, et al. Dysregulated iron homeostasis is strongly associated with multiorgan failure and early mortality in acute-on-chronic liver failure. Hepatology 2015;61(4):1306–20.

Thyroid Hormones in Critical Illness

Matthew J. Maiden, BSc, BMBS, PhD, FCICM, FACEM[a,b,c,*],
David J. Torpy, MBBS, PhD, FRACP[d]

KEYWORDS

- Critical illness • Thyroid hormone • Triiodothyronine • Low T3 syndrome
- Sick euthyroid • Non-thyroidal illness syndrom

KEY POINTS

- Thyroid hormone is pleiotropic and required for normal organ function.
- Illness precipitates a low triiodothyronine (T3) syndrome, where levels of the most active form of thyroid hormone are diminished in proportion to the severity of disease.
- Replacing T3 has been an attractive therapeutic target in many critical illnesses.
- Although many preliminary studies have suggested T3 replacement is beneficial, this has not been replicated in more controlled trials.
- The place of T3 replacement in critical illness requires further investigation, in particular, consideration given to the stage of disease.

The thyroid gland produces hormones that primarily regulate cellular metabolism, have wide-ranging pleiotropic effects, and are essential for life. During critical illness, the most active form of thyroid hormone (triiodothyronine [T3]) decreases. It remains controversial if this is an adaptive response to conserve energy or a pathologic state, particularly when intensive care supports are provided. To further understand this phenomenon, this article reviews the physiology of thyroid hormone how it alters during acute disease and summarizes studies that have supplemented these hormones during critical illness.

Disclosure Statement: The authors have no conflict of interest.
[a] Intensive Care Unit, Royal Adelaide Hospital, Port Road, Adelaide, South Australia 5000, Australia; [b] Intensive Care Unit, Barwon Health, Ryrie St, Geelong, Victoria 3220, Australia; [c] Discipline of Acute Care Medicine, University of Adelaide, Adelaide, South Australia 5005, Australia; [d] Endocrine and Metabolic Unit, Royal Adelaide Hospital, Port Road, Adelaide, South Australia 5000, Australia
* Corresponding author. Royal Adelaide Hospital, Port Road, Adelaide, South Australia 5000, Australia.
E-mail address: mjmaiden@ozemail.com.au

Crit Care Clin 35 (2019) 375–388
https://doi.org/10.1016/j.ccc.2018.11.012
criticalcare.theclinics.com

THYROID HORMONE PHYSIOLOGY
Thyroid Hormones

Thyroid follicle cells produce thyroglobulin, which contains tyrosine molecules that are iodinated to form monoiodotyrosine or diiodotyrosine (T2). These are subsequently coupled to form tetraiodothyronine (thyroxine) (T4) and T3 (**Fig. 1, Table 1**).

T4 is the most abundant thyroid hormone and is produced solely from the thyroid gland (approximately 100 μg per day). Plasma T3 is derived largely from extrathyroidal deiodination of T4, and 20% is directly from thyroid secretion. T3 is considered to have at least 10-times the biological activity of T4 and cells have higher affinity for this form of thyroid hormone. Reverse T3 (rT3) is also a product of T4 deiodination but is considered biologically inactive. The circulating half-lives of T4, T3, and rT3 are 7 days, 1 day, and 0.2 days, respectively.[1]

Control of Thyroid Hormone Secretion

Thyrotropin is synthesized by the thyrotroph cells of the anterior pituitary, is secreted in pulses with a slight circadian rhythm, and has a half-life of 1 hour. It activates all pathways involved in the synthesis and secretion of thyroid hormone. The hypothalamus releases thyrotropin-releasing hormone (TRH) into the hypophyseal-portal circulation to stimulate thyrotropin synthesis and release. Negative feedback of T4 and T3 on the hypothalamus and pituitary provides homeostasis of circulating thyroid hormone levels.

Protein Binding/Cellular Uptake

The iodothyronines are poorly soluble in water, and the extensive protein binding (>99.5%) serves to distribute the hormones throughout the circulation, prevent

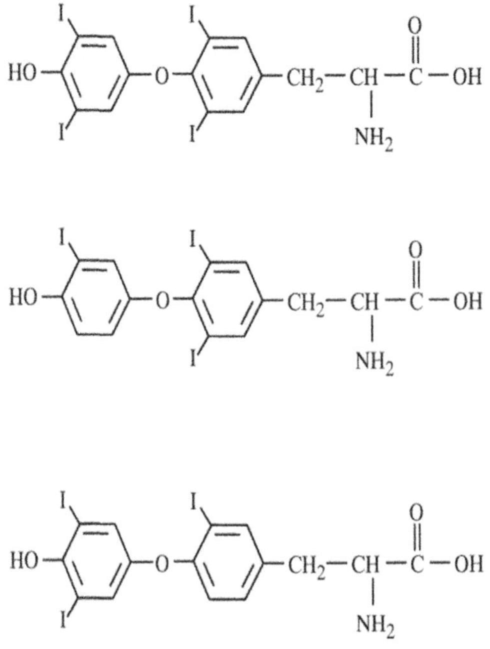

Thyroxine (T4)

3,5,3'-Triiodothyronine (T3)

3,3',5'-Triiodothyronine (rT3)

Fig. 1. Structure of the iodothyronines.

Table 1
Thyroid hormone kinetics in a euthyroid human

	Thyroxine	Triiodothyronine	Reverse Triiodothyronine
Daily production (μg)	110	50	45
Serum levels			
Total (nmol/L)	103	1.84	0.51
Free (pmol/L)	27	4.3	3.69
Total body hormone (nmol/L)	1023	71	62
Distribution (L)	10	38	98
Clearance rate (L/d)	1	22	90
Half-life (d)	7	1	0.2

Data from Greenspan FS. Basic and clinical endocrinology. 3rd edition. London: Prentice-Hall International; 1991.

renal clearance, and maintain a reservoir of thyroid hormone to be liberated when required. Most circulating T4 and T3 is bound to the high-affinity thyroxine binding globulin (TBG), with smaller a proportion bound to albumin and transthyretin (**Table 2**).[2] The iodothyronines (especially T3) are concentrated within the cell, and cellular hormone uptake occurs predominantly by energy-dependent carrier-mediated processes.[3]

Deiodinase System

Three deiodinase enzymes are found in most cells. The enzymes are structurally similar and contain selenocysteine that acts as the iodine acceptor during deiodination. Each deiodinase type differs according to which iodine it removes, location within the cell, distribution across the organs, antagonists, and their activity during illness (**Fig. 2**).[4,5]

Type 1 deiodinase (D1) is most effective at 5' deiodination (outer ring), and predominantly deiodinates rT3 (to T2). Propylthiouracil (PTU) inhibits D1 activity.

Type 2 deiodinase (D2) also catalyzes 5'-deidonation but preferentially deiodinates T4 rather than rT3 and is not inhibited by PTU. Located within the cell, most of the T3 destined for the nuclear thyroid receptors originates from D2.

Table 2
Thyroid hormone–binding proteins (euthyroid state)

	Thyroxine-Binding Globulin	Transthyretin	Albumin
Plasma concentration (μmol/L)	0.27	4.6	640
T4-binding capacity (μg/dL)	21	350	50,000
Binding sites occupied	0.31	0.02	<0.001
Distribution of iodothyronines (%)			
T4	68	11	20
T3	80	9	11

Data from Kronenberg H, Williams RH. Williams textbook of endocrinology. 11th edition. Philadelphia: Saunders Elsevier; 2008.

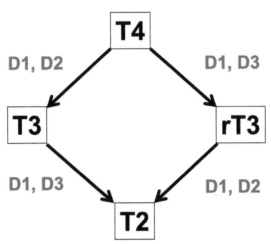

Fig. 2. Summary of the deiodinase enzyme pathways. D1 catalyzes all reactions but is most effective at clearing rT3. D2 primarily converts T4 to the more active T3. D3 metabolizes T4 and T3.

Type 3 deiodinase (D3) has only 5-deiodination (inner-ring) activity. Conceptually it is considered an inactivating enzyme because it metabolizes T3 (to T2) and T4 (to rT3). D3 is of low expression during health, whereas very high amounts are present in placental and fetal tissue to ensure independent thyroid hormone homeostasis of mother and fetus.

The iodothyronines themselves tightly regulate D2 and D3. T3 and T4 down-regulate D2 (limiting T3 synthesis) and up-regulate D3 (favoring T3 clearance). This reciprocal effect on D2 and D3 provides further regulation of thyroid hormone homeostasis.

Thyroid Hormone Cellular Action

Thyroid hormone exerts its effects by genomic and nongenomic mechanisms, leading to immediate and delayed cellular responses.[6–8] The iodothyronines can rapidly alter cell membrane channels (eg, Na^+, K^+, and Ca^{2+}), membrane pumps (eg, Na^+/K^+-ATPase pump, Na^+/H^+ exchange, and Ca^{2+}-ATPase), and protein kinases that act as second messengers. Thyroid hormones also bind to nuclear receptors and regulate gene expression of proteins involved with metabolism, cell proliferation, apoptosis, cellular immunity, and the cytoskeleton. Mitochondrial genome expression is also directly influenced by T3 (eg, ATPase, NADH dehydrogenase, and cytochrome-c oxidase).

PHYSIOLOGIC EFFECTS OF THYROID HORMONE
Metabolism and Thermogenesis

Thyroid hormone regulates multiple metabolic pathways and plays a pivotal role in thermogenesis.[9] T3 can increase oxygen consumption even before changes to thyrotropin occur.[10] Thyroid hormone also enhances provision of cellular glucose by up-regulating gluconeogenesis, promoting insulin clearance, and favoring cellular glucose uptake.[11]

Heat production is minimal without thyroid hormone. T3 increases obligatory heat production due to an increased rate of metabolic processes.[12] It also rapidly increases gene transcription of uncoupling protein that disengage mitochondrial oxidative phosphorylation, thereby favoring production of heat rather than ATP.[13]

Cardiovascular

Thyroid hormone has direct effects on the cardiovascular system to increase cardiac output. This incorporates a direct effect on chronotropy (heart rate), lusitropy (diastolic relaxation), inotropy (contractility), and relaxation of vascular smooth muscle.[14] The observed increase in myocardial work is higher than the increase in myocardial oxygen consumption, which suggests that thyroid hormone enhances myocardial efficiency (ie, enhanced diastolic function, reduced afterload, and improved coronary perfusion).[15]

Responsiveness to Catecholamines

Thyroid hormone increases sensitivity to α-agonists and β-agonists.[16] This may be mediated by an increase in receptor numbers, receptor sensitivity, second messenger coupling, pump activity, and synergism with other catecholamines.

Respiratory

Thyroid hormone is involved in the control of ventilation, surfactant production, and alveolar fluid clearance. T3 directly stimulates Na^+ pumps on the alveolar membrane and increases surfactant production, thereby enhancing water reabsorption and reducing alveolar surface tension.[17,18]

Renal

T3 favors renal reabsorption of sodium and water by stimulating release of renin and Na^+/K^+-ATPase activity in the proximal renal tubules.[19] Conversely, T3 also stimulates gene transcription of natriuretic peptides, leading to sodium and water excretion.

Immunologic

T3 can directly increase phagocytic activity of immune cells, lymphocyte proliferation, antibody production, cytokine production, cytokine receptor expression, and oxygen free radical generation.[20] Local release of the iodothyronines at sites of infection may have local antimicrobial effects due to liberated iodide ions.

Other Organs

Thyroid hormone is essential for neurologic development and normal cerebral function. It increases gastrointestinal motility and promotes synthesis of hepatic enzymes. In skeletal muscle, thyroid hormone transforms slow-twitch muscle fibers into fast-twitch and increases oxidative capacity, β-receptor density, and glycogenolysis.

LOW TRIIODOTHYRONINE SYNDROME

Levels of the thyroid hormones change during illness. Typically, there is an initial fall in circulating T3, reciprocal increase in rT3, and eventually a decline in T4. Despite the lower circulating levels of T3 and T4, thyrotropin usually remains within the normal range. This pattern of thyroid hormone changes has been well characterized during calorie restriction, after surgery, and in a variety of acute and chronic medical illnesses.[21]

These combinations of thyroid hormone changes have been referred to as

1. Sick euthyroid syndrome—normal thyrotropin during illness implies euthyroidism despite low T3 or T4.
2. Low T3 syndrome—low serum T3 is the most common thyroid hormone disturbance during illness.

3. Nonthyroidal illness syndrome—the changes in thyroid hormones during illness are unrelated to primary thyroid gland disease.

For this review, this phenomenon is referred to as the low T3 syndrome.

Critical Illness

The critically ill have been the most studied group of patients with low T3 syndrome.[22,23] In adults, children, and neonates, an elevated rT3 is seen within hours of admission to ICU. Low T3 is present in approximately half of patients at the time of admission to ICU and is nearly universal as acute illness progresses. A low T4 level is found in 10% of patients at ICU admission with up to 45% developing subnormal levels during their illness.[24–26] Tissue concentration of thyroid hormones seems proportional to the circulating levels during critical illness.[27,28]

The extent of change in thyroid hormone measured at any time during ICU admission is proportional to the severity of illness (eg, Acute Physiology And Chronic Health Evaluation II score), ICU length of stay, and mortality rate.[24–26,29,30] In the most extensive study of thyroid hormone changes in critical illness, 451 patients enrolled in a glycemic control trial had thyroid hormones measured at days 1, 5, and 15 and the last day of their ICU admission.[31] The group of patients who died in ICU had persistently lower T3 and T3:rT3 compared with those who survived. Although thyrotropin and T4 levels were within the normal range, nonsurvivors had lower serum levels than survivors.

Sepsis

Sepsis is associated with the greatest change in T3 and rT3, and the extent of disorder is associated with severity of disease and outcome.[32] The high rate of dopamine use (discussed later), and variable timing of thyroid hormone sampling limit interpretation of these studies.

Cardiac Surgery

There is a rapid and progressive decrease in T3 and increase of rT3 after cardiac surgery, which usually returns to baseline by the seventh postoperative day. Thyroid hormone changes are most marked in those with lower cardiac output or after complex cardiac surgery and are proportional to the extent of postoperative therapeutic intervention and hospital length of stay.[33]

Major Trauma/Burns

Major trauma patients have low T3 and elevated rT3 that is proportional to the severity of injury.[34] After severe burns, the alterations in thyroid hormones are proportional to burn size, persist with adequate nutrition, are exacerbated with intercurrent illness and are most marked in nonsurvivors.[35]

Hormone Assays During Illness

It remains controversial whether circulating bound (total) or unbound (free) thyroid hormone provides a better measure of overall hormone availability to the cells during illness. Although the rate of transcapillary transfer correlates best with free hormone concentration, bound hormone can be exchanged rapidly between circulating carrier proteins and cell-binding sites during transit through an organ. With many potential cofounders that may alter protein binding (eg, temperature, fatty acids, and medications) and variable performance of free hormone assays, changes in free thyroid hormone should be interpreted with caution during acute illness.

MECHANISM OF THE LOW TRIIODOTHYRONINE SYNDROME

The pattern of change in thyroid hormones is similar across a wide range of disease, which implies that there is a common process responsible. The mechanism is not precisely clear, however, and it likely involves complex interactions at all levels of the thyroid axis. The mechanism is not precisely clear, and likely involves complex interactions at all levels of the thyroid axis including hormone synthesis, control of circulating levels, protein binding, cellular uptake, receptor modulation, metabolism, and deiodination. The type of disease, duration of illness, certain medications, and the influence of calorie restriction[36] all may contribute.

The inflammatory cytokines (eg, interleukin 1, interleukin 6, tumor necrosis factor α, and interferon γ) can affect all components of the thyroid axis.[37] Although cytokine levels have been closely associated with the low T3 syndrome and can induce thyroid hormone changes in experimental studies,[38] not all patients with the low T3 syndrome have elevated cytokines,[39] and neutralizing these cytokines have not prevented the thyroid hormone changes.[40,41]

Cortisol suppresses secretion of thyrotropin and deiodination of T4 to T3.[42] The hypercortisolism of critical illness can contribute to the low T3 syndrome, comprising an integrated endocrine stress response.

Thyroid Hormone Metabolism During Illness

The decrease of serum T3 and increase of rT3 seen during illness imply altered deiodination of T4. Changes in deiodination pathways occur rapidly during fasting or disease and manifest well before disturbance to other components of the thyroid axis (**Fig. 3**).[28,31,43,44] D1 function in the liver is diminished during illness and primarily contributes to impaired clearance of rT3. Reduced expression and activity of D2 contributes to the T3 decrease and rT3 increase. D3 activity is not normally detected in healthy tissue but is significantly increased during illness and accounts for the clearance of T3 (and conversion of T4 to rT3). These changes in deiodination enzymes are proportional to the disturbance in thyroid hormone levels and severity of illness.

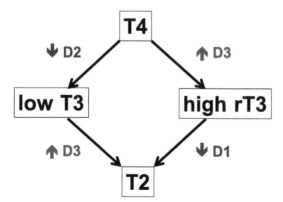

Fig. 3. Changes to the expression and activity of the deiodinase enzymes contribute to the low T3 syndrome. The predominant changes include down-regulation of D1 leading to accumulation of rT3, down-regulation of D2 limiting conversion of T4 to T3, up-regulation of D3 favoring conversion of T4 to rT3, and clearance of T3 to T2.

However, they do not entirely account for the hormonal changes in the low T3 syndrome.

Hypothalamus-Pituitary-Thyroid Axis During Illness

One of the hallmarks of the low T3 syndrome is that thyrotropin usually remains within the normal range. The failure of thyrotropin to increase as expected may represent pituitary dysfunction during illness. Dopamine is a potent inhibitor of the anterior pituitary,[45,46] and it profoundly influences thyrotropin levels. Other catecholamines do not have this effect on the thyrotroph.

Altered hypothalamic control of the thyroid axis may contribute to low T3. Hypothalamic TRH is reduced in many disease states, and, in human postmortem hypothalamic tissue, TRH mRNA expression was reduced in proportion to the decline in blood T3.[47,48] The hypothalamus also controls the pulsatility of thyrotropin, which is of smaller amplitude in prolonged critical illness.[49]

With protracted illness, thyroid follicle size is smaller than usual and may represent reduced thyrotropin stimulation, down-regulation of thyrotropin receptors, and impaired iodothyronine synthesis.[50] Some medications (eg, amiodarone) can alter thyroid function.

TRIIODOTHYRONINE TREATMENT IN CRITICAL ILLNESS

Some investigators argue that the decline in T3 is an important beneficial adaptation limiting metabolic demands during illness.[51–54] Proposals to test T3 replacement have been countered with concerns about negative effects on protein and fat metabolism, adverse effects on the myocardium, increased oxygen demand, coronary vascular spasm, arrhythmias, and death.[55] There is little evidence to support these claims.

Conversely, other investigators have concluded that assuming low T3 to be an adaptive response in critical illness is a "dangerous dogma."[56,57] The "teleological excuse" for low T3 may not apply to the critically ill patient in an ICU who is deteriorating despite receiving definitive treatment and optimized organ supports.[58] Despite the lack of clear evidence regarding the effect of T3 replacement in critical illness, some clinicians are supplementing this hormone in patients with multiorgan dysfunction.[43]

Coadministration of Corticosteroid

It has been advised that hydrocortisone be coadministered with T3 replacement in critical illness.[2,59] This is based on the known action of T3 stimulating β-hydroxysteroid dehydrogenase, which converts cortisol (hydrocortisone) to inactive cortisone.[42] Without a compensatory increase in cortisol production, glucocorticoid deficiency may ensue. It remains unclear if coadministration of corticosteroid is required for all critically ill patients without known pituitary-adrenal axis disease, when administering T3.

Triiodothyronine Treatment in Cardiac Disease

T3 has been tested in small open-label clinical trials in cardiac failure. A study in 23 cardiac transplant candidates suggested that T3 treatment increased cardiac output in a dose-dependent manner, without any adverse effects.[60] In 20 patients who had dilated cardiomyopathy, restoring serum T3 to normal levels seemed to increase stroke volume safely.[61]

Triiodothyronine Treatment in Cardiac Surgery

T3 replacement was seen to enhance cardiac function after cardiopulmonary bypass in experimental models, and early clinical studies suggested that T3 reduced mortality.[33] These studies were small, not blinded or randomized, and compared outcomes to historical controls. Placebo-controlled clinical trials in small groups of patients having coronary artery bypass graft surgery indicated that T3 treatment seemed safe but had only a slight effect on cardiac output.[62–65] There have since been larger clinical studies of T3 in adult patients undergoing cardiac surgery. Meta-analysis of these studies concluded that T3 slightly increases cardiac output without adverse effects but does not reduce inotrope requirement and has no impact on length of stay or mortality.[66] Similar findings were also seen in children undergoing cardiac surgery,[67–71] although, in some post hoc analyses, T3 seemed to have some efficacy in neonates and infants.

Triiodothyronine Treatment in Sepsis

Several preclinical sepsis studies have reported that providing T3 maintained surfactant composition, reduced pulmonary oedema, improved pulmonary compliance, increased myocardial contractility, increased antithrombin III levels, and supported gut barrier function.[72–75] The only report of T3 treatment in human sepsis was an observational study in 11 patients with septic shock who were mechanically ventilated and receiving dopamine.[76] Infusion of T3 was associated with a reduction of dopamine dose. Although these results support a therapeutic effect of T3 replacement, all studies were underpowered, unblinded, and subject to bias.

Recently, a randomized blinded placebo-controlled trial of T3 was conducted in an ICU model of septic shock. This controlled study indicated that T3 administered over 24 hours (with or without hydrocortisone) did not alter the amount of noradrenaline required or significantly change any of the 50 other physiologic endpoints.[77] Although this study suggested no benefit of supplemental T3 early in the treatment of septic shock, it also illustrated no signal of harm. The effects of a longer duration of T3 administration in critical illness remain unclear.

Triiodothyronine Treatment in Organ Donation

Low T3 levels have been proposed to contribute to cardiovascular instability of organ donors and impair the function of transplanted organs. Unblinded and uncontrolled studies suggested that a combination of hormones (eg, T3, T4, corticosteroids, insulin, and vasopressin) provided to the organ donor would improve organ function.[78] There is no correlation, however, between T3 level and organ function (before or after transplant),[79–81] and randomized blinded clinical trials have not identified any clinical benefit.[82–85] Meta-analysis of these studies highlighted the different conclusions based on the study design.[86]

Other Diseases

In acute kidney injury, T3 administration has favorable effects on renal physiology but yielded no difference in clinical outcomes.[87] Similarly, T3 provided to premature neonates led to a lower oxygen requirement but did not alter patient outcome.[88]

The role of hypothalamic impairment contributing to low T3 has been investigated in TRH replacement studies. In prolonged critically ill patients, TRH (with growth hormone–releasing hormone) restored thyrotropin pulsatility and T3 and T4 levels.[89] The combination of hypothalamic hormones has not been tested further in clinical trials.

SUMMARY

Thyroid hormone is pleiotropic and essential for life. Thyroid hormone homeostasis results in remarkably stable T3 levels during health. During illness, T3 levels fall, there is a reciprocal increase of rT3, and thyrotropin usually remains within the normal range. This low T3 syndrome is ubiquitous in critical illness and is associated with severity of disease. The place of restoring T3 levels in critical illness remains uncertain. Many uncontrolled studies have suggested T3 treatment has beneficial effects on specific physiologic parameters, yet randomized blinded studies have identified little or no efficacy of hormone replacement. Short-term provision of T3 seems safe, and further studies are required to determine if there is a stage of critical illness where hormone supplementation is advantageous.

REFERENCES

1. Greenspan FS. Basic and clinical endocrinology. 3rd edition. London: Prentice-Hall International; 1991.
2. Kronenberg H, Williams RH. Williams textbook of endocrinology. 11th edition. Philadelphia: Saunders Elsevier; 2008.
3. Visser WE, Friesema EC, Visser TJ. Minireview: thyroid hormone transporters: the knowns and the unknowns. Mol Endocrinol 2011;25:1–14.
4. Bianco AC, Salvatore D, Gereben B, et al. Biochemistry, cellular and molecular biology, and physiological roles of the iodothyronine selenodeiodinases. Endocr Rev 2002;23:38–89.
5. St Germain DL, Galton VA, Hernandez A. Minireview: defining the roles of the iodothyronine deiodinases: current concepts and challenges. Endocrinology 2009; 150:1097–107.
6. Davis PJ, Goglia F, Leonard JL. Nongenomic actions of thyroid hormone. Nat Rev Endocrinol 2016;12:111–21.
7. Brent GA. Mechanisms of thyroid hormone action. J Clin Invest 2012;122: 3035–43.
8. Cheng SY, Leonard JL, Davis PJ. Molecular aspects of thyroid hormone actions. Endocr Rev 2010;31:139–70.
9. Kim B. Thyroid hormone as a determinant of energy expenditure and the basal metabolic rate. Thyroid 2008;18:141–4.
10. al-Adsani H, Hoffer LJ, Silva JE. Resting energy expenditure is sensitive to small dose changes in patients on chronic thyroid hormone replacement. J Clin Endocrinol Metab 1997;82:1118–25.
11. Dimitriadis G, Baker B, Marsh H, et al. Effect of thyroid hormone excess on action, secretion, and metabolism of insulin in humans. Am J Physiol 1985;248: E593–601.
12. Silva JE. The thermogenic effect of thyroid hormone and its clinical implications. Ann Intern Med 2003;139:205–13.
13. Ledesma A, de Lacoba MG, Rial E. The mitochondrial uncoupling proteins. Genome Biol 2002;3(12). Reviews3015.
14. Klein I, Ojamaa K. Thyroid hormone and the cardiovascular system. N Engl J Med 2001;344:501–9.
15. Kahaly GJ, Dillmann WH. Thyroid hormone action in the heart. Endocr Rev 2005; 26:704–28.
16. Bilezikian JP, Loeb JN. The influence of hyperthyroidism and hypothyroidism on alpha- and beta-adrenergic receptor systems and adrenergic responsiveness. Endocr Rev 1983;4:378–88.
17. Folkesson HG, Norlin A, Wang Y, et al. Dexamethasone and thyroid hormone pretreatment upregulate alveolar epithelial fluid clearance in adult rats. J Appl Physiol 1985 2000;88:416–24.

18. Lei J, Nowbar S, Mariash CN, et al. Thyroid hormone stimulates Na-K-ATPase activity and its plasma membrane insertion in rat alveolar epithelial cells. Am J Physiol Lung Cell Mol Physiol 2003;285:L762–72.
19. Mariani LH, Berns JS. The renal manifestations of thyroid disease. J Am Soc Nephrol 2012;23:22–6.
20. De Vito P, Incerpi S, Pedersen JZ, et al. Thyroid hormones as modulators of immune activities at the cellular level. Thyroid 2011;21:879–90.
21. Pappa TA, Vagenakis AG, Alevizaki M. The nonthyroidal illness syndrome in the non-critically ill patient. Eur J Clin Invest 2011;41:212–20.
22. Van den Berghe G. Non-thyroidal illness in the ICU: a syndrome with different faces. Thyroid 2014;24:1456–65.
23. Fliers E, Bianco AC, Langouche L, et al. Thyroid function in critically ill patients. Lancet Diabetes Endocrinol 2015;3:816–25.
24. Plikat K, Langgartner J, Buettner R, et al. Frequency and outcome of patients with nonthyroidal illness syndrome in a medical intensive care unit. Metabolism 2007; 56:239–44.
25. Bello G, Pennisi MA, Montini L, et al. Nonthyroidal illness syndrome and prolonged mechanical ventilation in patients admitted to the ICU. Chest 2009;135: 1448–54.
26. Ray DC, Macduff A, Drummond GB, et al. Endocrine measurements in survivors and non-survivors from critical illness. Intensive Care Med 2002;28:1301–8.
27. Debaveye Y, Ellger B, Mebis L, et al. Effects of substitution and high-dose thyroid hormone therapy on deiodination, sulfoconjugation, and tissue thyroid hormone levels in prolonged critically ill rabbits. Endocrinology 2008;149:4218–28.
28. Peeters RP, van der Geyten S, Wouters PJ, et al. Tissue thyroid hormone levels in critical illness. J Clin Endocrinol Metab 2005;90:6498–507.
29. Rothwell PM, Lawler PG. Prediction of outcome in intensive care patients using endocrine parameters. Crit Care Med 1995;23:78–83.
30. Chinga-Alayo E, Villena J, Evans AT, et al. Thyroid hormone levels improve the prediction of mortality among patients admitted to the intensive care unit. Intensive Care Med 2005;31:1356–61.
31. Peeters RP, Wouters PJ, van Toor H, et al. Serum 3,3',5'-triiodothyronine (rT3) and 3,5,3'-triiodothyronine/rT3 are prognostic markers in critically ill patients and are associated with postmortem tissue deiodinase activities. J Clin Endocrinol Metab 2005;90:4559–65.
32. Angelousi AG, Karageorgopoulos DE, Kapaskelis AM, et al. Association between thyroid function tests at baseline and the outcome of patients with sepsis or septic shock: a systematic review. Eur J Endocrinol 2011;164:147–55.
33. Ranasinghe AM, Bonser RS. Thyroid hormone in cardiac surgery. Vascul Pharmacol 2010;52:131–7.
34. Mocchegiani E, Imberti R, Testasecca D, et al. Thyroid and thymic endocrine function and survival in severely traumatized patients with or without head injury. Intensive Care Med 1995;21:334–41.
35. Gangemi EN, Garino F, Berchialla P, et al. Low triiodothyronine serum levels as a predictor of poor prognosis in burn patients. Burns 2008;34:817–24.
36. Langouche L, Vander Perre S, Marques M, et al. Impact of early nutrient restriction during critical illness on the nonthyroidal illness syndrome and its relation with outcome: a randomized, controlled clinical study. J Clin Endocrinol Metab 2013; 98:1006–13.
37. de Vries EM, Fliers E, Boelen A. The molecular basis of the non-thyroidal illness syndrome. J Endocrinol 2015;225:R67–81.

38. Torpy DJ, Tsigos C, Lotsikas AJ, et al. Acute and delayed effects of a single-dose injection of interleukin-6 on thyroid function in healthy humans. Metabolism 1998; 47:1289–93.

39. Michalaki M, Vagenakis AG, Makri M, et al. Dissociation of the early decline in serum T(3) concentration and serum IL-6 rise and TNFalpha in nonthyroidal illness syndrome induced by abdominal surgery. J Clin Endocrinol Metab 2001; 86:4198–205.

40. Boelen A, Platvoet-ter Schiphorst MC, Wiersinga WM. Immunoneutralization of interleukin-1, tumor necrosis factor, interleukin-6 or interferon does not prevent the LPS-induced sick euthyroid syndrome in mice. J Endocrinol 1997;153: 115–22.

41. van der Poll T, Endert E, Coyle SM, et al. Neutralization of TNF does not influence endotoxininduced changes in thyroid hormone metabolism in humans. Am J Physiol 1999;276:R357–62.

42. Torpy DJ, Chrousos GP. Stress and critical illness: the integrated immune/ hypothalamic-pituitary-adrenal axis response. J Intensive Care Med 1997;12: 225–38.

43. Peeters RP, Wouters PJ, Kaptein E, et al. Reduced activation and increased inactivation of thyroid hormone in tissues of critically ill patients. J Clin Endocrinol Metab 2003;88:3202–11.

44. Rodriguez-Perez A, Palos-Paz F, Kaptein E, et al. Identification of molecular mechanisms related to nonthyroidal illness syndrome in skeletal muscle and adipose tissue from patients with septic shock. Clin Endocrinol (Oxf) 2008;68: 821–7.

45. Van den Berghe G, de Zegher F, Vlasselaers D, et al. Thyrotropin-releasing hormone in critical illness: from a dopamine-dependent test to a strategy for increasing low serum triiodothyronine, prolactin, and growth hormone concentrations. Crit Care Med 1996;24:590–5.

46. Schilling T, Grundling M, Strang CM, et al. Effects of dopexamine, dobutamine or dopamine on prolactin and thyreotropin serum concentrations in high-risk surgical patients. Intensive Care Med 2004;30:1127–33.

47. Helmreich DL, Parfitt DB, Lu XY, et al. Relation between the hypothalamic-pituitary-thyroid (HPT) axis and the hypothalamic-pituitary-adrenal (HPA) axis during repeated stress. Neuroendocrinology 2005;81:183–92.

48. Mebis L, Debaveye Y, Ellger B, et al. Changes in the central component of the hypothalamus-pituitary-thyroid axis in a rabbit model of prolonged critical illness. Crit Care 2009;13:R147.

49. Van den Berghe G, de Zegher F, Veldhuis JD, et al. Thyrotrophin and prolactin release in prolonged critical illness: dynamics of spontaneous secretion and effects of growth hormone-secretagogues. Clin Endocrinol (Oxf) 1997; 47:599–612.

50. De Jongh FE, Jobsis AC, Elte JW. Thyroid morphology in lethal non-thyroidal illness: a post-mortem study. Eur J Endocrinol 2001;144:221–6.

51. Stathatos N, Levetan C, Burman KD, et al. The controversy of the treatment of critically ill patients with thyroid hormone. Best Pract Res Clin Endocrinol Metab 2001;15:465–78.

52. Wartofsky L, Burman KD, Ringel MD. Trading one "dangerous dogma" for another? Thyroid hormone treatment of the "euthyroid sick syndrome". J Clin Endocrinol Metab 1999;84:1759.

53. Utiger RD. Decreased extrathyroidal triiodothyronine production in nonthyroidal illness: benefit or harm? Am J Med 1980;69:807–10.

54. Utiger RD. Altered thyroid function in nonthyroidal illness and surgery. To treat or not to treat? N Engl J Med 1995;333:1562–3.
55. Burman KD, Wartofsky L. Thyroid function in the intensive care unit setting. Crit Care Clin 2001;17:43–57.
56. De Groot LJ. Dangerous dogmas in medicine: the nonthyroidal illness syndrome. J Clin Endocrinol Metab 1999;84:151–64.
57. Degroot L. Non-thyroidal illness syndrome is a manifestation of hypothalamic-pituitary dysfunction, and in view of current evidence, should be treated with appropriate replacement therapies. Crit Care Clin 2006;22:57–86.
58. Fliers E, Alkemade A, Wiersinga WM. The hypothalamic-pituitary-thyroid axis in critical illness. Best Pract Res Clin Endocrinol Metab 2001;15:453–64.
59. Caplan RH. Comment on dangerous dogmas in medicine: the nonthyroidal illness syndrome. J Clin Endocrinol Metab 1999;84:2261–2.
60. Hamilton MA, Stevenson LW, Fonarow GC, et al. Safety and hemodynamic effects of intravenous triiodothyronine in advanced congestive heart failure. Am J Cardiol 1998;81:443–7.
61. Pingitore A, Galli E, Barison A, et al. Acute effects of triiodothyronine (T3) replacement therapy in patients with chronic heart failure and low-T3 syndrome: a randomized, placebo-controlled study. J Clin Endocrinol Metab 2008;93:1351–8.
62. Novitzky D, Cooper DK, Barton CI, et al. Triiodothyronine as an inotropic agent after open heart surgery. J Thorac Cardiovasc Surg 1989;98:972–7.
63. Teiger E, Menasche P, Mansier P, et al. Triiodothyronine therapy in open-heart surgery: from hope to disappointment. Eur Heart J 1993;14:629–33.
64. Vavouranakis I, Sanoudos G, Manios A, et al. Triiodothyronine administration in coronary artery bypass surgery: effect on hemodynamics. J Cardiovasc Surg 1994;35:383–9.
65. Spratt DI, Frohnauer M, Cyr-Alves H, et al. Physiological effects of nonthyroidal illness syndrome in patients after cardiac surgery. Am J Physiol Endocrinol Metab 2007;293:E310–5.
66. Kaptein EM, Sanchez A, Beale E, et al. Clinical review: thyroid hormone therapy for postoperative nonthyroidal illnesses: a systematic review and synthesis. J Clin Endocrinol Metab 2010;95:4526–34.
67. Bettendorf M, Schmidt KG, Grulich-Henn J, et al. Tri-iodothyronine treatment in children after cardiac surgery: a double-blind, randomised, placebo-controlled study. Lancet 2000;356:529–34.
68. Chowdhury D, Ojamaa K, Parnell VA, et al. A prospective randomized clinical study of thyroid hormone treatment after operations for complex congenital heart disease. J Thorac Cardiovasc Surg 2001;122:1023–5.
69. Portman MA, Fearneyhough C, Ning XH, et al. Triiodothyronine repletion in infants during cardiopulmonary bypass for congenital heart disease. J Thorac Cardiovasc Surg 2000;120:604–8.
70. Mackie AS, Booth KL, Newburger JW, et al. A randomized, double-blind, placebo-controlled pilot trial of triiodothyronine in neonatal heart surgery. J Thorac Cardiovasc Surg 2005;130:810–6.
71. Portman MA, Slee A, Olson AK, et al. Triiodothyronine supplementation in infants and children undergoing cardiopulmonary bypass (TRICC): a multicenter placebo-controlled randomized trial: age analysis. Circulation 2010;122: S224–33.
72. Raafat AM, Franko AP, Zafar R, et al. Effect of thyroid hormone (T3)-responsive changes in surfactant apoproteins on surfactant function during sepsis. J Trauma 1997;42:803–8.

73. Davidson SB, Dulchavsky SA, Diebel LN, et al. Effect of sepsis and 3,5,3'-triiodo-thyronine replacement on myocardial integrity during oxidant challenge. Crit Care Med 1996;24:850–4.
74. Chapital AD, Hendrick SR, Lloyd L, et al. The effects of triiodothyronine augmentation on antithrombin III levels in sepsis. Am Surg 2001;67:253–5.
75. Yang Z-L, Yang L-Y, Huang G-W, et al. Tri-iodothyronine supplement protects gut barrier in septic rats. World J Gastroenterol 2003;9:347–50.
76. Hesch RD, Hüsch M, Ködding R, et al. Treatment of dopamine-dependent shock with triiodothyronine. Endocr Res Commun 1981;8:229–37.
77. Maiden MJ, Chapman MJ, Torpy DJ, et al. Triiodothyronine administration in a model of septic shock: a randomized blinded placebo-controlled trial. Crit Care Med 2016;44:1153–60.
78. Cooper DK, Novitzky D, Wicomb WN, et al. A review of studies relating to thyroid hormone therapy in brain-dead organ donors. Front Biosci 2009;14:3750–70.
79. Powner DJ, Hendrich A, Lagler RG, et al. Hormonal changes in brain dead patients. Crit Care Med 1990;18:702–8.
80. Gramm HJ, Meinhold H, Bickel U, et al. Acute endocrine failure after brain death? Transplantation 1992;54:851–7.
81. Karayalcin K, Umana JP, Harrison JD, et al. Donor thyroid function does not affect outcome in orthotopic liver transplantation. Transplantation 1994;57:669–72.
82. Randell TT, Hockerstedt KA. Triiodothyronine treatment in brain-dead multiorgan donors - a controlled study. Transplantation 1992;54:736–8.
83. Goarin JP, Cohen S, Riou B, et al. The effects of triiodothyronine on hemodynamic status and cardiac function in potential heart donors. Anesth Analg 1996;83:41–7.
84. Perez-Blanco A, Caturla-Such J, Canovas-Robles J, et al. Efficiency of triiodothyronine treatment on organ donor hemodynamic management and adenine nucleotide concentration. Intensive Care Med 2005;31:943–8.
85. Venkateswaran RV, Steeds RP, Quinn DW, et al. The haemodynamic effects of adjunctive hormone therapy in potential heart donors: a prospective randomized double-blind factorially designed controlled trial. Eur Heart J 2009;30:1771–80.
86. Macdonald PS, Aneman A, Bhonagiri D, et al. A systematic review and meta-analysis of clinical trials of thyroid hormone administration to brain dead potential organ donors. Crit Care Med 2012;40:1635–44.
87. Acker CG, Flick R, Shapiro R, et al. Thyroid hormone in the treatment of post-transplant acute tubular necrosis (ATN). Am J Transplant 2002;2:57–61.
88. Amato M, Guggisberg C, Schneider H. Postnatal triiodothyronine replacement and respiratory distress syndrome of the preterm infant. Horm Res 1989;32:213–7.
89. Van den Berghe G, de Zegher F, Baxter RC, et al. Neuroendocrinology of prolonged critical illness: effects of exogenous thyrotropin-releasing hormone and its combination with growth hormone secretagogues. J Clin Endocrinol Metab 1998;83:309–19.

Hormonal Therapy in Organ Donors

Helen Ingrid Opdam, MD, MBBS, FCICM, FRACP

KEYWORDS

- Brain death • Organ donation • Donor management • Hormone therapy
- Thyroid hormone • Steroids • Vasopressin • Transplantation

KEY POINTS

- The provision of optimal supportive treatment of potential donors with brain death is important in maximizing donation opportunities and transplant recipient outcomes.
- Brain death is associated with physiologic changes that include activation of inflammatory pathways and loss of autoregulatory functions of the brain that may include autonomic and hypothalamic-pituitary dysfunction.
- Donor management includes careful hemodynamic and respiratory support, maintaining normal electrolytes and blood glucose levels, and specific treatment to counter the common sequelae of brain death that may include hypotension, hypothermia, and diabetes insipidus.
- In addition, the provision of specific hormonal therapies (thyroid hormone, steroids, and vasopressin) may be important for further optimization of the donor and function of transplanted organs although conclusive evidence for the efficacy of such treatments is lacking.

INTRODUCTION

Organs transplanted from deceased donors provide effective life-saving and life-enhancing treatment for many individuals with end-stage organ failure. Most of the donors have been determined dead using neurologic criteria that demonstrate the permanent loss of brain function, commonly referred to as "brain death".

Brain death is associated with physiologic changes that include cytokine release with activation of inflammatory and coagulation pathways, as well as the loss of autoregulatory functions of the brain. Loss of autonomic nervous system functions and hypothalamic-pituitary damage frequently lead to hypotension, loss of thermoregulation and hypothermia, and diabetes insipidus.

Disclosure Statement: The author does not have any commercial or financial conflicts of interest.
Department of Intensive Care, Austin Hospital, Melbourne, 145 Studley Road, Heidelberg, Victoria 3084, Australia
E-mail address: helen.opdam@austin.org.au

Crit Care Clin 35 (2019) 389–405
https://doi.org/10.1016/j.ccc.2018.11.013
0749-0704/19/Crown Copyright © 2018 Published by Elsevier Inc. All rights reserved.

The provision of optimal supportive treatment of potential donors with brain death is important in achieving the best outcomes for organ transplant recipients. This includes cardiorespiratory supportive treatment provided with the same care and attention as for other critically ill patients. In addition, the provision of hormonal supportive therapies in the setting of brain death may be important to further optimize donation and transplantation outcomes.

Such hormonal "therapies", also termed hormonal "resuscitation," "treatment," "support," and "replacement," commonly include thyroid hormone, vasopressin (antidiuretic hormone), and steroids.

This article reviews the evidence and current recommendations regarding the use of these agents in the setting of brain death and organ donation. Although some also consider insulin as part of hormonal treatment specific to brain death, others view it as part of general donor care. Insulin and glucose control will not be covered in this review.

BRAIN DEATH AND SEQUELAE

Permanent loss of brain function, also commonly referred to as brain death, develops after a devastating brain injury that results in marked elevation of intracranial pressure (ICP) and loss of adequate cerebral perfusion. Causes include hemorrhagic or ischemic stroke, traumatic brain injury, hypoxic-ischemic insults, infection, tumor, and other causes of cerebral edema. Given a consequence of devastating brain injury is inadequate spontaneous respiration leading to cardiorespiratory arrest, brain death is a phenomenon that is only possible since the advent of prolonged mechanical ventilation.

The pathophysiologic sequelae of brain death include hemodynamic changes, activation of inflammatory and coagulation pathways, and metabolic and endocrine effects, all of which can affect multiple organ systems.

During the development of brain death there is raised ICP and ischemia of the brain and brainstem that may be associated with classic physiologic responses first described by Cushing.[1] With increasing ICP there is compensatory arterial hypertension that may be associated with bradycardia. Marked sympathetic stimulation also results in intense vasoconstriction with increased afterload and tachycardia—the "autonomic storm." Acute myocardial ischemia with dysfunction, electrocardiographic changes, and myocyte necrosis has been demonstrated in animals and humans.[2,3] The vasoconstrictive effect of the autonomic storm compromises end-organ blood flow and its severity correlates with the rate of increase in intracranial pressure.[4] Raised pulmonary hydrostatic pressure may cause pulmonary edema, which is accentuated by capillary endothelial damage. After the autonomic storm, there is a loss of sympathetic tone with peripheral vasodilatation and hypotension resulting in inadequate organ perfusion and ischemia.

Hypothermia may develop from loss of hypothalamic function, vasodilation, and reduced heat production from absent cerebral metabolism.

An active inflammatory response is common in brain death. The damaged brain releases mediators that activate inflammatory pathways. Disseminated intravascular coagulation and coagulopathy may also occur, particularly when brain death follows trauma with release of tissue thromboplastin from necrotic brain.[5]

Endocrine and metabolic changes in brain death are variable in timing and severity. Animal models of brain death demonstrate loss of anterior and posterior pituitary function. Experimental studies in the 1980s using a baboon brain death model describe rapid declines in plasma levels of thyroid hormones, cortisol, and antidiuretic hormone.[6–8] Brain dead animals became unable to aerobically metabolize radiolabeled metabolites administered intravenously.[8,9] Replacement of certain hormones improved the metabolic and hemodynamic status of the brain dead animal.[9] Similar findings have been reported with more recent animal models of brain death.[10]

In human brain death, the profile of pituitary dysfunction is less consistent. Although posterior pituitary dysfunction is common as evidenced by the frequency of diabetes insipidus, anterior pituitary function may be preserved or only partially affected, perhaps because of preserved pituitary blood flow.[11,12]

The hormones most usually affected are vasopressin (also known as antidiuretic hormone [ADH]), thyroid hormones, and cortisol.

Vasopressin/Antidiuretic Hormone

In normal health, vasopressin (also known as ADH) is released by the posterior pituitary gland and has both vasopressor and antidiuretic effects (**Fig. 1**).[13]

There are multiple inputs regulating vasopressin release, with the most potent stimuli being increased plasma osmolality (osmotic regulation) and severe hypovolemia and hypotension (hypovolemic regulation). Vasopressin has a half-life of 10 to 35 min and is metabolized by liver and kidney vasopressinases.

Vasopressin receptors include V1 receptors on vascular smooth muscle that mediate vasoconstriction. In the setting of hypovolemia and at supraphysiologic blood levels, vasopressin has an accentuated effect on blood pressure, whereas in normal conditions at normal blood concentrations it affects blood pressure minimally. V2 receptors in the renal collecting duct epithelial cells promote water reabsorption and the antidiuretic effect. Vasopressin also binds on V3 receptors in the anterior pituitary

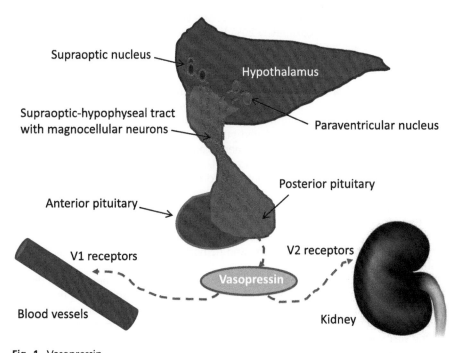

Fig. 1. Vasopressin.

gland to synergize with corticotropin-releasing hormone in increasing the production of adrenocorticotropic hormone (ACTH).

In brain death there is commonly but not universally a deficiency in ADH resulting in diabetes insipidus as evidenced by brisk hypoosmolar polyuria leading to hypovolemia, hyperosmolality, and hemodynamic instability if left untreated.[14,15]

Early human studies indicate that deficient vasopressin occurs in up to 80% of brain dead individuals.[11,12] Current outcome registries in Australia and New Zealand indicate that 77% of brain dead organ donors develop diabetes insipidus that requires treatment with vasopressin or synthetic desmopressin (1-d-amino-8-d-arginine vasopressin [DDAVP]).[16]

Thyroid Hormone

Thyroid hormones have a range of functions that include regulation of metabolic body processes; cellular respiration; total energy expenditure; turnover of hormones, substrates, and vitamins; and general growth and development. Dietary iodine is required for thyroid hormone synthesis, which occurs within the thyroid gland.

There are 2 thyroid hormones, the more potent and active triiodothyronine (T3) and its precursor thyroxine (T4). The thyroid gland contains large stored quantities of T4 and T3 incorporated in thyroglobulin, the protein within which the hormones are both synthesized and stored. Release of thyroid hormone into the circulation is through hydrolysis of thyroglobulin to T4 (80%) and T3 (20%). Most T3 is produced by extrathyroidal conversion of T4. Thyroxine-binding globulin is the primary protein that binds to T3 and T4 in the plasma. Unbound or free hormones are available to the tissue. T4 and T3 enter cells where the T4 is converted by deiodination to T3 where it may act in the cell or leave the cell providing much of the T3 that is produced in extrathyroidal tissues (**Fig. 2**).[17]

Approximately 80% of circulating T3 in humans is derived from extrathyroidal conversion of T4 to T3 and approximately 20% from direct thyroidal secretion. T3 acts by modifying gene transcription in virtually all tissues to alter rates of protein synthesis and substrate turnover. The metabolism of thyroid hormone is complex and by different pathways.

The thyroid gland is regulated by the hypothalamic-pituitary-thyroid axis. A low metabolic rate or decrease in thyroid hormone levels signals the hypothalamus to secrete thyrotropin-releasing hormone (TRH), which travels to the anterior pituitary gland and stimulates secretion of thyroid-stimulating hormone (TSH). TSH stimulates the thyroid gland to increase production and release stored T3 and T4. Elevated thyroid hormones inhibit release of TRH and TSH.

The presence of clinically significant thyroid hormone deficiency in human brain death is debated.

It has been claimed that brain death results in a deficiency in thyroid hormone with the effect of reduced mitochondrial function, metabolic dysfunction, loss of cellular homeostasis, and cell death. The clinical consequence is a decline in myocardial function, catecholamine unresponsiveness, and hemodynamic instability with cardiovascular collapse.[18]

Observational studies in human donors with brain death have almost always documented a reduction in the free plasma T3 concentration, but changes in the serum concentration of other hormone levels such as TSH and T4 are variable.[11,12,19,20] These changes in thyroid hormone levels and TSH in brain death may simply constitute the sick euthyroid syndrome, which is commonly seen in the critically ill patients without brain injury.

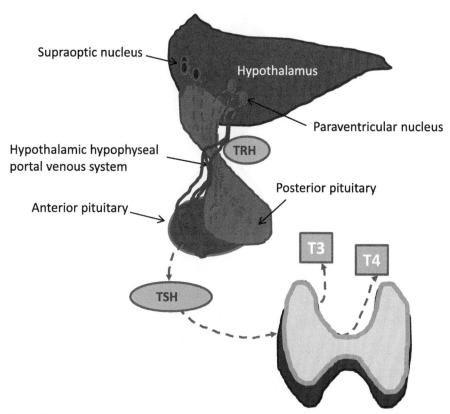

Fig. 2. Thyroid hormone.

Studies have also failed to identify a consistent association between circulating thyroid hormone concentrations in the brain dead donor and donor hemodynamic status, requirement for vasoactive drugs, or cardiac function.[19–22]

Adrenal Cortisol

Cortisol is one of the major glucocorticoids synthesized by the adrenal cortex and is integral in the control of most physiologic systems including regulation of the blood pressure, metabolism, the immune system, and inflammation.

Cortisol secretion is regulated by the hypothalamus and anterior pituitary. Basal input that demonstrates a circadian rhythm pattern as well as stress inputs to the hypothalamus lead to an increase in the release of corticotrophin-releasing hormone (CRH) into the hypophyseal portal veins that flow to the anterior pituitary and causes release of ACTH. ACTH stimulates the release of cortisol from the adrenal cortex (**Fig. 3**).

Only 5% to 6% of circulating cortisol is in the free active form with the rest being protein bound.

Cortisol binds to glucocorticoid receptors that are expressed in almost every cell in the body, leading to gene transcription to alter rates of protein synthesis that mediate multiple physiologic effects. Cortisol is cleared by conjugation in the liver and then urinary excretion.

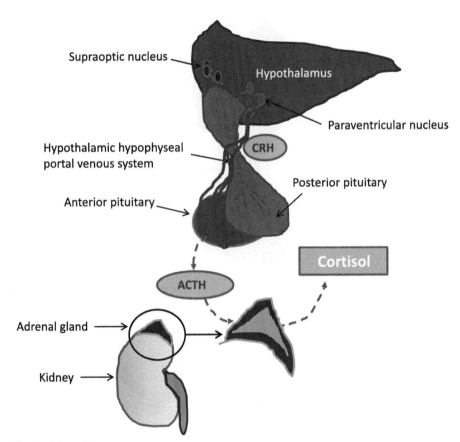

Fig. 3. Adrenal hormone.

Cortisol regulation includes negative feedback to reduce ACTH and CRH secretion.

As with thyroid hormone, there is controversy as to the occurrence of clinically significant adrenal hypofunction in human brain death.

Several small studies in potential donors with brain death have found normal or high levels of cortisol and ACTH levels or only a small proportion having low levels.[11,12,19] Some of these studies performed serial measurements with no change over time, including in some patients before brain death developed.[19] Potential donors with severe hypotension did not have significantly lower serum cortisol.[12]

In contrast, other small studies have found low cortisol levels in brain death along with poor response to ACTH stimulation.[23,24] A group of 17 patients with brain death, 10 of whom had measurements before and after the development of brain death, and a further 20 brain-injured patients who did not develop brain death, found significantly lower values for baseline and stimulated plasma cortisol in brain dead patients.[23] A study of 31 brain dead potential donors found that a high proportion (87%) lacked response to synthetic ACTH and that subsequent steroid administration led to a greater blood pressure improvement in ACTH nonresponders than in ACTH responders, 86% versus 50%, respectively.[24] A further study that included performing the ACTH stimulation test in 121 potential brain dead donors found insufficient response in 94 (78%) patients. This, however, was not associated with a hemodynamic response to subsequent steroid administration and the ability to wean vasopressors.[25]

Interpretation of these small studies is made difficult by the fact that critical illness may itself be associated with a "functional" or "relative" adrenal insufficiency. Furthermore, in critical illness total serum cortisol may be low due to decreased protein-bound cortisol and the free, active cortisol difficult to accurately measure due to the requirement for cumbersome techniques that are unlikely to be available in all hospital laboratories. Also, ACTH stimulation tests do not reliably predict response to glucocorticoid replacement therapy in critical illness.[26,27]

HORMONAL THERAPY

Hormonal therapy with combinations of thyroid hormones, steroids, and vasopressin remains controversial because there are few randomized trials and recommendations are predominantly derived from animal data, small clinical trials, and retrospective observational studies.

Human studies do not demonstrate a conclusive benefit from the routine use of hormonal support. Most studies that suggest a benefit are poorly controlled or include hormonal support as part of a broader approach to donor management, of which other components including close attention to cardiorespiratory care may be important in influencing outcomes in donation and transplantation.

Careful attentive monitoring and provision of care to potential donors with brain death is vital for optimizing organ function and transplantation outcomes. This is similar to the care provided routinely to critically ill patients with additional treatment to counter the known consequences of brain death, including hypotension, diabetes insipidus, and hypothermia.

This careful attention may be deficient in patients with brain death, perhaps more commonly so in the past. In these and other patients who have reached a point in their illness course when survival is deemed no longer possible, the focus on care may shift to provision of comfort, limitation of nonbeneficial treatments, and family support. Over recent decades there has been greater awareness of the vital importance of providing optimal physiologic management in patients with developing and established brain death in order to maximize donation opportunities and transplant outcomes.

In 1995 Wheeldon published the experience of their UK center of applying aggressive donor management instituted by the retrieval team on arrival at the donor hospital that included cardiorespiratory optimization assisted by the insertion of a pulmonary artery catheter.[28] The majority of donors were also at this time initiated on hormone replacement therapy by infusion. This led to the conversion of many of donors initially considered to be unacceptable based on hemodynamic parameters to acceptable donors with a resultant increase in the number of hearts and other organs procured and transplanted.

In 1999 in the United States the United Network for Organ Sharing (UNOS) introduced the Critical Pathway for the Organ Donor that recommended defined physiologic goals and a consistent and active approach to donor management. In a pilot introduction of the pathway, the number of organs transplanted per brain dead donor increased by 11.3%, including a 19.5% increase in hearts transplanted.[29]

Since that time various guidelines and bundles of care have been developed to guide the physiologic management of patients with the potential to donate organs for transplantation after brain death.[30–33] Many of these guidelines and care bundles include hormonal support, although it is impossible to tease out which components of the treatment approach are important for improved donation and transplantation outcomes.[34,35]

Studies have also confirmed that being able to meet prespecified donor management goals, including in more marginal or expanded criteria donors (ECDs), results in more organs transplanted per donor.[36,37]

Whether hormonal support in addition to excellent general intensive care treatment improves donation and transplantation outcomes it still an area of differing views.

Vasopressin/Antidiuretic Hormone Use in Brain Death

Hypotension and diabetes insipidus are common sequelae of brain death. Maintaining appropriate volume state, cardiac output, and blood pressure are all important for adequate organ perfusion.

Clearly treatment of diabetes insipidus is vital for donor stability. If left untreated, diabetes insipidus results in marked polyuria, hypovolemia, and hypernatraemia. Attempts to correct this with intravenous fluid alone lead to hypothermia due to the infusion of relatively cool fluids, electrolyte disturbance, and further donor instability. Hemodynamic instability, hypothermia, and hypernatraemia may prevent the determination of brain death by clinical examination due to the necessary preconditions not being met that make clinical examination reliable.

Hypernatraemia may be detrimental to organ transplant outcomes. An early database review showed worse outcomes for livers transplanted from hypernatremic donors (serum sodium >155 mmol/L).[38] More recent evidence suggests no difference in 1-year survival for liver recipients even with marked donor hypernatraemia.[39] There are also reports of donor hypernatraemia adversely effecting kidney graft function.[40] It may be that hypernatraemia is a marker of inadequate donor management rather than specifically injurious in itself.

Diabetes insipidus is best treated early before significant hypovolemia and metabolic derangement develop. Polyuria (urine output ≥ 3 mL/kg/h) and/or rising serum sodium are sufficient triggers to begin treatment, because formal confirmation with paired urinary and serum osmolarity can delay treatment resulting in donor instability.

Suitable agents include either vasopressin or the synthetic vasopressin analogue DDAVP. DDAVP is highly selective for the V2 renal receptor subtypes, has no significant vasopressor activity, and is the preferred agent to treat diabetes insipidus in the absence of hypotension. It may be given as an intravenous bolus of between 2 and 6 μg every 6 to 8 hours or as required because it has a much longer half-life than vasopressin.

DDAVP at higher doses (0.3 μg/kg) is used as a hemostatic agent due to its effect on increasing plasma factor VIII levels and causing platelet aggregation through stimulating endothelial release of von Willebrand factor.[41] Concern has been raised about the potential for the lower doses used in brain dead donors being procoagulant and detrimental to pancreatic and renal graft transplant function, although reports on any effect on transplant outcomes are inconsistent.[33]

Vasopressin may be used to treat both diabetes insipidus via its action of V2 renal receptors and also hypotension through its pressor effect by acting on V1 receptors on vascular smooth muscle. It must be given by infusion because of a short half-life (10–35 min). The usual dose range is 0.5 to 2.4 units per hour titrated to blood pressure and urine output (**Table 1**). Although some guidelines suggest dose ranges up to 4 units per hour,[30] there is concern that doses higher than 0.04 units per minute may cause potentially deleterious vasoconstriction of renal, mesenteric, pulmonary, and coronary vasculature.[13]

Table 1
Examples of hormonal therapy and doses in adults

Hormone Therapy	Dose in Adults
Vasopressin	0.5–2.4 units per hour by IV infusion
Triiodothyronine (T3)	4 µg IV bolus, then 3 µg/h by IV infusion
Thyroxine (T4)	20 µg IV bolus, then 10 µg/h by IV infusion
Methylprednisolone	15 mg/kg single IV bolus
Hydrocortisone	50 mg IV bolus every 6 h

Abbreviation: IV, intravenous.
Data from Refs.[30–33]

Whether vasopressin to treat hypotension provides any advantage over other vaso-active agents in brain death in terms of efficacy in donor support and transplant outcomes is not known. A retrospective registry analysis of US donor data found use of vasopressin to be associated with a higher number of organs recovered per donor.[42] In Australia and New Zealand, norepinephrine is the most commonly used agent to support blood pressure with more than 80% of donors administered norepinephrine in 2011.[16]

Both vasopressin and desmopressin can be administered concurrently in the potential organ donor to control diabetes insipidus and hypotension.

RECOMMENDATIONS

- For suspected diabetes insipidus (eg, polyuria of ≥ 3 mL/kg/h and/or rising serum sodium) administer DDAVP 4 µg (range 2–6 µg) by intravenous bolus. Repeat every 6 to 8 hours or with recurrence of polyuria as required. Correct hypovolemia and hypernatraemia with administration of low sodium intravenous fluids (eg, 5% glucose or sterile water infused into a large central vein). Correct electrolyte disturbances that may have occurred due to polyuria (eg, hypokalemia, hypophosphatemia, hypomagnesemia).
- If the potential donor is hypotensive and thought to have low systemic vascular resistance (and hypovolemia has been corrected and a low cardiac output state excluded or considered unlikely), start vasopressin by infusion at a rate of 0.5 to 2.4 units per hour. (see **Table 1**). Alternative agents include norepinephrine or inotropic agents.
- If the potential donor has both diabetes insipidus and hypotension, vasopressin may be the preferred agent because it conveniently treats both. Other vasoactive agents can be used in addition to support blood pressure and/or cardiac output. DDAVP can be used in addition to vasopressin if the vasopressin dose required for blood pressure support is not sufficient to also control diabetes insipidus.

Thyroid Hormone Use in Brain Death

There is controversy over the benefits of administrating thyroid hormone to brain dead potential organ donors. Despite this uncertainty, thyroid hormone, in conjunction with other hormonal therapies, remains part of the recommended management of cardiothoracic organ donors as per the UNOS Critical Pathway for the Organ Donor.[43]

UNOS first performed a retrospective analysis of all brain dead potential donors from January 2000 to September 2001 and found that multivariate analyses found hormone treatment was associated with a higher number of transplantable organs and a better 1-year posttransplant survival of kidneys and hearts when T3/T4 had been administered to the donor. Guidelines were developed recommending the inclusion of hormone "support" or "resuscitation."[35,44]

This practice was further reinforced by several early reviews of thyroid hormone in brain dead donors that concluded with recommendations that thyroid hormone be administered either routinely or as rescue treatment in the setting of hemodynamic instability in brain dead organ donors.[7,8,45]

The mechanism by which thyroid hormones are postulated to impart their beneficial effect on cardiac function and the hemodynamic state of brain dead donors is outlined by Novitzky who has published extensively of the effect of thyroid hormones in brain death in both animal models and humans.[6–9,18,46–49] It is suggested that replacement thyroid hormone improves the metabolic and hemodynamic status in brain death by reactivation of mitochondrial energy metabolism.

Two systematic reviews, which included meta-analyses of placebo-controlled randomized controlled trials, have concluded that thyroid hormone does not add hemodynamic benefits or result in an improved number or quality of organs procured for transplantation and cannot be recommended in the routine management of the brain dead potential organ donor.[50,51]

Almost without exception published case series and retrospective audits of the effect of thyroid hormone in brain dead donors tend to find a beneficial effect of thyroid hormone administration on donor hemodynamics, number of organs procured or transplanted, and/or on graft survival. For example, in a retrospective analysis of the UNOS database of donors in the United States in the 10-year period 2000 to 2009, the provision of T3/T4 to brain dead donors was associated with a higher number of organs procured per donor and greater numbers of overall organs procured, of all types except livers. Multivariate analysis suggested a beneficial effect of T3/T4 independent of other factors. There was also an association of T3/T4 use with improved posttransplantation graft survival but not recipient patient survival.[49]

In contrast, all randomized controlled trials have reported no benefit of thyroid hormone administration either alone or in combination with other hormonal therapies.[52–58] For example, in the largest and most recent randomized controlled study, which was double-blinded and involved 80 potential cardiac donors, 20 donors received T3, 19 methylprednisolone, 20 both drugs, and 21 placebo following initial hemodynamic assessment. Cardiac output–guided optimization then occurred, which included vasopressin use and weaning of norepinephrine and inotropes. Cardiac index increased significantly but administration of T3 and methylprednisolone alone or in combination did not affect this change or the heart retrieval rate.[58]

Clearly case series and retrospective audits are limited by factors such as the lack of controls, unblinded administration of thyroid hormone, concurrent administration of other hormones, provision of interventions that may affect the hemodynamic state, and inability to account for all variables that can influence outcome. Randomized controlled trials may also be limited by the small size of study groups, the inclusion of donors who may not benefit from thyroid hormone such as those with stable hemodynamics, and the lack of suitable study end points. A focus on hemodynamic variable outcomes is less relevant than, for example, number of organs procured, their function, and transplant outcome.

Only one human study has raised the possibility that thyroid hormone may be detrimental although this has also been proposed in animal research focusing on reperfusion injury to steatotic livers.[54,59]

Currently in the United States most of the organ procurement organizations use T3/T4 therapy with use varying between approximately 25% and 75% of potential donors.[49]

RECOMMENDATIONS

- The available evidence does not support the routine administration of thyroid hormone in potential organ donors with brain death.
- Thyroid hormone administration may provide benefit in donors who are hemodynamically unstable and/or heart donor candidates who have borderline cardiac function (eg, <45% left ventricular ejection fraction) despite optimization of volume state with fluid therapy, vasoactive agents, and other general supportive care including correction of electrolyte abnormalities. Although the use of thyroid hormone in these circumstances is based on low-level evidence, T3/T4 use may be justified in that there is little indication that thyroid hormone causes harm.
- Administration may be in the form of intravenous T3 (triiodothyronine) or T4 (thyroxine). (see **Table 1**).
- T3 may be initiated with a 4 μg intravenous bolus followed by infusion of 3 μg per hour.[30,33] Intravenous T3 may be preferable to other formulations due to its biological potency and immediate availability to tissues.
- Alternatively, T4 may be given initially with a 20 μg intravenous bolus followed by infusion of 10 μg per hour.[30,33] Thyroxine requires conversion to the biologically active T3 and so its onset of action and efficacy is less certain. Thyroxine may also be administered enterally if the intravenous formulation is not available although impaired enteral absorption may be further limit efficacy.

Steroids Use in Brain Death

Corticosteroids are the third component of hormone therapy and, as for thyroid hormone, there is uncertainty and varying views as to the potential benefit in administering steroids to brain dead potential donors.

Rationales for administering steroids to potential donors with brain death include to replace steroid that is deficient as a result of hypothalamic-pituitary-adrenal (HPA) dysfunction, to supplement steroid due to a "functional" or "relative" adrenal insufficiency, or for the immunomodulatory and antiinflammatory beneficial effects of steroids.

The lack of consistent findings of HPA dysfunction leading to reduced ACTH and cortisol levels in brain death does not provide strong evidence for treating potential donors with corticosteroids to replace deficient levels.

Steroids have, however, been observed to improve blood pressure and facilitate earlier weaning of vasopressor agents in many forms of shock. Two large double-blinded placebo randomized controlled trials on steroid use in critically ill patients with septic shock demonstrate an earlier resolution of shock in patients who received physiologic dose steroids (50 mg hydrocortisone every 6 hours).[60,61] Steroids may also improve blood pressure and responsiveness to vasopressors in nonseptic vasodilatory shock and hemorrhagic shock.[62,63]

Similar improvements in blood pressure have been demonstrated in brain dead donors who were administered steroids. In a prospective study of low-dose steroid use in brain dead potential donors in 22 intensive care units (ICUs) in France, 11 ICUs provided low-dose steroid treatment (50 mg intravenous bolus of hydrocortisone, then infusion of 10 mg/h until the organ retrieval), and 11 did not. Weaning of norepinephrine was more frequent in the 80 brain dead donors who received steroids than the 128 who did not, although there was no benefit observed in primary functional recovery of transplanted grafts.[25]

Brain death is associated with high levels of cytokines, higher than those that occur in patients with similar types of injury though without brain death.[64] Activation of inflammatory cascades in the donor may affect organ function and likelihood of rejection episodes in the recipient.[65–67] A neutrophilic pulmonary infiltration is observed in brain death and elevated concentrations of interleukin 8 (IL-8) in donor bronchoalveolar fluid correlate with early graft failure.[68,69] Higher plasma donor IL-6 concentrations are associated with fewer transplanted organs and reduced recipient survival.[70]

High-dose steroids may modulate immune function and decrease inflammation in the donor with the potential to improve recipient graft function. A study that randomized 50 of 100 brain dead donors to receive methyl prednisolone (250 mg intravenous bolus followed by an infusion of 100 mg/h until organ retrieval) found donors who received steroids to have significantly lower serum levels and liver biopsy expression of proinflammatory cytokines.[71] Recipients of donor livers who had received steroids had a posttransplant course with less ischemia-reperfusion injury and acute rejection.

In lung donors, treatment with high doses of methylprednisolone was reported to be associated with improved oxygenation in the donor and increased organ retrieval rates.[72]

Although other studies similarly demonstrate steroids to reduce inflammation in the donor, any benefit in recipient graft function is less certain. A double-blinded placebo controlled study of 1000 mg of methylprednisolone or placebo administered to brain dead kidney donors found suppressed inflammation and immune response on biopsies obtained at kidney procurement. However, there was no difference in posttransplantation acute renal failure that occurred in 52 of 238 recipients (22%) of kidneys from steroid-treated donors and 54 of 217 recipients (25%) of kidneys from placebo-treated donors.[73]

In randomized prospective studies evaluating the role of aggressive donor management strategies in potential heart and/or lung donors, whilst an active protocol-based approach to heart and lung donor management increased heart and lung retrieval rates, there was no additional benefit from high-dose steroid administration on the number of hearts and lungs retrieved, lung oxygenation, or levels of serum proinflammatory cytokines.[58,67,74]

If steroids are used, it has been suggested low-dose, as compared with high-dose, steroids may have no different effect in terms of organs retrieved and transplanted.[75]

RECOMMENDATIONS

- Physiologic stress dose steroids (eg, intravenous hydrocortisone 50 mg every 6 hours) may improve blood pressure and reduced vasopressor doses required (see **Table 1**).
- High-dose corticosteroid administration (eg, methylprednisolone, 1000 mg IV, 15 mg/kg IV, or 250 mg IV bolus, followed by infusion at 100 mg/h) may reduce the potential deleterious effects of the inflammatory cascade that follows brain death on donor organ function and improve transplant recipient outcomes. Blood for tissue typing should be collected before high-dose steroid administration because steroids have the potential to suppress human leukocyte antigen expression.

SUMMARY

The provision of excellent care to the potential organ donor with brain death is vital for optimizing donation and transplantation outcomes.

The approach to providing supportive care is similar to other critically ill patients managed in ICUs with close attention to hemodynamic support and respiratory care. In addition, specific treatment is usually required to counter the known consequences of brain death that include hypotension, diabetes insipidus, and hypothermia.

There remains uncertainty as to the efficacy of specific hormonal therapy provided based on hypothalamic-pituitary dysfunction and inflammation associated with brain death. Whether specifically vasopressin, thyroid hormone, or steroids provide any additional advantage in physiologic donor support and improving transplant recipient outcomes remains controversial.

REFERENCES

1. Cushing H. Some experimental and clinical observations concerning states of increased intracranial tension. Am J Med Sci 1902;124:375–400.
2. Novitzky D, Wicomb WN, Cooper DK, et al. Prevention of myocardial injury during brain death by total cardiac sympathectomy in the Chacma baboon. Ann Thorac Surg 1986;41(5):520–4.
3. Dujardin KS, McCully RB, Wijdicks EF, et al. Myocardial dysfunction associated with brain death: clinical, echocardiographic, and pathologic features. J Heart Lung Transplant 2001;20(3):350–7.
4. Shivalkar B, Van Loon J, Wieland W, et al. Variable effects of explosive or gradual increase of intracranial pressure on myocardial structure and function. Circulation 1993;87:230–9.
5. Hefty TR, Cotterell LW, Fraser SC, et al. Disseminated intravascular coagulation in cadaveric organ donors. Incidence and effect on renal transplantation. Transplantation 1993;55:442–3.
6. Novitzky D, Wicomb WN, Cooper DKC, et al. Electrocardiographic, hemodynamic and endocrine changes occurring during experimental brain death in the Chacma baboon. J Heart Transplant 1984;4:63.
7. Novitzky D, Cooper DK, Rosendale JD, et al. Hormonal therapy of the brain-dead organ donor: experimental and clinical studies. Transplantation 2006;82: 1396–401.
8. Cooper DK, Novitzky D, Wicomb WN, et al. A review of studies relating to thyroid hormone therapy in brain-dead organ donors. Front Biosci 2009;14:3750–70.
9. Novitzky D, Cooper DKC, Morrell D, et al. Change from aerobic to anaerobic metabolism after brain death, and reversal following triiodothyronine (T3) therapy. Transplantation 1988;45:32.
10. Chen EP, Bittner HB, Kendall SW, et al. Hormonal and hemodynamic changes in a validated animal model of brain death. Crit Care Med 1996;24:1352–9.
11. Gramm HJ, Meinhold H, Bickel U, et al. Acute endocrine failure after brain death? Transplantation 1992;54:851–7.
12. Howlett TA, Keogh AM, Perry L, et al. Anterior and posterior pituitary function in brain-stem-dead donors. Transplantation 1989;47:828–34.
13. Holmes CL, Patel BM, Russell JA, et al. Physiology of vasopressin relevant to management of septic shock. Chest 2001;120:989–1002.
14. Lagiewska B, Pacholczyk M, Szostek M, et al. Hemodynamic and metabolic disturbances observed in brain-dead organ donors. Transplant Proc 1996;28:165–6.

15. Finfer S, Bohn D, Colpitts D, et al. Intensive care management of paediatric organ donors and its effect on post-transplant organ function. Intensive Care Med 1996; 22:1424–32.

16. ANZOD Registry Report 2012 Australia and New Zealand Organ Donation Registry. Adelaide, South Australia. Editors: Leonie Excell, Violet Marion, Graeme Russ. Available at: http://www.anzdata.org.au/anzod/v1/reports.html. Accessed September 16, 2018.

17. White BA, Porterfield SP. The Thyroid Gland. Endocrine and Reproductive Physiology, 4th edition. Philadelphia: Elsevier/Mosby; 2013. p. 129–46.

18. Novitzky D, Mi Z, Videla LA, et al. Thyroid hormone therapy and procurement of livers from brain-dead donors. Endocr Res 2016;41(3):270–3.

19. Powner DJ, Hendrich A, Lagler RG, et al. Hormonal changes in brain dead patients. Crit Care Med 1990;18:702–8.

20. Masson F, Thicoïpe M, Latapie MJ, et al. Thyroid function in braindead donors. Transpl Int 1990;3:226–33.

21. Koller J, Wieser C, Gottardis M, et al. Thyroid hormones and their impact on the hemodynamic and metabolic stability of organ donors and on kidney graft function after transplantation. Transplant Proc 1990;22:355–7.

22. Robertson KM, Hramiak IM, Gelb AW. Endocrine changes and haemodynamic stability after brain death. Transplant Proc 1989;21(1 Pt 2):1197–8.

23. Dimopoulou I, Tsagarakis S, Anthi A, et al. High prevalence of decreased cortisol reserve in brain-dead potential organ donors. Crit Care Med 2003;31:1113–7.

24. Nicolas-Robin A, Barouk JD, Amour J, et al. Hydrocortisone supplementation enhances hemodynamic stability in brain-dead patients. Anesthesiology 2010;112: 1204.

25. Pinsard M, Ragot S, Mertes PM, et al. Interest of low-dose hydrocortisone therapy during brain-dead organ donor resuscitation: the CORTICOME study. Crit Care 2014;18(4):R158.

26. Hamrahian AH, Oseni TS, Arafah BM. Measurements of serum free cortisol in critically ill patients. N Engl J Med 2004;350:1629.

27. Annane D, Pastores SM, Rochwerg B, et al. Guidelines for the diagnosis and management of critical illness-related corticosteroid insufficiency (CIRCI) in critically ill patients (Part I): Society of Critical Care Medicine (SCCM) and European Society of Intensive Care Medicine (ESICM) 2017. Intensive Care Med 2017;43: 1751.

28. Wheeldon DR, Potter CD, Oduro A, et al. Transforming the "unacceptable" donor: outcomes from the adoption of a standardized donor management technique. J Heart Lung Transplant 1995;14:734–42.

29. Rosendale JD, Chabalewski FL, McBride MA, et al. Increased transplanted organs from the use of a standardized donor management protocol. Am J Transplant 2002;2:761–8.

30. Wood KE, Becker BN, McCartney JG, et al. Care of the potential organ donor. N Engl J Med 2004;351:2730.

31. Shemie SD, Ross H, Pagliarello J, et al. Organ donor management in Canada: recommendations of the forum on medical management to optimize donor organ potential. CMAJ 2006;174(6):S13–32.

32. McKeown DW, Bonser RS, Kellum JA. Management of the heartbeating brain-dead organ donor. Br J Anaesth 2012;108(Suppl 1):i96–107.

33. Kotloff RM, Blosser S, Fulda GJ, et al. Management of the potential organ donor in the ICU: Society of Critical Care Medicine/American College of Chest

Physicians/Association of Organ Procurement Organizations Consensus Statement. Crit Care Med 2015;43(6):1291–325.

34. Rosendale JD, Kauffman HM, McBride MA, et al. Aggressive pharmacologic donor management results in more transplanted organs. Transplantation 2003; 75:482–7.

35. Zaroff JG, Rosengard BR, Armstrong WF, et al. Consensus conference report: maximizing use of organs recovered from the cadaver donor: cardiac recommendations, March 28–29, 2001, Crystal City, Va. Circulation 2002;106:836–41.

36. Malinoski DJ, Patel MS, Daly MC, et al. The impact of meeting donor management goals on the number of organs transplanted per donor: results from the United Network for Organ Sharing Region 5 prospective donor management goals study. Crit Care Med 2012;40(10):2773–80.

37. Patel MS, Zatarain J, De La Cruz S, et al. The impact of meeting donor management goals on the number of organs transplanted per expanded criteria donor: a prospective study from the UNOS Region 5 Donor Management Goals Workgroup. JAMA Surg 2014;149:969–75.

38. Totsuka E, Dodson F, Urakami A, et al. Influence of high donor serum sodium levels on early postoperative graft function in human liver transplantation: effect of correction of donor hypernatremia. Liver Transpl Surg 1999;5:421–8.

39. Mangus RS, Fridell JA, Vianna RM, et al. Severe hypernatremia in deceased liver donors does not impact early transplant outcome. Transplantation 2010;90: 438–43.

40. Kazemeyni SM, Esfahani F. Influence of hypernatremia and polyuria of brain-dead donors before organ procurement on kidney allograft function. Urol J 2008;5(3):173–7.

41. Lethagen S. Desmopressin (DDAVP) and hemostasis. Ann Hematol 1994;69(4): 173–80.

42. Plurad DS, Bricker S, Neville A, et al. Arginine vasopressin significantly increases the rate of successful organ procurement in potential donors. Am J Surg 2012; 204:856–60 [discussion: 860–51].

43. United Network for Organ Sharing (UNOS) Critical Pathway for the Organ Donor. Available at: https://www.unos.org/wp-content/uploads/unos/Critical_Pathway. pdf. Accessed August 16, 2018.

44. Rosengard BR, Feng S, Alfrey EJ, et al. Report of the Crystal City Meeting to maximize the use of organs recovered from the cadaver donor. Am J Transplant 2002;2:701.

45. Powner DJ, Hernandez M. A review of thyroid hormone administration during adult donor care. Prog Transplant 2005;15:202–7.

46. Novitzky D, Cooper DKC, Reichart B. Value of triiodothyronine (T3) therapy to brain-dead potential organ donors. J Heart Transplant 1986;5:486.

47. Novitzky D, Cooper DKC, Reichart B. Hemodynamic and metabolic responses to hormonal therapy in brain-dead potential organ donors. Transplantation 1987;43: 852.

48. Novitzky D, Cooper DKC, Chaffin JS, et al. Improved cardiac allograft function following triiodothyronine therapy to both donor and recipient. Transplantation 1990;49:311.

49. Novitzky D, Mi Z, Sun Q, et al. Thyroid hormone therapy in the management of 63,593 brain-dead organ donors: a retrospective analysis. Transplantation 2014;98(10):1119–27.

50. Macdonald PS, Aneman A, Bhonagiri D, et al. A systematic review and meta-analysis of clinical trials of thyroid hormone administration to brain dead potential organ donors. Crit Care Med 2012;40:1635.
51. Rech TH, Moraes RB, Crispin D, et al. Management of the brain-dead organ donor: a systematic review and meta-analysis. Transplantation 2013;95:966.
52. Garcia-Fages LC, Antolin M, Cabrer C, et al. Effects of substitutive triiodothyronine therapy on intracellular nucleotide levels in donor organs. Transplant Proc 1991;23:2495–6.
53. Mariot J, Jacob F, Voltz C, et al. Value of hormonal treatment with triiodothyronine and cortisone in brain dead patients. Ann Fr Anesth Reanim 1991;10:321–8 [in French].
54. Randell TT, Hockerstedt KA. Triiodothyronine treatment in brain-dead multiorgan donors–a controlled study. Transplantation 1992;54:736–8.
55. Goarin JP, Cohen S, Riou B, et al. The effects of triiodothyronine on hemodynamic status and cardiac function in potential heart donors. Anesth Analg 1996;83:41–7.
56. Jeevanandam V. Triiodothyronine: spectrum of use in heart transplantation. Thyroid 1997;7:139–45.
57. Perez-Blanco A, Caturla-Such J, Canovas-Robles J, et al. Efficiency of triiodothyronine treatment on organ donor hemodynamic management and adenine nucleotide concentration. Intensive Care Med 2005;31:943–8.
58. Venkateswaran RV, Steeds RP, Quinn DW, et al. The haemodynamic effects of adjunctive hormone therapy in potential heart donors: a prospective randomized double-blind factorially designed controlled trial. Eur Heart J 2009;30(14):1771–80.
59. Ellett JD, Evans ZP, Fiorini JH, et al. The use of the Papworth cocktail is detrimental to steatotic livers after ischemia–reperfusion injury. Transplantation 2008;86:286–92.
60. Sprung CL, Annane D, Keh D, et al. Hydrocortisone therapy for patients with septic shock. N Engl J Med 2008;358:111–24.
61. Venkatesh B, Finfer S, Cohen J, et al. Adjunctive glucocorticoid therapy in patients with septic shock. N Engl J Med 2018;378(9):797–808.
62. Fuchs PCh, Bozkurt A, Johnen D, et al. Beneficial effect of corticosteroids in catecholamine-dependent septic burn patients. Burns 2007;33(3):306–11.
63. Hoen S, Mazoit JX, Asehnoune K, et al. Hydrocortisone increases the sensitivity to alpha1-adrenoceptor stimulation in humans following hemorrhagic shock. Crit Care Med 2005;33(12):2737–43.
64. Amado JA, Lopez-Espadas F, Vazquez-Barquero A, et al. Blood levels of cytokines in brain-dead patients: relationship with circulating hormones and acute phase reactants. Metabolism 1995;44:812–6.
65. Koo DD, Welsh KI, McLaren AJ, et al. Cadaver versus living donor kidneys: impact of donor factors on antigen induction before transplantation. Kidney Int 1999;56:1551–9.
66. Weiss S, Kotsch K, Francuski M, et al. Brain death activates donor organs and is associated with a worse I/R injury after liver transplantation. Am J Transplant 2007;7(6):1584–93.
67. Venkateswaran RV, Dronavalli V, Lambert PA, et al. The proinflammatory environment in potential heart and lung donors: prevalence and impact of donor management and hormonal therapy. Transplantation 2009;88:582–8.
68. Fisher AJ, Donnelly SC, Hirani N, et al. Enhanced pulmonary inflammation in organ donors following fatal non-traumatic brain injury. Lancet 1999;353:1412–3.

69. Fisher AJ, Donnelly SC, Hirani N, et al. Elevated levels of interleukin-8 in donor lungs is associated with early graft failure after lung transplantation. Am J Respir Crit Care Med 2001;163:259–65.
70. Murugan R, Venkataraman R, Wahed AS, et al. Increased plasma interleukin-6 in donors is associated with lower recipient hospital-free survival after cadaveric organ transplantation. Crit Care Med 2008;36:1810–6.
71. Kotsch K, Ulrich F, Reutzel-Selke A, et al. Methylprednisolone therapy in deceased donors reduces inflammation in the donor liver and improves outcome after liver transplantation: a prospective randomized controlled trial. Ann Surg 2008;248:1042–50.
72. Follette DM, Rudich SM, Babcock WD. Improved oxygenation and increased lung donor recovery with high-dose steroid administration after brain death. J Heart Lung Transplant 1998;17:423–9.
73. Kainz A, Wilflingseder J, Mitterbauer C, et al. Steroid pretreatment of organ donors to prevent post-ischemic renal allograft failure. Ann Intern Med 2010;153: 222–30.
74. Venkateswaran RV, Patchell VB, Wilson IC, et al. Early donor management increases the retrieval rate of lungs for transplantation. Ann Thorac Surg 2008; 85:278–86.
75. Dhar R, Cotton C, Coleman J, et al. Comparison of high- and low-dose corticosteroid regimens for organ donor management. J Crit Care 2013;28(1):111.e1-7.

Moving?

Make sure your subscription moves with you!

To notify us of your new address, find your **Clinics Account Number** (located on your mailing label above your name), and contact customer service at:

Email: journalscustomerservice-usa@elsevier.com

800-654-2452 (subscribers in the U.S. & Canada)
314-447-8871 (subscribers outside of the U.S. & Canada)

Fax number: 314-447-8029

Elsevier Health Sciences Division
Subscription Customer Service
3251 Riverport Lane
Maryland Heights, MO 63043

*To ensure uninterrupted delivery of your subscription, please notify us at least 4 weeks in advance of move.

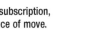

Printed and bound by CPI Group (UK) Ltd, Croydon, CR0 4YY

03/10/2024

01040404-0005